Neuroimaging

Editor

LASZLO L. MECHTLER

NEUROLOGIC CLINICS

www.neurologic.theclinics.com

Consulting Editor
RANDOLPH W. EVANS

February 2014 • Volume 32 • Number 1

ELSEVIER

1600 John F. Kennedy Boulevard • Suite 1800 • Philadelphia, Pennsylvania, 19103-2899

http://www.theclinics.com

NEUROLOGIC CLINICS Volume 32, Number 1
February 2014 ISSN 0733-8619, ISBN-13: 978-0-323-26670-3

Editor: Joanne Husovski
Developmental editor: Donald Mumford

Neurologic Clinics (ISSN 0733-8619) is published quarterly by Elsevier Inc., 360 Park Avenue South, New York, NY 10010–1710. Months of issue are February, May, August, and November. Periodicals postage paid at New York, NY, and additional mailing offices. Subscription prices are $300.00 per year for US individuals, $517.00 per year for US institutions, $145.00 per year for US students, $375.00 per year for Canadian individuals, $627.00 per year for Canadian institutions, $415.00 per year for international individuals, $627.00 per year for international institutions, and $210.00 for Canadian and foreign students/residents. To receive student/resident rate, orders must be accompanied by name of affiliated institution, date of term, and the *signature* of program/residency coordinator on institution letterhead. Orders will be billed at individual rate until proof of status is received. Foreign air speed delivery is included in all *Clinics* subscription prices. All prices are subject to change without notice. **POSTMASTER:** Send address changes to *Neurologic Clinics*, Elsevier Health Sciences Division, Subscription Customer Service, 3251 Riverport Lane, Maryland Heights, MO 63043. **Customer Service: Telephone: 1-800-654-2452 (U.S. and Canada); 314-447-8871 (outside U.S. and Canada). Fax: 314-447-8029. E-mail: journalscustomerservice-usa@elsevier.com (for print support); journalsonlinesupport-usa@elsevier.com (for online support).**

Reprints. For copies of 100 or more of articles in this publication, please contact the Commercial Reprints Department, Elsevier Inc., 360 Park Avenue South, New York, New York, 10010-1710; Tel.: +1-212-633-3874; Fax: +1-212-633-3820, and E-mail: reprints@elsevier.com.

Neurologic Clinics is also published in Spanish by Nueva Editorial Interamericana S.A., Mexico City, Mexico.

Neurologic Clinics is covered in *Current Contents/Clinical Medicine, MEDLINE/PubMed (Index Medicus), EMBASE/Excerpta Medica, and PsycINFO, and ISI/BIOMED.*

Printed and bound by CPI Group (UK) Ltd, Croydon, CR0 4YY

Transferred to digital print 2013

Contributors

CONSULTING EDITOR

RANDOLPH W. EVANS, MD
Clinical Professor, Department of Neurology, Baylor College of Medicine, Houston, Texas

EDITOR

LASZLO L. MECHTLER, MD
President, American Society of Neuroimaging; Professor, Department of Neurology and
Neuro-Oncology, State University of New York at Buffalo, Buffalo, New York; Medical
Director, Dent Neurologic Institute, Amherst, New York

AUTHORS

BELA AJTAI, MD, PhD
Attending Neurologist, Neuroimager, Dent Neurologic Institute, Amherst, New York

VERNICE E. BATES, MD
Medical Director, Dent Stroke/TIA Clinic, President, Dent Neurological Institute, Amherst,
New York

JOHN A. BERTELSON, MD
Assistant Professor, Department of Neurology and Neurotherapeutics, UT Southwestern
Medical Center; Clinical Assistant Professor, Department of Psychology, The University of
Texas at Austin, Austin, Texas

PATRICK M. CAPONE, MD, PhD
Director, Winchester Neuroimaging Fellowship, Adjunct Professor, Virginia Common-
wealth University, Richmond, Virginia; Department of Neurology and Medical Imaging,
Winchester Medical Center; Winchester Neurological Consultants, Inc, Winchester,
Virginia

KEVIN E. CRUTCHFIELD, MD
Director, Comprehensive Sports Concussion Program, The Sandra and Malcolm Berman
Brain and Spine Institute, Baltimore, Maryland

JÖRG DIETRICH, MD, PhD
Assistant Professor, Division of Neuro-Oncology, Department of Neurology,
Massachusetts General Hospital Cancer Center, Center for Regenerative Medicine,
Harvard Medical School, Boston, Massachusetts

TRAVIS M. DUMONT, MD
Clinical Assistant Professor of Neurosurgery, Endovascular Neurosurgery Fellow,
Department of Neurosurgery, Gates Vascular Institute-Kaleida Health, University at
Buffalo, State University of New York, Buffalo, New York

JOSEPH V. FRITZ, PhD
Chief Executive Officer, Dent Neurologic Institute, Amherst, New York

FERENC A. JOLESZ, MD
Division of MRI, National Center for Image-Guided Therapy, Department of Radiology, Brigham and Women's Hospital, Harvard Medical School, Boston, Massachusetts

JOSHUA P. KLEIN, MD, PhD
Assistant Professor, Departments of Neurology and Radiology, Harvard Medical School; Chief, Division of Hospital Neurology, Department of Neurology, Brigham and Women's Hospital, Boston, Massachusetts

JODY LEONARDO, MD
Assistant Professor of Neurosurgery, School of Medicine and Biomedical Sciences, University at Buffalo, State University of New York; Co-Director of Brain Endoscopy Center, University at Buffalo Neurosurgery, Buffalo, New York

ELAD I. LEVY, MD, MBA, FACS, FAHA, FAANS
Professor and Chair of Neurosurgery and Professor of Radiology, University at Buffalo, State University of New York; Director of Interventional Stroke Services, Director of Endovascular Neurosurgery Fellowship Education, Medical Director of Neuroendovascular Services, and Co-Director of Stroke Center, Gates Vascular Institute (GVI) at Kaleida Health, Buffalo, New York

DAVID S. LIEBESKIND, MD
Department of Neurology, David Geffen School of Medicine, University of California, Los Angeles, California

NATHAN J. McDANNOLD, PhD
Focused Ultrasound Laboratory, National Center for Image-Guided Therapy, Department of Radiology, Brigham and Women's Hospital, Harvard Medical School, Boston, Massachusetts

JENNIFER W. McVIGE, MD
Pediatric Neurology, Fellowship trained in Adult and Pediatric Headache, and Neuroimaging, Co-Director, Dent Concussion Center, Dent Neurologic Institute, Amherst, New York

LASZLO L. MECHTLER, MD
President, American Society of Neuroimaging; Professor, Department of Neurology and Neuro-Oncology, State University of New York at Buffalo, Buffalo, New York; Medical Director, Dent Neurologic Institute, Amherst, New York

MAXIM MOKIN, MD, PhD
Clinical Assistant Professor of Neurosurgery, Endovascular Neurosurgery Fellow, Department of Neurosurgery, Gates Vascular Institute-Kaleida Health, School of Medicine and Biomedical Sciences, University at Buffalo, State University of New York, Buffalo, New York

KAVEER NANDIGAM, MD
Director of Neuroimaging, Neurology and Stroke Associates, Lancaster, Pennsylvania; Former Neuroimaging Fellow, Dent Neurological Institute, Amherst, New York

MAY NOUR, MD, PhD
Department of Neurology, David Geffen School of Medicine; Department of Radiology, Division of Interventional Neuroradiology, University of California, Los Angeles, California

JOSEPH M. SCHELLER, MD
Neuroimaging Fellow, Department of Neurology and Medical Imaging, Winchester Medical Center; Winchester Neurological Consultants, Inc, Winchester, Virginia

KALYAN K. SHASTRI, MD, MS
Neuroimaging Fellow, Dent Neurologic Institute, Amherst, New York

JAMES G. SMIRNIOTOPOULOS, MD
Professor of Radiology, Neurology, and Bio Informatics, Uniformed Services University, Bethesda, Maryland

KENNETH V. SNYDER, MD, PhD
Assistant Professor of Neurosurgery, Radiology, and Neurology, Department of Neurosurgery, School of Medicine and Biomedical Sciences, University at Buffalo, State University of New York, Buffalo, New York

PAUL M. VESPA, MD, FCCM, FAAN
Professor of Neurology and Neurosurgery, Director of Neurocritical Care, David Geffen School of Medicine at University of California, Los Angeles, Los Angeles, California

Contents

course of ischemia—from acute onset to evolution. A thorough under-standing of imaging modalities, their strengths and their limitations, is essential for capitalizing on the benefit of this complementary source of information for understanding the mechanism of disease, making thera-peutic decisions, and monitoring patient response over time.

Critically ill neurologic patients are common in the hospital practice of neu-rology and are often in extreme states requiring accurate and specific information. Imaging, especially using advanced imaging techniques, can provide an important means of garnering this information. This article focuses on the clinical utilization of selective imaging methods that are commonly used in critically ill neurologic patients to render diagnoses, to monitor effects of treatment, or have contributed to a better understand-ing of pathophysiology in the intensive care unit.

Brain arteriovenous malformations (AVMs) are abnormal communications between arteries and veins characterized radiographically by the presence of a nidus and early venous drainage. Estimation of hemorrhage risk and determination of treatment strategy rely on the location and hemodynamic properties of the AVM. This article describes modern noninvasive approaches to diagnosing and evaluating AVMs, including dynamic 4-di-mensional computed tomographic and magnetic resonance angiography and perfusion imaging. The role and latest advances in digital subtraction angiography and intraoperative imaging are also described.

The introduction of computed tomography (CT) scanning in the 1970s rev-olutionized the way clinicians could diagnose and treat stroke. Subsequent advances in CT technology significantly reduced radiation dose, reduced metallic artifact, and achieved speeds that enable dynamic functional studies. The recent addition of whole-brain volumetric CT perfusion tech-nology has given clinicians a powerful tool to assess parenchymal perfu-sion parameters as well as visualize dynamic changes in blood vessel flow throughout the brain during a single cardiac cycle. This article reviews clinical applications of volumetric multimodal CT that helped to guide and manage care.

Transcranial MRI-guided focused ultrasound (TcMRgFUS) is an old idea but a new technology that may change the entire clinical field of the neurosciences. TcMRgFUS has no cumulative effect, and it is applicable for repeatable treatments, controlled by real-time dosimetry, and capable of immediate tissue destruction. Most importantly, it has extremely accurate targeting and constant monitoring. It is potentially more precise than proton beam therapy and definitely more cost effective. Neuro-oncology may be the most promising area of future TcMRgFUS applications.

NEUROLOGIC CLINICS

Preface

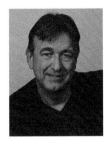

Laszlo L. Mechtler, MD
Editor

This issue of *Neurologic Clinics* is dedicated to the field of neuroimaging, and it is truly a joint effort by neurologists, neurosurgeons, and radiologists, who are at the forefront of this subspecialty. I am honored to have been asked to return as the guest editor for a follow-up to the 2009 *Neurologic Clinics*, Neuroimaging edition.

In this issue, we have attempted to strike a balance between exciting new technology and more conventional review articles. The future of neurologists in neuroimaging depend on increasing the understanding about the latest advances in this topic, as well as the development of greater participation by neurologists in academic and political organizations that are interested in neuroimaging. This edition of *Neurologic Clinics* devoted to the issue of neuroimaging is a testament to the awakening interest of neurologists.

Neuroimaging, over the years, has evolved beyond anatomic and basic tissue imaging into a field that offers exquisite information on the biological processes on central nervous system disease. A spectrum of subspecialists in the field of neuroimaging has worked together to provide a rational approach for the evaluation and multidisciplinary care of neurological disorders. The imaging of the central nervous system is a shared science, and it should never be exclusive of any one subspecialty. In the end, our patients will reap the benefits of this practice.

I have the utmost gratitude for the time and effort that the authors have spent on preparing this issue. I believe that you will be impressed with the outstanding contributions from these authors.

I would like to take the opportunity to thank Randolph Evans, MD, for his encouragement, faith, and support of the field of neuroimaging. I would also like to thank Donald Mumford, developmental editor of *Neurologic Clinics* at Elsevier, for his professionalism, patience, and guidance.

Last, I would like to thank my parents, Stephen and Gizella Mechtler, for always nurturing my passion for medicine.

Neurol Clin 32 (2014) xiii–xiv
http://dx.doi.org/10.1016/j.ncl.2013.09.001
0733-8619/14/$ – see front matter © 2014 Elsevier Inc. All rights reserved.

neurologic.theclinics.com

In the words of Hippocrates, "Wherever the art of medicine is loved, there is also a love of humanity."

Laszlo L. Mechtler, MD
Dent Neurologic Institute
3980A Sheridan Drive, Suite 101
Amherst, NY 14226, USA

E-mail address:
lmechtler@dentinstitute.com

Neuroimaging Trends and Future Outlook

Joseph V. Fritz, PhD

KEYWORDS

- Diagnostic neuroimaging • Imaging trends • Functional imaging
- Quantitative imaging

KEY POINTS

- Imaging equipment continues to experience advances in speed, sensitivity, safety, and workflow.
- Fast acquisition methods increasingly take advantage of advances in hardware and algorithms, particularly sparse sampling methods to minimize data collection.
- There is an increasing trend toward physiologic imaging and quantitation, requiring greater consistency across manufacturers and clinics.
- The Human Connectome Project is symbolic of the drive toward combining multimodality anatomic and functional imaging with quantitation and sophisticated atlases to understand the complex circuitry of the central nervous system.
- Advanced visualization methods derived from the computer graphics and entertainment industries have become essential in the evaluation of large multidimensional data sets.
- Hybrid imaging blends advantages from multiple modalities to provide a comprehensive anatomic, functional, physiologic, and metabolic data set.
- Breakthrough clinical neuroimaging applications are derived from an alignment of scientific, engineering, clinical, and business conditions.

INTRODUCTION

Magnetic resonance (MR), computed tomography (CT), nuclear medicine, and ultrasound have been the foundation for modern noninvasive diagnostic neuroimaging during the past 4 decades. Research and innovations in engineering, algorithms, computer processing, pharmaceuticals, and the understanding of biophysical mechanisms have propelled each individually and collectively toward sophisticated visualization and quantification of disease processes. It is often the case that core ideas are developed before commercialization, subject to sometimes unpredictable solutions to nontechnical hurdles such as clinical reimbursement. Despite these

Disclosures: None.
Dent Neurologic Institute, 3980A Sheridan Drive, Suite 101, Amherst, NY 14226, USA
E-mail address: jfritz@dentinstitute.com

Neurol Clin 32 (2014) 1–29
http://dx.doi.org/10.1016/j.ncl.2013.07.007   **neurologic.theclinics.com**

inherent risks in prognostication, this article offers an outlook on some promising technologies that may affect clinical neuroimaging in the near future.

COMMON DEVELOPMENTS

Historical reviews[1–4] offer insights into the complex interplay of inventions and collaborations across disciplines and generations that factor into product evolution. **Table 1** summarizes general trends in neuroimaging that are common to the development and integration of individual imaging systems.

An important goal of medical imaging is preclinical detection of disease or disease progression. For example, the diagnosis of multiple sclerosis in radiologically isolated syndrome is now acceptable in the absence of clinical findings.[5] There is an increasing trend toward using more numeric data to supplement or highlight conventional image analysis because quantitative comparisons with normal ranges may detect more subtle variations that may arise early in a disease. Variability caused by the lack of robust standardization across technologists, physicians, centers, and vendors must be minimized in order to fully exploit the benefits of quantitation.[6] Automation in volume positioning, technique selection, workflow, and display processing will continue to be a development focus for the purpose of reducing variability.

The computer graphics and movie industries have accelerated the evolution of visualization tools in medical imaging. Very-high-resolution three-dimensional (3D), four-dimensional (4D) (dynamic), and multimodal data sets that are now obtained within reasonable scan times combine with interactive rendering, fly-through, and morphing algorithms and computer graphics engines to produce views of the human body that previously were unattainable. Visualization tools have become essential given the large volume of raw data collected. Obstacles to the use of sophisticated visualization

Table 1 General trends	
Feature	**Innovations**
Connectomics	Merging functional and anatomic data from multiple modalities; large disease databases and atlases; connectivity informatics applied to understanding brain circuitry, and its relationship to cognition, development, and disease characteristics
Quantitation	Standardization and testing across vendors; age-matched controls; improved sensitivity and consistency in acquisitions; measurement and visualization of physiologic characteristics
Visualization	Multimodality fusion; integrated numerical analysis; sophisticated computer graphics to manipulate multidimensional data sets
Simplicity and repeatability	Automatic positioning and acquisitions; intervendor standardization
Patient comfort	Faster acquisitions; motion correction; gantries designed for comfort
Acquisition speed	Hardware speed; sparse sampling
Hybrid systems	PET/MR/EEG, photoacoustic, MR/HIFU

Abbreviations: EEG, electroencephalogram; HIFU, high-intensity focused ultrasound; PET, positron emission tomography.

include medicolegal issues (is it possible to reconstruct and review every possible view?), workflow required for complex data interaction, expense associated with delivering services that are insufficiently reimbursed, and standardization required to determine normal variants.

As the health care industry has become more consumer-driven, reducing patient anxiety and minimizing the patient's time spent in the medical setting have become important goals. This trend has translated into the development of diagnostic imaging equipment that is less intimidating and accomplishes more in less time. To address this need, gantries have been modified in appearance and size, communication and entertainment systems are better integrated, and scan speed has been increased to minimize the duration of the procedure.

Improved acquisition speed is also essential to minimizing motion artifacts and for assessing physiology that requires high temporal sampling rates, such as blood flow and perfusion. Physical approaches to speed enhancement (faster gantry rotations, stronger magnets and gradients, better detectors) are increasingly supplemented by improvements in reconstruction algorithms that permit more efficient data collection. Sparse sampling methods take advantage of known information to fill in for acquired data, accomplishing orders of magnitude speedup factors.

Hybrid acquisition technology has been gaining momentum since the introduction of positron emission tomography (PET)/CT systems. Fused data sets that overlay metabolic, physiologic, and anatomic information offer more complete insights into the disease process. Data fusion may be performed on independently acquired data sets, but there is growing appreciation of the advantages to the simultaneous acquisition of coregistered data sets from complimentary modalities. PET/MR, therapy/imaging, electroencephalogram (EEG)/MR are some examples.

The Human Connectome Project is a unification of anatomic, functional, white matter circuitry, atlases, and database projects designed to develop a more thorough understanding of normal and pathologic variants to brain processing and its complex neural network.[7-9] Initiated in 2005, it is now a National Institutes of Health (NIH)–funded program based at the University of California Los Angeles, Harvard University/Massachusetts General Hospital, Washington University, and the University of Minnesota. Its clinical effectiveness fundamentally relies on the collection of precise, quantifiable data and reference atlases that can be linked to functional attributes (**Fig. 1**).[10-13]

MR

MR imaging (MRI) and spectroscopy (referred to in this article as MR to represent its breadth beyond imaging) is unique in its programmability and collaborative development efforts. Sophisticated software-based pulse sequence programming tools permit rapid prototyping and extremely productive alliances between industry, clinics, and academia. Commercial updates occur multiple times per year, ranging from subtle sequence improvements to major innovations. These methods can be complex, and build on core principles that the reader may wish to review in order to gain a full understanding of the topics discussed herein.[14] **Table 2** summarizes recent trends in MR.

Magnet Hardware

Current standard 1.5-T and 3-T clinical systems and commercial research systems operating at 7 T and 9.4 T would not have been possible without Heike Onnes' discovery of superconductivity in 1911 and George Yntema's 1954 production of the first 4°K

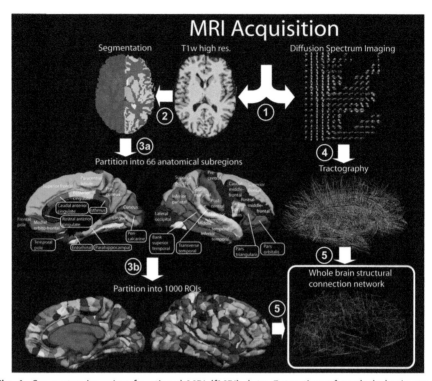

Fig. 1. Connectomics using functional MRI (fMRI) data. Extraction of a whole-brain structural connectivity network. (1) High-resolution T1-weighted and diffusion spectrum MRI (DSI) is acquired. DSI is represented with a zoom on the axial slice of the reconstructed diffusion map, showing an orientation distribution function at each position represented by a deformed sphere whose radius codes for diffusion intensity. Blue codes for the head-feet, red for left-right, and green for anterior-posterior orientations. (2) White and gray matter segmentation is performed from the T1-weighted image. (3a) Sixty-six cortical regions with clear anatomic landmarks are created and then (3b) individually subdivided into small regions of interest (ROIs), resulting in 998 ROIs. (4) Whole-brain tractography is performed providing an estimate of axonal trajectories across the white matter. (5) ROIs identified in step (3b) are combined with the result of step (4) in order to compute the connection weight between each pair of ROIs. The result is a weighted network of structural connectivity across the brain. (*From* Hagmann P, Cammoun L, Gigandet X, et al. Mapping the structural core of human cerebral cortex. PLoS Biol 2008;6(7):e159.)

superconducting magnet using niobium wire. Ultrahigh field strength MRI systems operating up to 26.8 T have been made possible by the discovery of high-temperature superconductors in 1986 by Georg Bednorz and Karl Muller, and more recently the 2007 development of yttrium barium copper oxide (YBCO)–based superconductors. The US Food and Drug Administration currently permits clinical scanners to operate up to 4 T. It is possible that this limit could be increased given an established safety record for commercial high-field systems and promising research in very-high-resolution and functional imaging achievable at ultrahigh field strength. Issues such as siting expense (eg, massive steel shielding), safety, and artifacts have created barriers for ultrahigh-field system commercialization into the clinical market. Attempts to address these impracticalities of ultrahigh-field systems range

Table 2
MRI trends

Feature	Research Innovations
Magnet design	Maturity of 7-T research systems; high-temperature superconductors for ultrahigh field strengths; multiple configurations that balance patient comfort with hardware specifications
Quiet MRI	Silent sequences (eg, SWIFT); gradient mounting strategies
Parallel transmit	Independent control of multiple RF transmitters; efficient acquisition of small FOV with high resolution; improved homogeneity and transmit power control at 3 T
Digital receivers	High-density coil arrays with fiberoptic connection; high parallel imaging speedup factor; can be autoconfigured for optimum signal and less variability
Compressed sensing	Sparse k-space sampling that increases acquisition speedup to match information content
fMRI	Integration of paradigm generator and acquisition; resting state fMRI without paradigms; higher density head coils for improved signal; MR connectomics visualization and interpretation
Diffusion tensor imaging	High Angular Resolution Diffusion Imaging (HARDI); improved spine tractography using parallel transmit
SWI	Quantitative phase mapping; explosive growth in applications: blood products, venous visualization, white matter microarchitecture, myelin imaging, iron concentration, amyloid marker
Perfusion	ASL maturing as quantitative noncontrast perfusion, dynamic flow visualization, and identification of vascular territories; improved contrast-based perfusion and permeability modeling
Spectroscopy	Fast acquisitions using parallel imaging; 3D chemical shift imaging; identification of hidden metabolites using spectral editing; ultrahigh-field research with other nuclei
Other	Nanoparticle-targeted contrast agents and therapy delivery; ultrashort TE; uniform fat suppression at high field/large FOV

Abbreviations: ASL, arterial spin labeling; fMRI, functional MRI; FOV, field of view; HARDI, high angular resolution diffusion imaging; RF, radiofrequency; SWI, susceptibility-weighted imaging; SWIFT, sweep imaging with Fourier transform; TE, echo time.

from self-shielding magnet designs to prepolarized MRI in which a large net magnetization is created by a pulsed magnetic field rather than an ultrahigh static field.[15]

3T has become the de facto standard for neuroimaging and the focus for most industry-based research. Work at higher field strength often produces insights that are useful at 3 T and 1.5 T. The cost for clinical MR systems in the United States has steadily declined as a result of economy of scale and designed cost cutting that directly targets the strained US health care market. Systems using 1.5 T retain a strong clinical presence because of favorable price points, sufficient quality for routine work, and safety advantages for patients with certain implants. The popularity of open-sided and stand-up scanners has faded because of their association with lower field strength and poorer gradient performance. Much research emphasis has been on finding the optimum trade-off between signal quality and bore dimensions (patient comfort, greater room for therapy planning), and overcoming artifacts and patient comfort issues that worsen with field strength. For example, the signal to noise advantage of high-field systems is compromised by the requirement for greater radiofrequency (RF) power deposition, dielectric effects that cause nonuniformities, and less tissue contrast with certain conventional sequences. The more comfortable wide, short-bore magnets are technically more challenging in terms of gradient linearity (eg, spatial precision may depend on distortion correction algorithms), RF power control, and homogeneity.

Acoustic noise is also more problematic with increasing field strength and wider bore systems. Vacuum containment and cushioned gradient mounting are among the approaches used to reduce the loud banging sounds that cause patient anxiety and induce motion either by startling the patient or from sonic vibrations.[16,17] Pulse sequences may also be modified to soften the sharp transitions in gradient switching used for spatial localization.[18,19] In the past, such methods have been less useful in fast imaging, which typically collects data by rapid transitions through k-space. A novel recent method uses a swept RF excitation and incremental rather than abrupt adjustments to spatial encoding gradients, thereby eliminating the source of acoustic noise.[20] These sequences result in virtually silent acquisitions. Research activities include understanding and controlling the artifacts, resolution, and contrast associated with these radically different methods of data acquisition.

Parallel Transmission

Modern magnet designs now incorporate multiple fully controllable transmit coils that help generate a uniform excitation and optimize the use of RF power.[21] This parallel transmit technology helps overcome specific absorption rate (SAR) limitations with high-field sequences and also creates interesting possibilities for focused imaging. Freely tailored regions of excitation offer the possibility to target excitation to a small field of view (FOV) and eliminate phase aliasing. Thus high-resolution imaging can be accomplished with fewer phase encode steps, less RF power deposition, and greatly improved scan time (**Fig. 2**).[22]

Manufacturers have so far implemented this technology using 2 independent, freely controllable RF transmit channels, incorporating hardware that is similar to standard quadrature coils. This technology will continue to evolve as more transmit coils are added, creating the possibility for more precise control of small and arbitrarily shaped excitation patterns.[23,24] Important advances include the development of appropriate

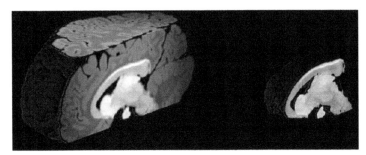

Fig. 2. Using parallel transmit to excite a small FOV. The figure compares full and zoomed FOV gradient recalled echo images obtained after global and 3D selective excitation. Both volumes were acquired within the identical measurement time whereby the zoomed image exhibits a spatial resolution that is a factor of 2 better in all 3 dimensions. (*From* Shah NJ, Oros-Peusquens AM, Arrubla J, et al. Advances in multimodal neuroimaging: Hybrid MR–PET and MR–PET–EEG at 3 T and 9.4 T. J Magn Reson 2013;229:9; with permission.)

safety mechanisms that ensure excessive RF power is not transmitted in the event of the failure of one or more channels.

Array Coils and Parallel Imaging

By digitizing the MR signal directly at the coil, a single flexible fiberoptic cable can replace the bulky collection of individual wires that place practical limits on the number of receive channels. The ability to conduct information to and from a limitless number of receiver elements creates the possibility of very-high-density coil arrays and enhanced parallel imaging factors. Multiple small coils can be electronically enabled, calibrated, and combined to produce the effect of an optimally oriented and positioned large coil, and create the optimum compromise between the coil size required to maximize signal/noise ratio (SNR) versus necessary penetration depth. It is possible to imagine replacing special-purpose coils with an electronically configurable body sleeve embedded with many small elements, thus removing the variability and setup time that are inherent in patient positioning.

Fast k-space Sampling

In general, fast data acquisition can be accomplished by several approaches, including rapid collection of raw data (k-space) in a single repetition time (TR) interval using high gradient amplitudes and switching rates; undersampling k-space data (eg, half Fourier, parallel imaging); and short repetition time. The ability to rapidly traverse k-space with clever trajectories is possible through continuing advances in digital electronics and gradient and receiver engineering. Because of patient safety and comfort (heating, neurostimulation, acoustic noise) as well as equipment expense, there is a limit to the speedup achievable by hardware alone.

Recent innovations in fast scanning have emphasized sparse sampling. Early concepts simply eliminated the edges of k-space and accepted some loss in resolution. Keyhole methods accelerate dynamic imaging by sampling the contrast-sensitive center of k-space more frequently than the edges. Parallel imaging uses knowledge of coil sensitivity profiles to unwrap undersampled k-space. New methods generalize this sparse sampling concept using principles of information content and compression.

Compressed sensing or compressed sense offers the promise of orders of magnitude acceleration by using known image characteristics to minimize the amount of data collected.[25] The currently accepted practice of compressing images for Picture Archiving and Communication System (PACS) storage and transmission implies that there is redundant information content in the acquired data. For example, consider MR angiogram source images that contain few nonzero pixels. Dynamic images similarly have significant frame-to-frame similarities.[26] The principle is applicable to general images as well. Although undersampling is normally associated with a wraparound artifact, a random distribution of k-space samples produces an image that looks like the original with structured noise added. Then iterative reconstruction using known constraints is used to remove the noise produced. The combination of compressed sense, parallel RF transmission, and multicoil receiver technologies offers opportunities for very short acquisition times or very fast dynamic sampling (**Fig. 3**).

Accelerated acquisition methods offer benefits beyond reducing overall scan time, including subsecond imaging that produces acceptable-quality images despite patient motion; tighter echo spacing that results in less opportunity for artifact caused by T2 decay or susceptibility-induced dephasing; shorter echo times (TEs) to improve visibility of very short T2 tissue; dynamic acquisitions with high temporal sampling rates that permit visualization and functional quantification of physiologic processes

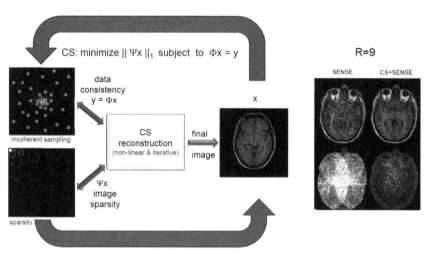

Fig. 3. Compressed sensing (CS). Compressed sensing has 2 fundamental premises: signal sparsity and incoherent sampling. A nonlinear sparsity promoting reconstruction enables accurate signal recovery from highly undersampled data. Such a reconstruction is iterative, minimizing image sparsity under data consistency constraint (y, measured data; x, image; Φ, encoding matrix; Ψ, sparsity transform) (*left*). A basic flow chart of such a reconstruction is shown (*right*). Example: CS is advantageous at high reduction factors. A comparison between SENSE and a combination of CS and SENSE is shown for an 8-channel head coil, reduction factor of 9. SENSE breaks down because the problem is underdetermined. CS can better handle this missing data problem. (*Courtesy of* Peter Börnert, PhD, and Mariya Doneva, PhD, Philips Research Laboratories, Hamburg, Germany.)

such as blood perfusion, vascular or cerebrospinal fluid (CSF) flow, and motion tracking.

Functional MRI

Functional imaging, including MR spectroscopy (MRS), diffusion tensor imaging (DTI), susceptibility-weighted imaging (SWI), arterial spin labeling (ASL), and blood oxygen level dependent (BOLD) functional MRI (fMRI), has entered into clinical practice.[27] An overview of some recent advances and trends in fMRI follows.

BOLD fMRI and DTI

Improvements to the magnet (higher field strength, homogeneity), gradients (higher amplitude, slew rate, linearity and eddy current control, stability), RF transmit design (stability, higher power), RF receiver design (many element array coils, parallel imaging) and algorithms (parallel imaging, statistical processing, motion compensation) have combined to increase sensitivity and temporal sampling rate, reduce artifacts, and improve the statistics that correlate regions of signal change with function.[28] Stimulation paradigms and the methods of presenting the stimuli have also evolved, and the process of probing cognitive relationships is at least as important as the acquisition itself.[29] Greater integration between the paradigm generator and the scanner both in terms of synchronization and presentation will continue to improve the workflow. Resting-state fMRI uses BOLD imaging without stimulus to assess baseline brain activity.[30] It is simpler to acquire in that there is no need to coordinate a paradigm, but noncommercial postprocessing is needed to produce connectivity maps representing cross-correlations between brain regions. As visualization of these connectivity maps is standardized and normal variants determined, this tool is expected to become diagnostically meaningful in the understanding of cognitive processes.

DTI is currently achieved using multidirectional diffusion acquisitions. The fractional anisotropy associated with diffusion restriction outlines fiber tracts. High-order diffusion acquisitions (eg, probing hundreds of diffusion directions and processing using DTI variants such as diffusion spectral imaging) in a reasonable scan time are beginning to move from research to clinical implementation, resulting in more accurate representation of complex axonal routing. Longitudinal tracking of white matter tract characteristics is expected to be important in assessing neurodegenerative processes. The fractional anisotropy value has been shown to correlate with local trauma, perhaps as a result of the development of varicosities stemming from structural injury to the axon.[31]

DTI and BOLD imaging, together with anatomic imaging, are useful in planning surgical pathways.[32] Overall brain function represented by the combination of connecting circuitry from DTI and cellular activity from paradigm-driven or resting state BOLD or other fMRI variants offers the promise of understanding cognitive processing, the impact of brain injury, autism, multiple sclerosis, dementia, psychiatric disorders, and brain plasticity.

Susceptibility imaging

Susceptibility imaging applies additional processing to gradient (field) echo sequences that are sensitive to local changes in magnetic field homogeneity. These regional distortions may occur as the result of oxygenation changes, the presence of iron, or blood products. Phase information that is normally discarded from typical magnitude reconstructions is used to enhance the visualization of these field changes and the quantification of local magnetic susceptibility (**Fig. 4**).

Typical applications have been in Alzheimer disease and trauma (eg, microbleeds resulting from shearing injury or stroke).[33] It has also been applied to tumor imaging and deep vein visualization in relation to multiple sclerosis plaques. Quantitative susceptibility is an extension of modern qualitative imaging that could have a revolutionary effect on functional imaging. More sophisticated processing of the phase data is revealing myelin distribution, white matter microarchitectures, and iron concentration levels associated with neurodegenerative disease and oxygen saturation (**Fig. 5**).[34–36]

ASL

ASL is a noninvasive way to measure brain perfusion using RF pulses to produce a contrast bolus that affects distal image slices in a manner similar to dynamic contrast enhancement or dynamic susceptibility contrast perfusion.[37,38] It is a safe alternative to gadolinium-based methods in patients with compromised kidney function, and offers improved workflow and the potential for absolute quantification. The general concept is to subtract images obtained while saturating inflowing blood from images collected without the application of such tagging. Absolute perfusion measurements are achievable, resulting in a broad range of applications including stroke, hydrocephalus, dementia, oncology, neuropsychiatric disorders, and as a biomarker for pharmacologic actions.[39–42]

ASL methods have evolved to better account for such variables as T1 relaxation and off-resonance effects, as well as providing improvements in SNR and using targeted RF stimulation to probe individual vascular territories. Dynamic spin labeling acquisitions can also be created by introducing cardiac gating and multiple time delay acquisitions, permitting the visualization of blood or CSF flow (**Fig. 6**).[43–46]

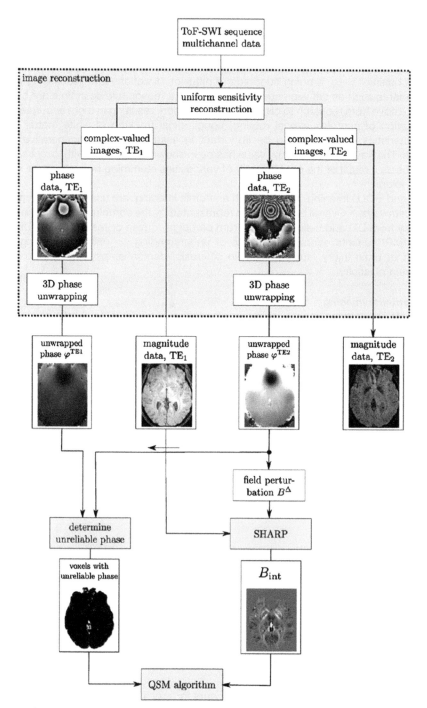

Fig. 4. The quantitative susceptibility mapping (QSM) framework for quantitative SWI. (*Reprinted from* Schweser F, Deistung A, Lehr BW, et al. Quantitative imaging of intrinsic magnetic tissue properties using MRI signal phase: an approach to in vivo brain iron metabolism. Neuroimage 2011;54(4):2791; with permission from Elsevier.)

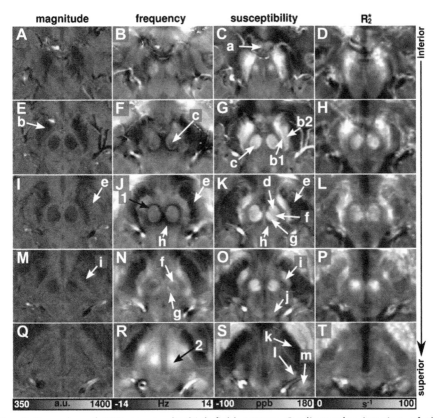

Fig. 5. Examples of SWI in an ultrahigh-field system: Gradient-echo imaging of the midbrain. Average intensity projections (projection length, 1.2 mm) of magnitude, frequency, susceptibility, and R2* images are displayed in the first, second, third, and fourth columns from the left, respectively. The rows from top to bottom sample the midbrain from an inferior to superior direction with a slice separation of 1.2 mm. Average intensity projections were computed to cover tissue variations typically visible in images with slice thicknesses of 1.2 mm. The white arrows indicate a, mammillary body; b, substantia nigra; b1, substantia nigra pars reticulata; b2, substantia nigra pars compacta; c, red nucleus pars caudalis; d, red nucleus pars oralis; e, crus cerebri; f, medullary lamella of red nucleus; g, red nucleus pars dorsomedialis; h, central tegmental tract; i, subthalamic nucleus; j, superior colliculus; k, internal capsule; l, medial geniculate nucleus; m, lateral geniculate nucleus. Nonlocal signal contributions on frequency maps are marked by black arrows (1, 2). (*Reprinted from* Deistung A, Schäfer A, Schweser F, et al. Toward in vivo histology: a comparison of quantitative susceptibility mapping (QSM) with magnitude-, phase-, and R2*-imaging at ultra-high magnetic field strength. Neuroimage 2013;65:303; with permission from Elsevier.)

Spectroscopy

Proton spectroscopy is a mature technology and can readily be applied to neurologic applications.[47,48] Single-voxel, two-dimensional (2D), and 3D chemical shift imaging; fast and automated acquisitions; and short TE sequences are readily available to produce reliable spectra for the most abundant metabolites (N-acetyl aspartate, choline, creatine, myoinositol, and lactate). Direct measurement of neurotransmitters is improved using spectral editing methods. Research systems offer phosphorous and fluorine spectroscopy. Sodium spectroscopy is also available, but is best performed

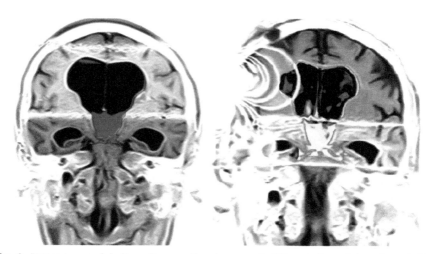

Fig. 6. Dynamic spin labeling. By sampling images at different time delays from inflow tagging, ASL methods conventionally used for noncontrast perfusion imaging can also be applied to visualizing cerebrospinal fluid flow dynamics. (*Left*) Normal-pressure hydrocephalus with visible flow obstruction. (*Right*) After surgery, with restored communication of flow. (*Courtesy of* Shinya Yamada, MD, PhD, TOSHIBA Rinkam Hospital, Kanagawa, Japan.)

on ultrahigh-field research systems (eg, 7 T or 9.4 T).[22] In the past, the technologic capabilities of spectroscopy have outpaced its clinical acceptance. Reducing variability across practices and vendors is an important component of education and development activities.[49] Semiautomatic shimming, vendor-to-vendor comparison studies, automatic peak labeling, fast acquisitions of 2D and 3D maps that overcome sampling error, and payer reimbursement have contributed to greater clinical use of MRS.

Other Methods

Various methods have been used to correct for metal and flow artifacts that result from field inhomogeneity or turbulence-related spin dephasing.[50] Pulse sequences have been developed using radial k-space acquisitions and partial echo techniques to produce images with TEs on the order of tens of microseconds, thereby revealing tissues otherwise invisible on conventional MRI because of very short T2 decay characteristics, such as ligaments or cortical bone. For neuroimaging applications, ultrashort TE (UTE) may become to be useful for artifact reduction and improved tissue discrimination.[51–53]

Uniform fat suppression is an essential requirement in routine MRI. High-field and wide-bore systems burden classic chemical shift saturation methods, whereas T1-based methods (short tau inversion recovery) are inappropriate for postcontrast studies. New, efficient implementations that combine Dixon-based methods (using multiple TEs acquired when water is in and out of phase with fat) and adiabatic RF pulses are promising alternatives that improve fat saturation at high field strength and large FOVs (**Fig. 7**).[54]

There is a growing number of other examples of functional/quantitative imaging, including use of diffusion coefficient values in characterizing tumor cellularity, segmented volumetrics of 3D data sets to evaluate cortical thickening or regional atrophy,[55] and permeability mapping using dynamic perfusion series subjected to pharmacokinetic modeling.[56] Automatic slice and patient positioning algorithms help to improve consistency and longitudinal tracking of measurements. As precision

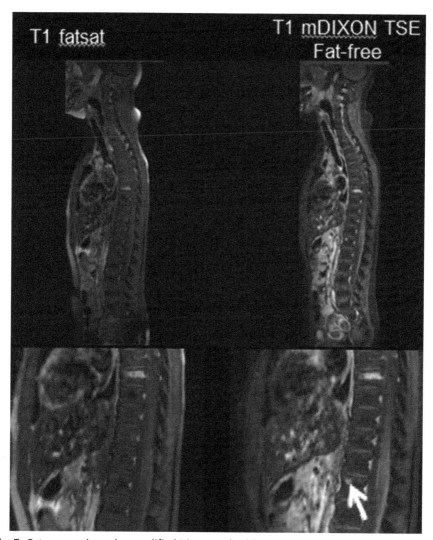

Fig. 7. Fat suppression using modified Dixon method (mDIXON). Images on the right using a more uniform fat suppression mDIXON method show greater conspicuity for a contrast-enhancing lesion (*arrow*) than the images on the right collected using conventional fat suppression. (*Courtesy of* Jeffrey H. Miller, MD, Phoenix Children's Hospital, Phoenix, AZ.)

across vendors improves and normal databases and atlases become integrated within the clinical practice, quantitative analysis will offers a greater sensitivity to subtle abnormalities, and those changes will be associated with early detection of disease processes.[57,58]

Contrast Agents

Research in new forms of contrast agents is promising, ranging from modest upgrades to gadolinium formulations for increased safety and greater enhancement, to molecular imaging agents and drug delivery. Biocytin-based contrast agents that may specifically enhance white matter tracts are in the early stages of preclinical research.[59]

Targeted nanoparticles are analogues to PET tracers,[60,61] and also can function as payloads for therapeutic delivery or optical tumor marking for surgical guidance.[62,63]

CT

Steady improvements in CT tube engineering (heat capacity, collimation, fast voltage, and current switching), detector (size, coverage, sensitivity), and reconstruction processing (computers, algorithms) continue to speed up acquisitions and improve resolution.[64] As the acquired slice thickness reached submillimeter proportions, CT transformed from an axial slice imager to an isotropic volume acquisition, thereby eliminating a fundamental disadvantage compared with MRI. New volume-rendering and display methods that borrow from computer graphics enable 3D and fly-through views that have radically changed CT imaging. Scan time has steadily declined as well, thus the time required to collect a volume of data has reached a temporal resolution threshold in which dynamic imaging can adequately sample physiologic processes. For example, repeatedly acquiring a 16-cm volume comprising isotropic voxels at a resolution of 0.5 mm × 0.5 mm × 0.5 mm every 0.3 seconds enables a level of functional assessment that is not achievable by early CT scans, which could only produce a single 5-mm slice every few seconds. Clinical examples such as dynamic CT angiography, perfusion, permeability, and kinematic imaging are discussed in the article by Snyder and Colleagues elsewhere in this issue. **Table 3** summarizes recent trends in CT.

Acquisition Speed

Gantry rotation times have declined over the past 2 decades from several seconds to 300 milliseconds. It is difficult to imagine this trend continuing given the enormous inertial forces on precision components such as the x-ray tube(s) and detector arrays. Alternatives to gantry speed are needed to realize significant improvements in temporal resolution.

Two other methods for collecting more data in less time are to acquire more volume per rotation, and to collect a sufficient amount of data using less than a full 360° rotation. Wide detector arrays enable the acquisition of a long longitudinal FOV in fewer

Table 3 CT trends	
Feature	**Research Innovations**
Dynamic volume acquisition	Fast gantry rotation; wide detector arrays with thin-slice detectors; high heat unit tubes; cone beam reconstruction algorithms
Dose reduction	Model-based iterative 3D reconstruction methods; fewer gantry rotations using wider detector arrays; adaptive tube modulation and collimation
High spatial resolution	Detector/flat-panel technology; interior tomography for zoom mode imaging; flying focal spot/anode control
High temporal resolution	Dual source; interior tomography with multiple tube/detector pairs; asynchronous gated sampling
Multienergy	Dual-energy image sets at different peak kilovolt (kVp) setting; tube switching or dual source; layered detectors for multienergy; artifact reduction; single-dose CTA bone removal; new tissue contrast control

Abbreviation: CTA, CT angiography.

rotations. Single organs, such as the brain and heart, can now be imaged in a single rotation. Current detector arrays consist of thousands of discrete detector elements. X-ray angiography systems are now capable of fast-rotation, high-resolution imaging using flat-panel arrays (FPA), showing the potential use of FPAs in conventional CT systems to achieve higher resolution and wider coverage. At present, FPAs do not offer adequate low-contrast performance for tissue imaging, but research continues. X-ray tubes are able to generate wide 3D cone beams that uniformly irradiate the detector array, and their high heat capacity, achieved by efficient dissipation of anode heat, permits the continuous exposure required for dynamic imaging. CT scanners with 2 x-ray tubes oriented perpendicular to each other can acquire a complete data set in half the time of a conventional scanner using less radiation.[65] Coupled with algorithms that reconstruct images from partial rotations, acquisition times on the order of one-fourth that of the gantry rotation can be attained.

In theory, the total acquisition time can be reduced by a factor equal to the number of tube/detector pairs. However, the amount of space in the gantry creates a practical limit. The azimuthal extent of the detector array is determined by the cone beam angle that is required to irradiate the full FOV (eg, FOV = 50 cm). Using conventional reconstruction algorithms, it is essential that the FOV completely contains the axial anatomy inside the gantry; a smaller FOV results in incomplete and inconsistent projections. Interior tomography uses iterative reconstruction algorithms that incorporate a priori information to permit the imaging within a small portion of the anatomy, thereby allowing for very-high-resolution imaging in faster scan times (**Fig. 8**).[66,67]

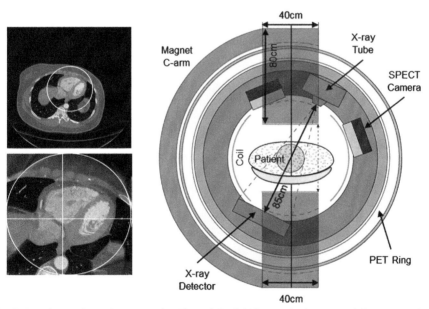

Fig. 8. Interior and omnitomography. The original CT image in the upper left was acquired with conventional FOV. The CT image in the lower right was reconstructed using a narrow cone beam. The diagram on the right illustrates a concept of merging multiple modalities each capable of a zoom mode of imaging using interior tomography concepts. The CT fan beam includes only a portion of the anatomy. (*Adapted from* Wang G, Zhang J, Gao H, et al. Towards omni-tomography—grand fusion of multiple modalities for simultaneous interior tomography. PLoS One 2012;7(6):e39700; with permission. http://dx.doi.org/10.1371/journal.pone.0039700.)

In addition to enabling a high-resolution zoom mode, interior tomography also allows the implementation of many tube/detector pairs, each responsible for narrower arcs, and allowing for complete data acquisition in a fraction of gantry rotation. For example, a gantry with 5 tube/detector pairs rotating at 300 milliseconds per rotation would reach 30 milliseconds temporal resolution.

Slice Resolution

Slice resolution is directly related to the size of individual detector elements. However, smaller surface area and interdetector collimation can reduce the amount of incident radiation captured, making it difficult for hardware alone to improve slice resolution much further than the current status of 0.5 mm. Hardware solutions seek to improve the sensitivity of the detector, including adjusting the orientation of the detectors to better align with incident cone beam radiation, using materials that convert absorbed radiation to greater light output and ultimately increased signal, and minimizing the area of the detector collimation grid.

In conjunction with radiation source manipulation, the effective slice resolution may be improved beyond the limitations of the detector. An example is the flying focal spot method, in which the angle of the anode is changed during one-half of the gantry rotation, offsetting the focal spot of the irradiated x-ray beam by half the detector width.[68] As a result, a single rotation produces 2 sets of data shifted by half the slice thickness. Although the resolution is unchanged, the half-thickness spacing results in improvements similar to those attained with smaller detectors (less streaking or windmill artifact, higher quality multiplanar reconstruction and volume rendering) at approximately the same dose requirements. Variations of the flying focal spot technology, such as the use of a rotating anode to produce saddle-line cone beam radiation patterns, may offer advantages in cardiac or interior tomography imaging.

Dose Reduction

Manufacturers have been placing increased emphasis on reducing and reporting doses. Some studies have suggested that growing CT use is responsible for an increase in cancer rates, especially in children.[69] Radiation burns have also been reported when CT is operated in dynamic mode. It is important to understand some fundamentals about dose measurement in order to gauge the potential risk of a CT scan. Effective dose is measured in millisieverts (mSV), and is calculated as a product of the CT Dose Index, which measures the amount of radiation produced by the x-ray tube, the total length of the radiated anatomy, and a k-factor that accounts for tissue absorption as a function of factors such as organ and age. Background radiation from all sources in nature is on the order of 3 mSV per year. Radiology professionals are limited to 50 mSv exposure per year. Clinical scans had historically delivered dose in the tens of millisieverts, but a wide variety of methods have been developed to reduce doses to submillisievert levels for many scans. Improved detector sensitivity implies that less radiation is required for a desired contrast/noise ratio; wide detector arrays minimize the degree of overlapping radiation caused by multiple gantry rotations, tube current modulation automatically optimizes radiation in real time as a function of anatomic position, and advanced iterative reconstruction algorithms are able to substantially reduce image noise in very-low-dose acquisitions.

Reconstruction processing is a particularly aggressive area of development in dose reduction. The newest algorithms iteratively apply known information to 3D cone beam reconstructions, and have enabled most neuroimaging techniques to be reduced to less than natural background levels, even for pediatric patients.[70] The dose is reduced in dynamic CT angiography and perfusion scanning by using temporal sampling that is greatest during the initial arrival of the contrast bolus and less frequent during washout. The full technique is not required for each dynamic sample because the goal of the dynamic acquisition is to generate parametric maps. Therefore, even perfusion scanning can be performed at dose levels near or less than background radiation, with further improvements likely in the coming years.

Multienergy

In conventional single-energy CT scanners, the x-ray tube emits an energy spectrum in which the peak kilovolt (kVp) parameter sets the maximum delivered energy. The detector then integrates the energy spectrum to yield a single number representing the attenuation along each projection line. A multiple-energy approach repeats the scan with a different energy spectrum. Because tissue attenuation is a function of the incident energy spectrum, additional contrast information can be obtained. In particular, iodine, bone, and calcium have different values, permitting combinations of the two data sets to remove or isolate bone, assess plaque, remove or retain contrast in filled blood vessels, and reduce artifact from implanted hardware (**Fig. 9**).[71]

A simple approach for dual energy is to acquire a second set of images at a different kVp which results in a different energy spectrum. Image registration, dose reduction, and expansion from dual to multienergy are among the improvements in development. Several more sophisticated approaches have been developed for multienergy acquisitions.[72] Image registration can be improved by quickly switching kVp during the gantry rotation. As an alternative, systems that already use multiple tube/detector subsystems can apply different techniques to each tube. A third approach is to use

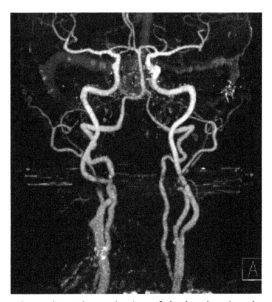

Fig. 9. Thick-slab maximum intensity projection of the head and neck vessels in a 62-year-old patient after dual-energy bone removal. The postprocessing was fully automated and did not require user interaction. Note the almost complete removal of osseous structures of the skull base. Because of dental artifacts, segmentation errors occurred at the level of the artifacts. (*Reprinted from* Thomas C, Korn A, Krauss B, et al. Automatic bone and plaque removal using dual energy CT for head and neck angiography: feasibility and initial performance evaluation. Eur J Radiol 2010;76:63; with permission from Elsevier.)

layered detectors that are each sensitive to a different energy band. This approach has the advantages of perfect registration, simultaneous detection, and the ability to detect multiple nonoverlapping energy bands using a single kVp. Combinations of the multiple images offer the opportunity for improved tissue discrimination using conventional single-scan doses.

ULTRASOUND

Current clinical systems have benefited from regular updates in the design of transducers (eg, array configurations, comfort, frequency, sensitivity), algorithms (eg, 3D and 4D reconstructions, spectral processing), system portability (eg, handheld units), and workflow.[4,73,74] **Table 4** summarizes recent trends in ultrasound imaging.

A primary use of ultrasound in neuroimaging is to assess the carotid arteries for stenosis and wall thickness.[75] Methods are being developed that make use of multielement high-frequency transducer designs to improve resolution.[76] New techniques generate double oscillating fields parallel and perpendicular to the surface to permit accurate flow measurements in all directions; quantification of wall strain may then be estimated. Furthermore, 3D and 4D reconstructions can be created using electronic and mechanical beam-steering techniques. New display strategies include the overlay of flow vectors. Together, these strides in carotid ultrasound offer the potential to more fully visualize, measure, and characterize the carotids and plaque evolution (**Fig. 10**).[77]

Standard ultrasound remains limited in its tissue contrast and spatial resolution relative to MR or CT, but new techniques have been developed that offer novel contrast characteristics. For example, harmonic imaging after bubble contrast injection can be used to assess the vasa vasorum through detection of adventitial enhancement.[78–80] Ultrasound elastography has been used to assess brain stiffness to detect edematous changes and tumors.[81] Also, MRI elastography combines the mechanical insonation properties of ultrasound with MR phase imaging to measure elastic properties.[82] Photoacoustic imaging research offers the possibility of providing greater

Table 4 Ultrasound trends	
Feature	**Research Innovations**
Color Doppler	Transducer arrays, beam steering, and transverse oscillation for multidirectional sensitivity; vector display visualization; quantification of wall strain for plaque stiffness characterization
3D acquisition	Mechanical linear scanning transducers; speckle filtering using spatial compounding
Contrast imaging	Harmonic imaging of the vasa vasorum for plaque characterization; perfusion imaging improvements with dynamic registration methods; microbubble payloads for imaging and therapy
Photoacoustic imaging	Hybrid laser/ultrasound for high-resolution, high-contrast imaging
Continuous wave Doppler	High-resolution Fourier-based method to decode Doppler effect from moving transducer
Functional TCD	Flow velocity spectrum vs functional paradigm; noninvasive motion tolerant language lateralization test

Abbreviation: TCD, transcranial Doppler.

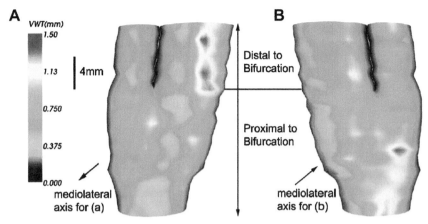

Fig. 10. 3D vessel wall plus plaque thickness (VWT) map of the patient who did not receive any treatment, obtained by analyzing the 3D carotid ultrasound image at baseline. The VWT map is visualized from (*A*) the near side (ie, the mediolateral axis points out of the page), and (*B*) the far side from the transducer (ie, the mediolateral axis points into the page). (*Reprinted from* Chiu B, Egger M, Spence DJ, et al. Area-preserving flattening maps of 3D ultrasound carotid arteries images. Med Image Anal 2008;12:679; with permission from Elsevier.)

specificity than conventional ultrasound imaging.[83] Improvements continue to overcome deficiencies in penetration depth and laser technology. Applications include plaque characterization when combined with intravascular imaging, visualization of microvasculature if the probe can be positioned sufficiently close, blood oxygenation, and temperature monitoring in focused ultrasound therapy.

Methods for improved resolution include improvements in high-frequency probes, intravascular ultrasound in an interventional setting, and new approaches using continuous wave imaging. Continuous wave imaging uses the concept of Doppler frequency shift, but applied to decoding the effect of a moving probe relative to the tissue being imaged.[84]

Functional imaging is possible by monitoring middle cerebral artery (MCA) velocities bilaterally during stimulus paradigms.[85] Harmonic reflections occur as a result of functionally induced vasoreactivity in distal branches, and are detectable by a spectroscopic analysis of the velocity measurements. The harmonics correspond to standing waves formed at distances to successive branches. Thus temporal changes to harmonics that are correlated with the functional paradigm localize associated brain activity. Transcranial Doppler spectroscopy is a safe alternative to other methods for assessing language lateralization in children, and is not prone to the motion artifacts, expense, and anxiety that may be associated with fMRI.

Transcranial imaging is also evolving as a convenient neuroimaging tool for observing the hyperechogenicity of the substantia nigra, with potential application in Parkinson disease.[86] Molecular imaging in ultrasound is similar to molecular MR. It is achievable using labeled microbubbles that are targeted to receptors and locally ruptured to release their contents by high-energy insonation.[87]

NUCLEAR MEDICINE

As with MR and CT, Positron Emission Tomography (PET) and single-photon emission computed tomography (SPECT) scanner specifications such as resolution, coverage, acquisition time, SNR, and contrast to noise continue to improve as a result of engineering innovations in detector materials, gantry design, and reconstruction algorithms.[88] The integration with CT improved PET acquisition times by replacing slower attenuation scanning with fast CT acquisition, and led to simultaneous anatomy and functional imaging. Advances in radiopharmacy have driven an expansion in the development of new tracers. **Table 5** summarizes trends in nuclear medicine.

Hardware

PET image reconstruction relies on the detection of coincident events in opposing detectors. Detector crystals materials such as $Lu_2SiO_5[Ce]$ (LSO) and lutetium yttrium orthodilicate (LSO) have higher light output and shorter decay times than earlier bismuth germanium oxide (BGO) based crystals, resulting in improved signal and better time sensitivity. SNR is also increased using the recently commercialized time-of-flight method, which takes advantage of more precise determination of arrival time to identify the approximate location of the source isotope.[89] This information is then used by iterative reconstruction algorithms to determine precise localization. SNR is improved by applying the full projection data set to resolving smaller regions than can be assumed using non-TOF methods. For example, a temporal resolution of 500 picoseconds is currently achievable, and the SNR gain compared with non-TOF systems is on the order of a factor of 2, with further improvements on the horizon. Additional dose and scan time reductions can be derived from 3D iterative reconstruction and compressed sensing algorithms, as described earlier. The combination of these and other hardware advances suggest that PET scans currently requiring several minutes of acquisition time will likely be completed in less than a minute in the near future, with improved spatial resolution.

Unlike PET, SPECT requires the use of physical collimation rather than the virtual collimation associated with coherence detection, resulting in decreased detector efficiency, less sensitivity, and poorer resolution. Despite these disadvantages, SPECT hardware and its longer half-life radiopharmaceuticals are less expensive and radiosynthesis is more practical. Also, image quality can be improved by imaging longer because of the longer half-life, allowing washout of nonspecific signals. An important engineering focus for SPECT has been the development of new types of collimation.

Hybrid imaging is commercially available and in wide clinical use. For example, additional sensitivity and anatomic reference is achieved through the subtraction of preictus and intraictus SPECT scans of patients with epilepsy; when overlaid on MR

Table 5	
Nuclear medicine trends	
Feature	**Research Innovations**
PET	Dose reduction and faster scan times using iterative reconstruction algorithms, increased crystal time and energy sensitivity; improved time-of-flight resolution opportunities for dramatic increase in SNR
SPECT	SISCOM to reveal seizure focus; collimator designs to improve SNR
Tracers	Radiochemistry advances for efficient, high-yield production; improved selectivity of tracers: amyloid, acetylcholinesterase, angiogenesis, white matter, neurotransmitters
PET/MR	Simultaneous hybrid acquisition; motion and partial volume correction; integration with EEG for complete functional assessment

Abbreviation: SISCOM, subtraction ictal SPECT coregistered to MRI.

images, this technique, known as subtraction ictal SPECT coregistered to MRI (SIS-COM), has been useful in surgical planning and electrode placement in children with seizure disorders.[90–92] Physically combined PET/CT and SPECT/CT systems offer advantages compared with single-modality nuclear medicine in the precision with which high-resolution anatomic and metabolic images can be aligned. Attenuation correction using CT data also resulted in faster PET imaging. These benefits have motivated the investment in prototype hybrid MR-PET.[93] Such systems permit the overlay of DTI, fMRI, ASL, and other structural/functional imaging from MRI with PET and even EEG acquisitions obtained simultaneously during a single stimulus paradigm and identical physiologic conditions.[22] PET-MR systems are now commercially available, having overcome many barriers that forced the redesign of fundamental components of each system. MR-compatible PET detectors, low-attenuation MR coils, MR-based PET attenuation correction algorithms using ultrashort TE sequences, and many other engineering challenges had to be addressed in creating such a system.[22,93] Progress continues with the goal of leveraging the advantages of one modality to address the disadvantages of another, resulting in more complete information content, motion-corrected functional imaging, and minimum scan time (**Fig. 11**).

PET Tracers

In general, imaging probes used in nuclear medicine must have high affinity and selectivity for the target receptor and good pharmacokinetic properties so as to minimize the amount of agent required to a precise, well-defined dose that easily crosses the cell membrane. Flourine-18 has been the mainstay of PET imaging for several reasons: its long half-life obviates an on-site cyclotron, and more complex radiosynthesis is possible. F18 replaces hydrogen to produce an imaging agent that is indistinguishable from its nonradioactive counterpart, and the strong carbon-fluorine bond results in a ligand that is not easily metabolized. Radioisotopes based on C11 result in agents that also possess these desired pharmacologic properties (the radioisotope formulation substitutes for the naturally occurring C-12). Because of its short half-life, use of C11 tracers has been restricted to institutions with cyclotrons.

Although fluorodeoxyglucose has long been the standard radiopharmaceutical used in PET, it has limitations. For example, its high uptake in normal brain tissue restricts its use in gliomas and inflammatory conditions. In general, fast and efficient generation of tracers and high radiochemical yields have resulted in advances in radiochemistry that promise significant breakthroughs in neuroimaging during the coming years.[94]

Significant research in radiochemistry has been applied to the development of new isotopes that are more sensitive for brain tumors.[95] F18-tagged derivatives of myoinositol have been developed, although currently their low brain penetration has made these more appropriate for breast imaging. Another approach recognizes that alpha amino acids, nutrients for cell proliferation by protein synthesis, are upregulated in tumors; there are now efficient synthesis techniques for both C11 and F18 versions of such radioisotopes. Examples include F18-fluoro-L-dopa (F18-DOPA), fluoroethyl-L-tyrosine (F18-FET), and 11C-methionine (C11-MET). A third strategy for ligand development aligns with the development of anticancer drugs that inhibit cell proliferation. Examples include [18F]-2′-Fluoro-5-methyl-1-beta-D-arabinofuranosyluracil (18F-FMAU), which measures DNA synthesis, and galacto labeled arginine-glycine-aspartic acid (RGD) containing peptides, which identifies $\alpha V\beta 3$ integrin expression to identify angiogenesis in malignant gliomas.[96,97]

Neurodegenerative and neuropsychiatric conditions are best assessed using noradrenaline, serotonin, and dopamine transporters labeled with either C11 or F18. These radiotracers are inherently suited to receptor studies. Expression of the

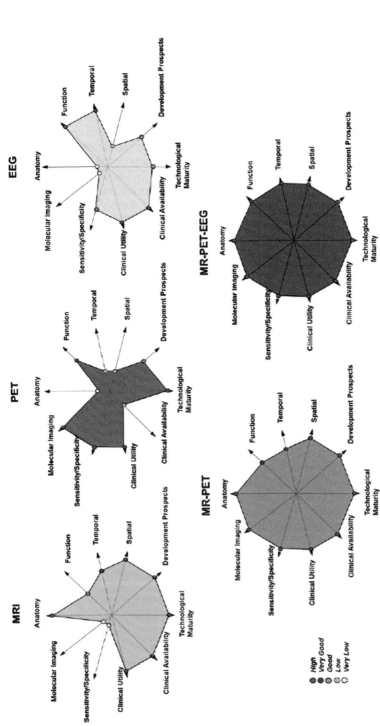

Fig. 11. Hybrid multimodality imaging. Fingerprint diagrams giving an overview of the strengths of MRI, PET, and hybrid MR-PET, and hybrid MR-PET-EEG. Starting at the origin, the further the movement along a given axis, the better that particular attribute is fulfilled. MRI can provide exquisite spatial resolution and the technology is widely available. However, MRI is not strong in the area of molecular imaging and its specificity is also limited. In contrast, PET has poorer spatial and temporal resolution than MRI but it is extremely specific(an attribute conferred on it by the choice of radiolabeled tracer) and also very sensitive. Both MRI and PET have poor temporal resolution regarding mapping of brain function, for example. In a hybrid scanner capable of simultaneous measurement of all three datasets, all the chosen attributes are fulfilled. (*Reprinted from* Shah NJ, Oros-Peusquens AM, Arrubla J, et al. Advances in multimodal neuroimaging: hybrid MR-PET and MR-PET-EEG at 3 T and 9.4 T. J Magn Reson 2013;229:2. Available at: http://dx.doi.org/10.1016/j.jmr.2012.11.027. Accessed March 12, 2013; with permission from Elsevier.)

translocator protein (TSPO) is increased by reactive glial cells in ischemia, epilepsy, nerve injury, and neurodegeneration. Radiolabeling of this ligand with C11 was initially limited by its nonspecific binding, low brain uptake, and low sensitivity, but new versions offering higher uptake look promising. Alzheimer disease plaques are characterized by a mixture of insoluble β-amyloid peptides (most prevalent) and neurofibrillary tangles. Thioflavin-T derivatives bind to insoluble but not soluble forms of amyloid, and are the basis for the preclinical detection of amyloid using tracers such as Pittsburgh compound B, 2-(1-{6-[(2-[fluorine-18]fluoroethyl)(methyl)amino]-2-naphthyl}-ethylidene)malono nitrile ([18F] FDDNP) developed at the University of California, Los Angeles, and Avid Pharmaceutical's 18F-AV-45.[98] C11 raclopride targets the D2 receptors in the striatum, with application to Parkinson disease and schizophrenia. C11-based amyloid probes have also been developed to monitor acetylcholinesterase levels using 1-[11C]methylpiperidin-4-yl propionate ([11C]PMP) in Alzheimer disease.

SPECT Tracers

Tc-99m has been the mainstay of SPECT imaging, in part because its parent Mo-99 has a half-life of 67 hours, thereby allowing on-site synthesis using commercially available kits. It had been restricted from imaging specific targets because the chelating agent produces a metal complex rather than generating a direct substitution of a hydrogen atom as in I-123 and F18. For neuroimaging, Tc-99m is mostly used to measure cerebral blood flow by binding with small lipophilic compounds that cross the blood-brain barrier by simple diffusion. Recent developments have created novel, target-specific Tc-99m radioisotopes using bifunctional chelating agents that link to biologically active molecules.

Unlike Tc-99m, I-123 bonds with carbon, and is easier to incorporate into small molecules. Advances in SPECT neuroimaging have made use of serotonin and noradrenaline transporters and acetylcholine receptors using I-123. 123I-*N*-fluoropropyl-2β-carbomethoxy-3β-(4-iodophenyl)nortropane (123I-FP-CIT) is a cocaine derivative that binds to the dopamine receptors in the basal ganglia. It can be used in Parkinson disease and Lewy body dementia.

Noradrenaline transporter (NAT) is a radiolabeled derivative of the noradrenaline selective reuptake inhibitor, reboxetine, with research focused on both PET and SPECT imaging of Alzheimer and Parkinson disease. Probes of the acetylcholine system have overcome early issues with toxicity and have progressed to human imaging studies (eg, 5-[I-123]-A85380), offering the opportunity to investigate α4β2 nicotinic acetylcholine receptor (nAChR) in Alzheimer disease, Lewy body dementia, and nicotine addiction.

A cyclotron is required to generate I-123, but its long half-life allows affordable regional transportation. Advances in radiochemistry using iodine have had to address issues of stability, toxicity, ease of synthesis, and purification. As with PET tracer development, SPECT tracer progress has benefited from new methods and approaches for the design and rapid and efficient synthesis and radiosynthesis of precursors using technology such as solid phase chemistry, microreactors, and flow chemistry. Research also continues into the development of dual-tracer imaging for neurodegenerative disease, such as Tc-99m–labeled perfusion agent and an I-123 neurotransmitter agent.[88]

SUMMARY

Individual modalities will continue to improve in sensitivity, specificity, and speed. A strong movement toward quantitation and sophisticated visualization supports early detection. Efforts are underway to reduce variability and develop normal references driven by complex database projects. Data from multiple modalities are being fused visually, and combined to create greater insights into the human disease process, especially in brain function assessment. The Human Connectome Project represents a movement toward a complete understanding of biologic and disease processes.

Workstation and PACS development is an essential component to the practical handling and interpretation of the high-resolution, multimodality, multidimensional datasets arising from the scanners. Integration of quantitative analysis and visualization must consider workflow efficiency for increasingly busy clinical settings. Digital Imaging and Communications in Medicine (DICOM) standards must evolve continuously to keep up new acquisition parameters. Integration with databases and atlases representing normal and pathologic variances will lead to improvements in computer-assisted diagnostic tools.

There are several technologies beyond those discussed earlier that deserve recognition. Diffuse optical imaging is available in various forms, including portable near-infrared detection systems that may be useful in acute trauma. For seizure focus and functional activity mapping, magnetic source imaging offers improved cortical spatial localization compared with EEG, and retains its temporal resolution advantages compared with PET and fMRI. The relationship between diagnostic neuroimaging technologies and intervention is an important area of evolution. Flat-panel detector technology and fast C-arm rotation has allowed interventional x-ray angiography to produce CT-like 3D and 4D images that surpass the temporal and spatial resolution of CT. Intravascular ultrasound and optical coherence tomography support stent planning, aneurysm rupture risk assessment, and plaque vulnerability. Surgical or fluoroscopic guidance is possible with fast MR, CT, or ultrasound units. Transcranial neurostimulation, ablation, or drug delivery can be performed with magnetic, ultrasonic, and electrical energy sources typically used in imaging.

Many advances in neuroimaging actively occur as incremental improvements to commercial products that are already cleared for clinical use. Others are early in research and require fundamental or practical breakthroughs before their potential can be realized. A substantial number of innovations are in between, sufficiently mature for clinical use but implementation slowed by economic, regulatory, and other peripheral factors. Many issues cloud any technology forecast, but history is a good indicator that imaging will continue to add anatomic, physiologic, functional, and metabolic insights that will enable earlier diagnosis, individualized therapy, and increased understanding of cognitive processing.

ACKNOWLEDGMENTS

I am grateful to Tom Perkins, PhD, and Steve Mitchell of Philips Medical Systems, Mark Stoez of GE Medical Systems, Bernd Stoeckel PhD of Siemens Medical Solutions, and Guy Poloni PhD of Toshiba Medical Systems for their valuable insights.

REFERENCES

1. Blamire AM. The technology of MRI–the next 10 years? Br J Radiol 2008; 81(968):601–17.
2. Mishra SK, Singh P. History of neuroimaging: the legacy of William Oldendorf. J Child Neurol 2010;25(4):508–17.
3. Geva T. Magnetic resonance imaging: historical perspective. J Cardiovasc Magn Reson 2006;8(4):573–80.

4. Powers J, Kremkau F. Medical ultrasound systems. Interface Focus 2011;1(4): 477–89.
5. Granberg T, Martola J, Kristoffersen-Wiberg M, et al. Radiologically isolated syndrome - incidental magnetic resonance imaging findings suggestive of multiple sclerosis, a systematic review. Mult Scler 2012;19(3):271–80.
6. Dani KA, Thomas RG, Chappell FM, et al. Systematic review of perfusion imaging with computed tomography and magnetic resonance in acute ischemic stroke: heterogeneity of acquisition and postprocessing parameters: a translational medicine research collaboration multicentre acute stroke imaging study. Stroke 2012;43(2):563–6.
7. Hagmann P, Cammoun L, Gigandet X, et al. MR connectomics: principles and challenges. J Neurosci Methods 2010;194(1):34–45.
8. Hagmann P, Grant PE, Fair DA. MR connectomics: a conceptual framework for studying the developing brain. Front Syst Neurosci 2012;6:43.
9. Sporns O. From simple graphs to the connectome: networks in neuroimaging. Neuroimage 2012;62(2):881–6.
10. Xing W, Nan C, ZhenTao Z, et al. Probabilistic MRI brain anatomical atlases based on 1,000 Chinese subjects. PLoS One 2013;8(1):e50939.
11. D'Haese PF, Pallavaram S, Kao C, et al. Effect of data normalization on the creation of neuro-probabilistic atlases. Stereotact Funct Neurosurg 2013;91(3): 148–52.
12. Oishi K, Faria A, Jiang H, et al. Atlas-based whole brain white matter analysis using large deformation diffeomorphic metric mapping: application to normal elderly and Alzheimer's disease participants. Neuroimage 2009;46(2):486–99.
13. Mazziotta J, Toga A, Evans A, et al. A probabilistic atlas and reference system for the human brain: International Consortium for Brain Mapping (ICBM). Philos Trans R Soc Lond B Biol Sci 2001;356(1412):1293–322.
14. Plewes DB, Kucharczyk W. Physics of MRI: a primer. J Magn Reson Imaging 2012;35(5):1038–54.
15. Matter NI, Scott GC, Venook RD, et al. Three-dimensional prepolarized magnetic resonance imaging using rapid acquisition with relaxation enhancement. Magn Reson Med 2006;56(5):1085–95.
16. Katsunuma A, Takamori H, Sakakura Y, et al. Quiet MRI with novel acoustic noise reduction. MAGMA 2002;13(3):139–44.
17. Hamaguchi T, Miyati T, Ohno N, et al. Acoustic noise transfer function in clinical MRI a multicenter analysis. Acad Radiol 2011;18(1):101–6.
18. de Zwart JA, van Gelderen P, Kellman P, et al. Reduction of gradient acoustic noise in MRI using SENSE-EPI. Neuroimage 2002;16(4):1151–5.
19. Segbers M, Rizzo Sierra CV, Duifhuis H, et al. Shaping and timing gradient pulses to reduce MRI acoustic noise. Magn Reson Med 2010;64(2):546–53.
20. Idiyatullin D, Corum C, Park JY, et al. Fast and quiet MRI using a swept radiofrequency. J Magn Reson 2006;181(2):342–9.
21. Zhu Y. Parallel excitation with an array of transmit coils. Magn Reson Med 2004; 51(4):775–84.
22. Shah NJ, Oros-Peusquens AM, Arrubla J, et al. Advances in multimodal neuroimaging: hybrid MR-PET and MR-PET-EEG at 3T and 9.4T. J Magn Reson 2012; 229:101–15.
23. Ke F, Hollingsworth NA, McDougall MP, et al. A 64-channel transmitter for investigating parallel transmit MRI. IEEE Trans Biomed Eng 2012;59(8):2152–60.
24. Wright SM, McDougall MP, Feng K, et al. Highly parallel transmit/receive systems for dynamic MRI. Conf Proc IEEE Eng Med Biol Soc 2009;2009:4053–6.

25. Liu F, Duan Y, Peterson BS, et al. Compressed sensing MRI combined with SENSE in partial k-space. Phys Med Biol 2012;57(21):N391–403.

26. Hansen MS, Baltes C, Tsao J, et al. k-t BLAST reconstruction from non-Cartesian k-t space sampling. Magn Reson Med 2006;55(1):85–91.

27. Gillard JH, Waldman AD, Barker PB, editors. Clinical MR neuroimaging. 2nd edition. Cambridge (UK): Cambridge University Press; 2010.

28. Wald LL. The future of acquisition speed, coverage, sensitivity, and resolution. Neuroimage 2012;62(2):1221–9.

29. Hasson U, Honey CJ. Future trends in neuroimaging: neural processes as expressed within real-life contexts. Neuroimage 2012;62(2):1272–8.

30. Lowe MJ. A historical perspective on the evolution of resting-state functional connectivity with MRI. MAGMA 2010;23(5–6):279–88.

31. Tang-Schomer MD, Johnson VE, Baas PW, et al. Partial interruption of axonal transport due to microtubule breakage accounts for the formation of periodic varicosities after traumatic axonal injury. Exp Neurol 2012;233(1):364–72.

32. Dimou S, Battisti RA, Hermens DF, et al. A systematic review of functional magnetic resonance imaging and diffusion tensor imaging modalities used in presurgical planning of brain tumour resection. Neurosurg Rev 2012;36(2):205–14.

33. Edlow BL, Wu O. Advanced neuroimaging in traumatic brain injury. Semin Neurol 2012;32(4):374–400.

34. Fujima N, Kudo K, Terae S, et al. Non-invasive measurement of oxygen saturation in the spinal vein using SWI: quantitative evaluation under conditions of physiological and caffeine load. Neuroimage 2011;54(1):344–9.

35. Schweser F, Deistung A, Lehr BW, et al. Quantitative imaging of intrinsic magnetic tissue properties using MRI signal phase: an approach to in vivo brain iron metabolism? Neuroimage 2011;54(4):2789–807.

36. Deistung A, Schäfer A, Schweser F, et al. Toward in vivo histology: a comparison of quantitative susceptibility mapping (QSM) with magnitude-, phase-, and R2*-imaging at ultra-high magnetic field strength. Neuroimage 2013;65:299–314.

37. Pfefferbaum A, Chanraud S, Pitel AL, et al. Volumetric cerebral perfusion imaging in healthy adults: regional distribution, laterality, and repeatability of pulsed continuous arterial spin labeling (PCASL). Psychiatry Res 2010;182(3):266–73.

38. Jung Y, Wong EC, Liu TT. Multiphase pseudocontinuous arterial spin labeling (MP-PCASL) for robust quantification of cerebral blood flow. Magn Reson Med 2010;64(3):799–810.

39. Jain V, Duda J, Avants B, et al. Longitudinal reproducibility and accuracy of pseudo-continuous arterial spin-labeled perfusion MR imaging in typically developing children. Radiology 2012;263(2):527–36.

40. Wolk DA, Detre JA. Arterial spin labeling MRI: an emerging biomarker for Alzheimer's disease and other neurodegenerative conditions. Curr Opin Neurol 2012;25(4):421–8.

41. Binnewijzend MA, Kuijer JP, Benedictus MR, et al. Cerebral blood flow measured with 3D pseudocontinuous arterial spin-labeling MR imaging in Alzheimer disease and mild cognitive impairment: a marker for disease severity. Radiology 2012;267(1):221–30.

42. Hernandez DA, Bokkers RP, Mirasol RV, et al. Pseudocontinuous arterial spin labeling quantifies relative cerebral blood flow in acute stroke. Stroke 2012;43(3):753–8.

43. Yamada S, Miyazaki M, Kanazawa H, et al. Visualization of cerebrospinal fluid movement with spin labeling at MR imaging: preliminary results in normal and pathophysiologic conditions. Radiology 2008;249(2):644–52.

44. Wu H, Turski PA, Mistretta CA, et al. Noncontrast-enhanced three-dimensional (3D) intracranial MR angiography using pseudocontinuous arterial spin labeling and accelerated 3D radial acquisition. Magn Reson Med 2013;69(3):708–15.

45. Koktzoglou I, Gupta N, Edelman RR. Nonenhanced extracranial carotid MR angiography using arterial spin labeling: improved performance with pseudo-continuous tagging. J Magn Reson Imaging 2011;34(2):384–94.

46. Detre JA, Wang DJ, Chen YF, et al. Applications of arterial spin labeled MRI in the brain. J Magn Reson Imaging 2012;35(5):1026–37.

47. Lin A, Ross BD, Harris K, et al. Efficacy of proton magnetic resonance spectroscopy in neurological diagnosis and neurotherapeutic decision making. NeuroRx 2005;2(2):197–214.

48. Tran T, Ross B, Lin A. Magnetic resonance spectroscopy in neurological diagnosis. Neurol Clin 2009;27(1):21–60, xiii.

49. Currie S, Hadjivassiliou M, Wilkinson ID, et al. Magnetic resonance spectroscopy of the normal cerebellum: what degree of variability can be expected? Cerebellum 2013;12(2):205–11.

50. Hargreaves BA, Worters PW, Pauly KB, et al. Metal-induced artifacts in MRI. AJR Am J Roentgenol 2011;197(3):547–55.

51. Gatehouse PD, Bydder GM. Magnetic resonance imaging of short T2 components in tissue. Clin Radiol 2003;58(1):1–19.

52. Hiwatashi A, Yoshiura T, Yamashita K, et al. Ultrashort TE MRI: Usefulness after percutaneous vertebroplasty. AJR Am J Roentgenol 2010;195(5):W365–8.

53. Kadbi M, Wang H, Negahdar M, et al. A novel phase-corrected 3D cine ultra-short TE (UTE) phase-contrast MRI technique. Conf Proc IEEE Eng Med Biol Soc 2012;2012:77–81.

54. Lee MH, Kim YK, Park MJ, et al. Gadoxetic acid-enhanced fat suppressed three-dimensional T1-weighted MRI using a multiecho Dixon technique at 3 tesla: emphasis on image quality and hepatocellular carcinoma detection. J Magn Reson Imaging 2013;38(2):401–10.

55. Garcia-Lorenzo D, Francis S, Narayanan S, et al. Review of automatic segmentation methods of multiple sclerosis white matter lesions on conventional magnetic resonance imaging. Med Image Anal 2013;17(1):1–18.

56. Leigh R, Jen SS, Varma DD, et al. Arrival time correction for dynamic susceptibility contrast MR permeability imaging in stroke patients. PLoS One 2012;7(12): e52656.

57. Kassubek J, Ludolph AC, Muller HP. Neuroimaging of motor neuron diseases. Ther Adv Neurol Disord 2012;5(2):119–27.

58. Kloppel S, Abdulkadir A, Jack CR Jr, et al. Diagnostic neuroimaging across diseases. Neuroimage 2012;61(2):457–63.

59. Mishra A, Schuz A, Engelmann J, et al. Biocytin-derived MRI contrast agent for longitudinal brain connectivity studies. ACS Chem Neurosci 2011;2(10):578–87.

60. Wagner S, Schnorr J, Ludwig A, et al. Contrast-enhanced MR imaging of atherosclerosis using citrate-coated superparamagnetic iron oxide nanoparticles: calcifying microvesicles as imaging target for plaque characterization. Int J Nanomedicine 2013;8:767–79.

61. Li A, Zheng Y, Yu J, et al. Superparamagnetic perfluorooctylbromide nanoparticles as a multimodal contrast agent for US, MR, and CT imaging. Acta Radiol 2013;54(3):278–83.

62. Chen PY, Liu HL, Hua MY, et al. Novel magnetic/ultrasound focusing system enhances nanoparticle drug delivery for glioma treatment. Neuro Oncol 2010; 12(10):1050–60.

63. Olson ES, Jiang T, Aguilera TA, et al. Activatable cell penetrating peptides linked to nanoparticles as dual probes for in vivo fluorescence and MR imaging of proteases. Proc Natl Acad Sci U S A 2010;107(9):4311–6.

64. Wang G, Yu H, De Man B. An outlook on x-ray CT research and development. Med Phys 2008;35(3):1051–64.

65. Pan CJ, Qian N, Wang T, et al. Adaptive prospective ECG-triggered sequence coronary angiography in dual-source CT without heart rate control: image quality and diagnostic performance. Exp Ther Med 2013;5(2):636–42.

66. Wang G, Yu H, Ye Y. A scheme for multisource interior tomography. Med Phys 2009;36(8):3575–81.

67. Wang G, Zhang J, Gao H, et al. Towards omni-tomography–grand fusion of multiple modalities for simultaneous interior tomography. PLoS One 2012;7(6): e39700.

68. Flohr T, Stierstorfer K, Raupach R, et al. Performance evaluation of a 64-slice CT system with z-flying focal spot. Rofo 2004;176(12):1803–10.

69. Chodick G, Ronckers CM, Shalev V, et al. Excess lifetime cancer mortality risk attributable to radiation exposure from computed tomography examinations in children. Isr Med Assoc J 2007;9(8):584–7.

70. Hutton BF. Recent advances in iterative reconstruction for clinical SPECT/PET and CT. Acta Oncol 2011;50(6):851–8.

71. Thomas C, Korn A, Krauss B, et al. Automatic bone and plaque removal using dual energy CT for head and neck angiography: feasibility and initial performance evaluation. Eur J Radiol 2010;76(1):61–7.

72. Fornaro J, Leschka S, Hibbeln D, et al. Dual- and multi-energy CT: approach to functional imaging. Insights Imaging 2011;2(2):149–59.

73. Liang H, Noble J, Wells P. Recent advances in biomedical ultrasonic imaging techniques. Interface Focus 2011;1(4):475–6.

74. Wells PN. Ultrasound imaging. Phys Med Biol 2006;51(13):R83–98.

75. Fenster A, Parraga G, Bax J. Three-dimensional ultrasound scanning. Interface Focus 2011;1:503–19.

76. Brown JA, Foster FS, Needles A, et al. Fabrication and performance of a 40-MHz linear array based on a 1-3 composite with geometric elevation focusing. IEEE Trans Ultrason Ferroelectr Freq Control 2007;54(9):1888–94.

77. Chiu B, Egger M, Spence DJ, et al. Area-preserving flattening maps of 3D ultrasound carotid arteries images. Med Image Anal 2008;12(6):676–88.

78. Partovi S, Loebe M, Noon GP, et al. Detection of adventitial vasa vasorum and intraplaque neovascularization in carotid atherosclerotic lesions with contrast-enhanced ultrasound and their role in atherosclerosis. Methodist Debakey Cardiovasc J 2011;7(4):37–40.

79. Staub D, Schinkel AF, Coll B, et al. Contrast-enhanced ultrasound imaging of the vasa vasorum: from early atherosclerosis to the identification of unstable plaques. JACC Cardiovasc Imaging 2010;3(7):761–71.

80. Magnoni M, Coli S, Marrocco-Trischitta MM, et al. Contrast-enhanced ultrasound imaging of periadventitial vasa vasorum in human carotid arteries. Eur J Echocardiogr 2009;10(2):260–4.

81. Xu ZS, Lee RJ, Chu SS, et al. Evidence of changes in brain tissue stiffness after ischemic stroke derived from ultrasound-based elastography. J Ultrasound Med 2013;32(3):485–94.

82. Johnson CL, McGarry MD, Van Houten EE, et al. Magnetic resonance elastography of the brain using multishot spiral readouts with self-navigated motion correction. Magn Reson Med 2012;70(2):404–12.

83. Beard P. Biomedical photoacoustic imaging. Interface Focus 2011;1(4):602–31.
84. Liang HD, Tsui CS, Halliwell M, et al. Continuous wave ultrasonic Doppler tomography. Interface Focus 2011;1(4):665–72.
85. Bishop DV, Badcock NA, Holt G. Assessment of cerebral lateralization in children using functional transcranial Doppler ultrasound (fTCD). J Vis Exp 2010;(43). pii:2161.
86. Vivo-Orti MN, Tembl JI, Sastre-Bataller I, et al. Evaluation of the substantia nigra by means of transcranial ultrasound imaging. Rev Neurol 2013;56(5):268–74 [in Spanish].
87. Liang HD, Blomley MJ. The role of ultrasound in molecular imaging. Br J Radiol 2003;76(Spec No 2):S140–50.
88. Rahmim A, Zaidi H. PET versus SPECT: strengths, limitations and challenges. Nucl Med Commun 2008;29(3):193–207.
89. Conti M. State of the art and challenges of time-of-flight PET. Phys Med 2009; 25(1):1–11.
90. Lee JY, Joo EY, Park HS, et al. Repeated ictal SPECT in partial epilepsy patients: SISCOM analysis. Epilepsia 2011;52(12):2249–56.
91. Kim S, Mountz JM. SPECT imaging of epilepsy: an overview and comparison with F-18 FDG PET. Int J Mol Imaging 2011;2011:813028.
92. O'Brien TJ, So EL, Cascino GD, et al. Subtraction SPECT coregistered to MRI in focal malformations of cortical development: localization of the epileptogenic zone in epilepsy surgery candidates. Epilepsia 2004;45(4):367–76.
93. Zaidi H, Del Guerra A. An outlook on future design of hybrid PET/MRI systems. Med Phys 2011;38(10):5667–89.
94. Pimlott SL, Sutherland A. Molecular tracers for the PET and SPECT imaging of disease. Chem Soc Rev 2011;40(1):149–62.
95. Lopci E, Nanni C, Castellucci P, et al. Imaging with non-FDG PET tracers: outlook for current clinical applications. Insights Imaging 2010;1(5–6):373–85.
96. Haubner R, Weber WA, Beer AJ, et al. Noninvasive visualization of the activated alphavbeta3 integrin in cancer patients by positron emission tomography and [18F]Galacto-RGD. PLoS Med 2005;2(3):e70.
97. Schnell O, Krebs B, Carlsen J, et al. Imaging of integrin alpha(v)beta(3) expression in patients with malignant glioma by [18F] galacto-RGD positron emission tomography. Neuro Oncol 2009;11(6):861–70.
98. Matsuda H, Imabayashi E. Molecular neuroimaging in Alzheimer's disease. Neuroimaging Clin N Am 2012;22(1):57–65, viii.

Advanced Neuroimaging of Mild Traumatic Brain Injury

Laszlo L. Mechtler, MD[a,b,]*, Kalyan K. Shastri, MD, MS[b],
Kevin E. Crutchfield, MD[c]

KEYWORDS

- Mild traumatic brain injury • Concussion • Diffuse axonal injury
- Diffusion tensor imaging • Susceptibility-weighted imaging
- Magnetic resonance spectroscopy

KEY POINTS

- Traumatic brain injury (TBI) is an important cause of death and disability in the United States, with annual incidence of approximately 1.7 million and overall annual costs estimated to be $76.5 billion.
- 75% of all TBIs can be classified as mild TBI (mTBI), defined as Glasgow Coma Scale score of 13 or more. Concussion, a term commonly used in sports-related injuries, is a form of mTBI.
- The goals of neuroimaging in TBI are to identify treatable injuries, assist in the prevention of secondary damage, and provide useful prognostic information on a patient's long-term clinical condition.
- Advanced neuroimaging of mTBI includes anatomic/structural imaging techniques, such as diffusion tensor imaging and susceptibility-weighted imaging, and functional imaging techniques such as functional MRI, perfusion-weighted imaging, MR spectroscopy, and positron emission tomography.

INTRODUCTION

Traumatic brain injury (TBI), a major public health concern at the beginning of the 21st century, has been called a "silent epidemic"[1] because it is underreported, often remains undiagnosed, and its long-term consequences are generally underrecognized. However, owing to growing experience with combat-related TBI among military personnel, media focus on TBI-related long-term disability in professional athletes,

The authors have no financial conflicts to disclose.
[a] Department of Neurology and Neuro-Oncology, State University of New York at Buffalo, 3435 Main Street, Buffalo, NY 14223, USA; [b] Dent Neurologic Institute, 3980A Sheridan Drive, Suite 101, Amherst, NY 14226, USA; [c] Comprehensive Sports Concussion Program, The Sandra and Malcolm Berman Brain & Spine Institute, 5051 Greenspring Avenue, Baltimore, MD 21209, USA
* Corresponding author. Dent Neurologic Institute, 3980A Sheridan Drive, Suite 101, Amherst, NY 14226.
E-mail address: lmechtler@dentinstitute.com

Neurol Clin 32 (2014) 31–58
http://dx.doi.org/10.1016/j.ncl.2013.08.002
0733-8619/14/$ – see front matter © 2014 Elsevier Inc. All rights reserved.

neurologic.theclinics.com

educational initiatives, such as the "Heads Up" program of the Centers for Disease Control and Prevention,[2] and the voices of patients and affected families, the silence is beginning to be broken.

Approximately 75% of all reported TBIs can be classified as mild TBI (mTBI).[3] Although most patients with mTBI become asymptomatic within days to weeks, some develop persistent troubling symptoms that have been referred to as "persistent postconcussive syndrome."[4,5] One of the inherent challenges in applying neuroimaging to predict clinical outcome in mTBI is that patients who develop persistent symptoms typically have no detectable abnormalities on conventional neuroimaging, such as computed tomography (CT) and magnetic resonance imaging (MRI) of the brain. Novel structural and functional neuroimaging techniques have emerged that have the sensitivity to identify hitherto undetected brain abnormalities in mTBI. This article focuses on advancements in neuroimaging techniques, compares the advantages of each of the modalities in the evaluation of mTBI, and discusses their contribution to our understanding of the pathophysiology as it relates to prognosis.

MTBI: BRIEF OVERVIEW
Terminology

"Traumatic brain injury" refers to an alteration in brain function or other evidence of brain pathology caused by external force[6] and traditionally is classified as mild, moderate, and severe based on the Glasgow Coma Scale (GCS).[7] TBI with GCS score of 13 or more is classified as mild, 9 to 12 as moderate, and 8 and lower as severe.[8] mTBI is defined as a traumatically induced physiologic disruption of brain function as manifested by at least 1 of the following: (1) any period of loss of consciousness up to 30 minutes, (2) any loss of memory for events before or after the accident not exceeding 24 hours, (3) any alteration in mental state at the time of the accident, and (4) focal neurologic deficits that may or may not be transient.[9,10] Concussion is a form of mTBI, and "concussion" is a term commonly used in sports, whereas "mTBI" is used more often in the medical context.[11]

Pathophysiology

Pathophysiologically, TBI involves 2 phases of tissue injury: primary and secondary. Whereas primary injuries are almost immediate and generally irreversible, secondary injuries are delayed and can continue for an extended period of time and thereby provide an opportunity for therapy.[12] The primary injury phase involves direct and indirect mechanical damage from impact and acceleration/deceleration that could result in cortical contusions, subdural or epidural hematomas, axonal shearing, and microvascular injury. Secondary injury is the nonmechanical damage that results from a complex metabolic cascade set off by neuronal cell membrane disruption and axonal stretch.[13] Neuronal membrane deformity leads to ionic flux and release of excitatory neurotransmitters. Attempts to restore homeostasis lead to a cellular energy crisis. Depletion of cellular energy stores leads to initiation of apoptosis and neuronal death. Impaired cerebrovascular autoregulation that leads to decreased cerebral blood flow (CBF), inflammatory response with activation of microglia,[14] and release of free radicals are additional mechanisms of tissue damage during the secondary injury phase of TBI.

Diffuse axonal injury (DAI) is best described after severe TBI and is characterized by axonal stretching leading to axolemmal disruption, ionic flux, neurofilament compaction, and microtubule disassembly. The effect of these pathophysiologic processes is axonal swelling and eventual disconnection.[15,16] Although best described in severe TBI, DAI occurs in mTBI as well and is recognized as an important determinant of long-term cognitive and neuropsychiatric outcome in mTBI.[17,18] As discussed in subsequent sections, key advances in neuroimaging of mTBI involve newer techniques that can detect disruption of axonal integrity.

Symptomatology

mTBI can lead to a wide range of symptoms, including loss of consciousness, if any, at the time of injury and memory loss, if any, for events before and after the injury. Post-concussion syndrome refers to symptoms from multiple "symptom categories" that develop within a maximum of 4 weeks following head trauma.[19] Broad symptom categories include somatic, cognitive, affective, and sleep-related. Typical symptoms include headache, dizziness, memory impairment, difficulty concentrating, insomnia, mood alteration, and anxiety. Most people with mTBI recover within a few days to weeks with rest and minimal symptomatic treatment. Approximately 15% of patients with mTBI suffer from long-term complications.[4,5]

Chronic traumatic encephalopathy (CTE) is a rare progressive degenerative condition that is thought to be a consequence of repetitive TBI. First described as *dementia pugilistica* in boxers,[20] CTE is equally concerning for other professional athletes who are at risk for repeated concussions. For instance, retired professional football players with history of 3 or more concussions are 5 times more likely to develop mild cognitive impairment.[21] From the autopsy studies of 3 professional athletes with CTE, we know that it is related to deposition of tau protein in neurons and resultant progressive degeneration of the central nervous system.[22]

CONVENTIONAL NEUROIMAGING OF TRAUMATIC BRAIN INJURY
General Considerations

The goals of neuroimaging of TBI are to identify treatable injuries, assist in prevention of secondary damage, and provide prognostic information about long-term clinical outcome. Conventional neuroimaging continues to play a crucial role in the initial management of TBI. CT is generally the imaging modality of choice for initial screening to exclude serious intracranial injury in patients who present with head injury. MRI, particularly at 3 T strength, improves structural sensitivity and is indicated in acute TBI when neurologic findings cannot be explained by CT. MRI is also recommended for evaluation of TBI-related symptoms in the subacute and chronic phases of injury.[23]

Standard questions in this area are as follows: which patients with TBI should be imaged, when, and how? The general consensus is that moderate and severe TBI should be imaged with CT immediately.[24] At present, consensus is lacking regarding the imaging of mTBI. Various guidelines that address the use of CT for initial assessment of TBI have been proposed, including the National Institute of Health and Clinical Excellence guidelines in the United Kingdom,[25] the Canadian CT Head Rule,[26] the American College of Emergency Physicians clinical policy,[27] and the New Orleans Criteria.[28] Some of these guidelines have been validated.[29,30] Overall, implementation of the guidelines in emergency departments (EDs) has proven to be cost effective, owing primarily to a decrease in hospital admission rates. However, an estimated 10% to 35% of CT scans obtained in EDs for mTBI (GCS≥13) are not compliant with the guidelines.[31]

In 2012, the American College of Radiology published revised appropriateness criteria for imaging in head trauma.[32] In cases of minor or mild acute closed-head injury (GCS≥13) without risk factors or neurologic deficits, the study of choice is CT of the head without contrast, despite its low yield. Among patients who present to EDs with GCS scores of 15, 6% to 7% have positive findings on head CT scans.

The rates of intracranial abnormalities and subsequent neurosurgical intervention are higher in pediatric patients.[33,34] In moderate TBI (GCS 9–12), the incidence of CT abnormalities is approximately 61%.[35]

CT

In patients with head injury, CT can help to detect intracranial hemorrhage, mass effect, midline shift, ventricular distortion, skull fractures, displaced bone fragments, foreign bodies, and intracranial air. CT scans offer several advantages: scanner-equipped facilities are widely available, they generally offer convenient hours of operation,[36] and scanning is extremely fast, typically requiring only a few seconds to obtain a head CT. Faster scan times minimize the risk of image degradation from motion artifact, which could be a significant concern, for instance, in the disoriented patient or a young child. Multidetector CT scanners have multiple rows of detectors (eg, 16, 64, 128, 256, 320 "slices") that permit greater coverage per rotation, high resolution, and faster scanning times. Slices degraded by motion artifact can easily be repeated. A 320-slice CT scanner can image a 16-cm (6.3-inch) volume in less than 1 second. Scan times on the higher-slice CT scanners can actually reduce radiation dose, which is very advantageous, especially in the pediatric population. CT datasets can be post-processed to yield 2-dimensional (2D) or 3-dimensional (3D) reformatted images (**Fig. 1**). 2D-reformatted images in either the coronal or sagittal plane in addition to the axial plane have become a standard in many EDs.

Following neurologic deterioration, patients with closed-head injuries should undergo repeat head CT with clinical neurologic assessment to determine if a surgically

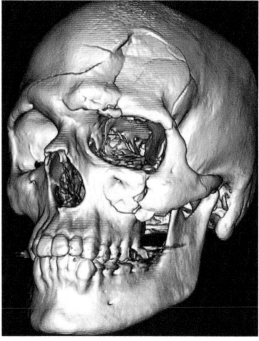

Fig. 1. Depressed frontal fracture: 3D surface-rendered images of the skull and face are useful for depicting displaced fractures before repair. (*From* Kubal WS. Updated imaging of traumatic brain injury. Radiol Clin North Am 2012;50(1):15–41; with permission.)

correctable lesion is present, as is the case in more than one-third of patients. Scheduling repeat head CTs within 24 hours for patients with mild head injury is a standard practice in many trauma centers. However, recent studies have shown that it is unnecessary to routinely schedule repeat CT scans when patients are unchanged or improving neurologically.[37–39]

CT angiography (CTA) has a role in the diagnosis and management of traumatic vascular injury, such as pseudoaneurysm, dissection, or uncontrolled hemorrhage. Vascular injuries typically occur with penetrating trauma, skull base fractures, or neck trauma. In these cases, CTA is best performed with a multidetector scanner and a rapid bolus of contrast injection using vessel tracking.[40] Although conventional angiography remains the gold standard for detecting arterial dissections, carotid or vertebral dissections can be detected by CTA of the aortic arch and neck. Independent predictors of arterial injury in blunt trauma include cervical facet subluxation or dislocation, fracture lines approaching an artery, and high-impact injury mechanisms.[41]

CT Overuse and Radiation Exposure

The number of CT scans performed annually in the United States has markedly increased, rising from 3 million in 1980 to 20 million in 1995 and to more than 60 million in 2005.[42] Studies show that in excess of 30% of patients had more than 3 CT examinations, 7% had more than 5 examinations, and 4% had more than 9 examinations,[43] and that between 10% and 35% of CTs obtained in EDs for minor or mild head injury are not guideline compliant.[31] An obvious consequence of overuse of CT scanning is excessive health care expenditure. It is believed that ensuring strict compliance with published guidelines could potentially save $394 million annually.

The other major concern related to CT overuse is radiation exposure and risk of cancer. Up to 2% of all cancers in the United States may be attributable to radiation from CT.[42] The typical radiation dose for head CT is 3 mSv. The risk of cancer associated with this ionizing radiation dose is age and gender dependent, but it is approximately in the order of magnitude of 1 radiation-induced cancer per 10,000 CTs performed in adult patients.[44] The lifetime risk of mortality from leukemia or solid-organ malignancy from a single pediatric head CT ranges from approximately 1:2000 for infants to 1:5000 for older children.[45] Certain characteristics render the pediatric population particularly susceptible to the harmful effects of ionizing radiation. Children have rapidly dividing cells that are more sensitive to the effect of radiation. Compared with an equivalent dose in an adult, radiation exposure in a child is associated with a 10-fold increase in neoplastic potential.[46] In addition, children have a longer lifetime during which radiation-related cancers can develop. Finally, until the past few years, most CT scans were not performed with due consideration to the smaller size of children, resulting in children receiving a higher relative radiation dose than did adults.[47] The acronym ALARA (as low as reasonably achievable) highlights an important principle in radiation safety that is also a regulatory requirement, that of minimizing the radiation exposure by using all reasonable measures.[48] Measures that help to reduce the radiation dose associated with CT are listed in **Box 1**.

Overuse of health care resources can be largely attributed to the practice of defensive medicine, whereby tests or services of marginal or no medical value are ordered out of fear of litigation. CT imaging rates for head injury are lowest in EDs in those states that have passed tort reform laws.[44] Ultimately, the decision to perform a CT scan for a minor or mild head injury is a clinical decision based on weighing the risk of serious underlying intracranial injury or skull fracture against the risk of harm from radiation exposure.[49]

Box 1
Reasonable measures for reduction of radiation exposure associated with CT

Appropriately justify CT examinations for clinical need

Develop weight-based protocols

Improve shielding

Perform focused and/or limited-view studies when clinically appropriate

Avoid "routine" repeat CT studies

Consider alternative nonradiation modalities, such as ultrasound or MRI

MRI

MRI has better resolution and can detect structural abnormalities earlier than did CT. However, historically, MRI use in the assessment of head trauma has been hindered by its limited availability in the acute trauma setting and EDs, longer scan times, sensitivity to patient motion, and relative insensitivity to subarachnoid hemorrhage. Other factors include need for MRI-compatible monitoring equipment and ventilators, contraindications (such as most cardiac pacemakers and some cerebral aneurysm clips), and risk of occult foreign bodies.

Over time, many of these limitations have been addressed, and technological advancements have made this imaging modality more readily available and quite popular in the acute trauma setting. Advances such as open-bore geometry, rapid-scan sequences, motion-correction algorithms, and improved patient-monitoring equipment have allowed a greater role for MRI in closed-head injury. MRI is particularly valuable in the assessment of pathology in the brainstem, posterior fossa, and brain parenchyma adjacent to the calvaria.[50] As mentioned previously, it is also the imaging modality of choice when neurologic findings in patients with acute TBI cannot be explained by CT, and it is the recommended modality for evaluation of TBI-related symptoms in the subacute or chronic phase of injury.[23,50]

Structural MRI in mTBI

Standard T1-weighted imaging provides excellent resolution of the more striking anatomic findings in TBI, such as mass effect, midline shift, and ventricular distortion. The addition of gadolinium-based contrast offers no significant advantage for lesion detection or characterization when compared with noncontrast MRI in patients with head injury. More subtle structural abnormalities in mTBI are best seen with key MRI sequences, such as gradient-recalled echo (GRE) for hemorrhagic DAI and contusions, and fluid-attenuated inversion-recovery (FLAIR) for nonhemorrhagic DAI and subarachnoid hemorrhage.

Routine GRE images are sensitive to the presence of blood breakdown products, including deoxyhemoglobin, intracellular (but not extracellular) methemoglobin, ferritin, and hemosiderin. In GRE pulse sequences, the 180° refocusing pulse is omitted and a flip angle smaller than 90° is used, thereby significantly reducing scan time. Echo-planar imaging uses rapid gradient switching instead of repeated radiofrequency excitations, resulting in much shorter scan times than those of conventional GRE.

FLAIR produces T2-weighted images with attenuated cerebrospinal fluid signal by using an inversion prepulse placed at the cerebral spinal fluid null point, followed by a long echo time readout. As a result, periventricular and cerebral cortical lesions become more conspicuous. Compared with conventional T2-weighted images, FLAIR is far superior in its sensitivity for cortical contusions, DAI, and subarachnoid hemorrhage.[51]

Short tau (or TI) inversion recovery (STIR) uses an inversion prepulse that selectively suppresses the fat signal and improves long-T1/long-T2 lesion conspicuity. It is particularly useful in avoiding chemical shift artifacts[52] and is commonly used to differentiate lipomas from hemorrhage and, in the setting of trauma, for the evaluation of optic nerve injury and vertebral body compression fractures. However, its usefulness in TBI is somewhat limited. STIR should not be used to evaluate for gadolinium-contrast enhancement, as the short tau of gadolinium will also be suppressed by the inversion prepulse. Chemical, fat-suppressed, T1-weighted images are preferable for the evaluation of contrast enhancement when fat suppression is desired, such as in the orbits.

Magnetization transfer imaging (MTI) uses off-resonance prepulses that reduce signal from semisolid tissue, such as brain parenchyma, relative to the signal from more fluid tissue, such as blood. Typically, MTI has been shown to be sensitive in the detection of white matter abnormalities in such disorders as multiple sclerosis, progressive multifocal leukoencephalopathy, and wallerian degeneration.[53] Magnetization-transfer ratio provides a quantitative measure of the structural integrity of tissue. Studies have shown that a reduction of magnetization-transfer ratio correlates with worse clinical outcome in patients with TBI.[54,55]

ADVANCED STRUCTURAL NEUROIMAGING OF MTBI

DAI occurs in both direct- and indirect-impact TBI and is the most common cause of long-term disability and functional deficits in patients. Even mTBI can be associated with significant DAI. Hemorrhagic and nonhemorrhagic shearing lesions are located in the major white matter tracts, spreading from the surface to deeper structures, such as corpus callosum, internal capsule, and brainstem. Conventional neuroimaging is insensitive to DAI.[56]

Susceptibility-Weighted Imaging

One of the key advancements in the imaging of mTBI has been susceptibility-weighted imaging (SWI), which is a technique that exploits differences in magnetic susceptibility between tissues. The particular advantage that SWI confers is detection of microhemorrhages that are not seen on conventional MRI (**Fig. 2**). In the setting of TBI, microhemorrhages are thought to be neuroimaging markers of hemorrhagic DAI. SWI is up to 3 to 6 times more sensitive than is GRE in detecting hemorrhagic DAI.[57] SWI is also very sensitive for hemorrhagic DAI in the cerebellum and brainstem.

Detection of microhemorrhages depends on a number of factors, including pulse sequence, echo time, slice thickness, spatial resolution, and, possibly, imaging plane.[58] SWI is best obtained at higher field strengths, as the echo time is much longer in low fields and acquisitions need to be longer at higher field strengths.[59] The signal-to-noise ratio is also higher. With the advent of parallel imaging and the greater availability of clinical 3-T scanners, it is now possible to image the entire brain with SWI in approximately 4 minutes.[60]

In a study of TBI in the pediatric population,[61] SWI lesions were detected in children at all injury severity levels, indicating that the technique can be useful not only for diffuse/severe axonal injuries, but also for identification of mild and focal injuries. Nineteen percent of patients with mTBI who had either not undergone a clinical CT or had negative CT findings were found to have SWI lesions. Most injuries were located in the

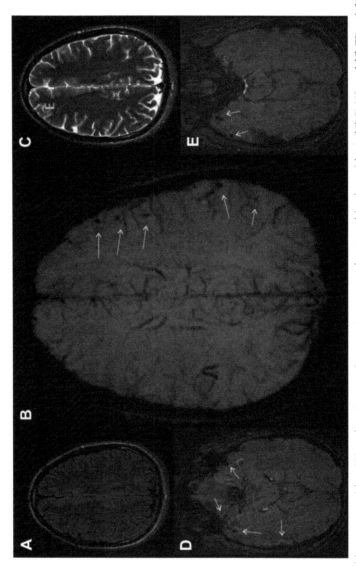

Fig. 2. A 14-year-old teenager with mTBI and postconcussive symptoms secondary to a bicycle accident. (*A*) FLAIR and (*C*) T2-weighted images were unremarkable. (*B, D, E*) SWI images show microhemorrhages (*arrows*) in juxtacortical locations and in orbitofrontal and temporal lobes.

frontal lobes, often in combination with lesions in the temporal, parietal, and occipital lobes. The study found that the greater the number of SWI lesions, the worse the intellectual functioning. This finding is indicative of an association between SWI lesions and intellectual functioning that can be detected as early as 6 months after injury.[61–63] SWI has detected microhemorrhages in amateur boxers that were not detected with T2 fast spin echo or T2* GRE sequences.[64] Although CT may be important for early classification of brain injury, MRI in combination with SWI is superior for accurate diagnosis and assessment of need for neurosurgery. SWI can play an important role in accurately diagnosing the degree of injury and in determining the aggressiveness of management and rehabilitation.

Diffusion-Weighted Imaging

Mobility of water molecules is the essential contrast mechanism exploited in diffusion-weighted imaging (DWI), reflecting a measure of the apparent diffusion coefficient (ADC). Areas with a high degree of diffusion, such as the cerebrospinal fluid, will be hypointense on DWI and display a high ADC value. Areas with restricted diffusion (eg, protons within the gray and white matter) will be hyperintense on DWI and display a low ADC value. This technique allows differentiation between cytotoxic edema (restricted diffusion) and vasogenic edema (increased diffusion). Focal areas of restricted diffusion are often seen in patients with TBI and have been associated with DAI or cerebral edema. Acute DAI lesions appear bright on DWI and dark on ADC because of restricted diffusion from acute cell death. DWI reveals a greater extent and degree of abnormality than do T2-weighted and FLAIR images, and the measured ADC values of the white matter are lower in patients with more severe injuries.[65] Decreased ADC can be demonstrated in the acute phase of DAI and may persist into the subacute phase for a period of time beyond that described for cytotoxic edema. Mean ADC in the whole brain is the best predictor of outcome among all degrees of TBI.[66] Lower ADC scores were found to be predictive of the duration of coma or functional outcome in patients with severe TBI. DWI may be especially useful in assessing nonaccidental injury in children.[67]

Diffusion Tensor Imaging

An extension of the DWI technique is diffusion tensor imaging (DTI), in which diffusion data are acquired in 6 or more directions. A tensor is used to describe diffusion in an anisotropic system. DTI allows visualization of the location, orientation, and anisotropy of the brain's white matter tracts. A fractional anisotropy (FA) value of zero means that the diffusion is isotropic (ie, free diffusion in all directions), whereas an FA value of 1 indicates that diffusion occurs only along one axis and is fully restricted along all other directions. Color coding the various axonal projections in a 2D representation produces a color FA map. The standard convention for color coding the FA map is that green represents anterior-posterior pathways, red represents commissural (lateral) pathways, and blue represents cranial-caudal (ascending and descending) pathways. A 3D representation is referred to as diffusion tractography (eg, **Fig. 3**).[68]

Three major approaches are used to examine microstructure damage from DTI data: (1) whole-brain voxel-based analysis, (2) region-of-interest analysis, and (3) in vivo tractography.[69,70] Briefly, whole-brain voxel-based DTI analysis is an operator-independent approach that allows the analysis of entire brain volume. Another approach consists of finding a region of interest to identify between-group differences and correlations in a specific brain region. DTI also provides opportunity to perform in vivo tractography, or virtual dissections, of major white matter pathways.

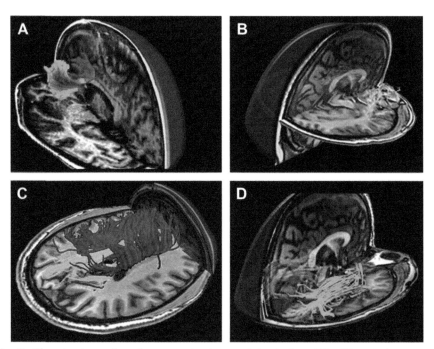

Fig. 3. Fiber tractography of commonly damaged tracts in mTBI: (*A*) anterior corona radiata and genu of corpus callosum, (*B*) uncinate fasciculus, (*C*) cingulum bundle in green and body of corpus callosum in red, and (*D*) inferior longitudinal fasciculus. (*From* Niogi SN, Mukherjee P. Diffusion tensor imaging of mild traumatic brain injury. J Head Trauma Rehabil 2010;25(4):241–55; with permission.)

Over the past decade, the literature has grown significantly regarding the use of DTI in mTBI. Cases have been reported of mTBI with normal CT and GCS score of 15 in adolescents who were found to have increased FA and decreased diffusivity in the corpus callosum within 6 days after injury.[71] Cognitive, affective, and somatic post-concussion symptoms were all related to DTI indices of corpus callosum integrity, including FA. Furthermore, DTI measures of white matter fiber tract integrity were assessed in varsity-level college athletes who had sports-related concussion without loss of consciousness and experienced symptoms for at least 1 month after injury.[72] Notable abnormalities in structural integrity were present in subjects after they sustained concussion. The structures most affected were the left temporal lobe, the retrolenticular part of the internal capsule, and the posterior thalamic radiation, which contains fibers that connect the frontal and occipital lobes as well as the temporal and occipital lobes. Affected patients were found to have increased mean diffusivity and decreased FA compared with controls.

Two major patterns of DTI changes have emerged in mTBI. Decreased FA or increased mean diffusivity in patients with mTBI compared with age-matched healthy controls has been shown, indicating loss of directional diffusivity or anisotropy, suggesting microstructural disruption of white matter.[73,74] Other studies have demonstrated seemingly contradictory increases in FA in patients with mTBI compared with controls.[71,75] However, these patients were, in general, imaged sooner after injury than those in the comparative studies. Unlike the previously mentioned studies, the investigators suggested that increases in FA may be caused by acute axonal injury that results in overall reduction and diffusivity akin to cytotoxic edema. Decreased FA in mTBI may represent chronic structural injuries and correlate with postconcussion symptoms. DTI images from 72 veterans of the Iraq and Afghanistan wars who had mTBI were compared with DTI images from 21 veterans with no TBI during deployment.[76] Several years after the trauma, veterans with a history of mTBI had a higher number of diffusely distributed areas of decreased FA (potholes) than did the veterans without history of TBI. DTI abnormalities of the corpus callosum have been consistently associated with decreased cognitive function in TBI. Potholes were also observed in patients who experienced mTBI in civilian settings and were examined within 90 days after the trauma. White matter potholes may constitute a sensitive biomarker of axonal injury that can be identified in mTBI at acute and chronic stages of its clinical course. DTI holds promise as a method by which to objectively assess abnormal cerebral connectivity underlying cognitive deficits in mTBI.

Voxel-based Morphometry

Voxel-based morphometry (VBM) is a method of voxel-by-voxel analysis of 3D MRI data. It is a statistical method that compares regional differences in the concentration of gray matter between 2 groups of individuals. VBM has traditionally been used to assess brain atrophy in Alzheimer disease. This method uses high-resolution images that are spatially normalized into the same stereotactic space. Gray matter is segmented and smoothed, and statistical parametric tests are used to assess differences in gray matter between groups.[77,78] Whole-brain atrophy can be evident 11 months after trauma.[79] It has also been found that all patients with TBI show decreased gray matter concentration in the frontal and temporal cortices, subcortical gray matter, cingulate gyrus, and the cerebellum.[77] The reported gray matter atrophy may have 2 potential mechanisms, one of which could be cortical involvement, as the brain strikes the cranial vault in a coup-contrecoup manner. Next, DAI can cause axonal damage, leading to retrograde degeneration and neuronal somatic loss.[80] The use of VBM in TBI is unique among brain disorders in that the exact time of onset of injury is known. For this reason, longitudinal studies of MRI brain volume in mTBI are more important than cross-sectional analyses. In comparison with a cross-sectional design, a longitudinal study design may be preferable for understanding the progression of brain atrophy after injury and understanding its association with important clinical variables.[81] A recent study demonstrated, via automated volumetric analysis, whole-brain longitudinal changes in global and regional volume in patients 1 year after mTBI. These changes specifically affected the anterior part of the cingulate white matter bilaterally, the left cingulate gyrus isthmus white matter, and the precuneal gray matter.[82]

ADVANCED FUNCTIONAL NEUROIMAGING OF MTBI
Magnetic Resonance Spectroscopy

Magnetic resonance spectroscopy (MRS) is a powerful noninvasive imaging technique that can provide information about metabolic alterations in patients with mTBI, including and especially in the absence of obvious injury on conventional neuroimaging. The most common brain metabolites measured using proton MRS include N-acetyl aspartate (NAA), creatine (Cr), choline (Cho), glutamate/glutamine (Glx), lactate (Lac), and myoinositol (Ins).[83,84] The ability to quantify neuronal and glial metabolites makes MRS a particularly useful tool for repeated studies in survivors of TBI. Higher-field-strength MRI has increased the ability to accurately determine concentrations of a broader range of metabolites, including neurotransmitters like gamma-amino butyric acid (GABA) and glycine. Very briefly, NAA is synthesized in mitochondria and is a marker in neuronal integrity, Cr is involved in cellular energy metabolism and is assumed to be more or less constant, Cho is a marker of a membrane turnover, Ins is found in glial cells, Glx are excitatory neurotransmitters, and Lac is a marker of anaerobic metabolism and, indirectly, ischemia and hypoxia. The common neurometabolite alterations in mTBI that can be measured using MRS are summarized in **Table 1**.

An extensive body of research indicates that NAA levels (eg, **Fig. 4**) and NAA/Cr ratios are reduced in TBI as a result of neuronal loss and/or dysfunction.[85] Reduced NAA levels have been shown to be predictive of long-term functional outcomes in TBI. Twelve intercollegiate varsity athletes who had sustained sports-related concussions were compared with healthy age-matched controls within 6 days of injury. The NAA/Cr levels were significantly reduced in the primary motor cortex and, to a lesser extent, in the dorsolateral prefrontal cortex in the concussed athletes.[86] Sports-related concussion was the primary focus in another study of 14 individuals in whom MRS was obtained at 3 to 4 days, 15 days, and 30 days after injury. Decreased NAA/Cr ratio was observed at 3 to 4 days following concussion, modest recovery was seen at 15 days postinjury, and normalization of the NAA/Cr ratio was noted by 30 days postinjury. It is of interest that these athletes reported resolution of postconcussive symptoms by day 3, despite abnormal MRS findings.[87] These studies suggest that quantification of neurochemicals with MRS could offer a noninvasive and safe approach to assessing brain cellular injury and response.[88]

Functional MRI

Functional MRI (fMRI) allows assessment of brain function in a noninvasive manner. Neuronal function is inferred from a blood oxygen level–dependent (BOLD) signal that reflects magnetic field inhomogeneity brought about by changes in the oxygenation state of hemoglobin. Neuronal activation results in a local increase in CBF in the area out of proportion to the cerebral oxygen consumption, thereby resulting in net reduction in the amount of deoxyhemoglobin. As neuronal activity increases, blood flow overcompensates such that the local blood oxygenation actually increases. Because deoxyhemoglobin is an endogenous paramagnetic contrast agent, a decrease in its concentration is reflected as an increase in BOLD signal. fMRI can be performed at either 1.5 T or 3.0 T, but higher field strength is generally preferred. To accentuate the differences, this test is usually performed while the patient completes a neurocognitive task, which places an increased demand on the brain, and differences in local perfusion are measured in real time.[89] fMRI holds great potential for

Table 1		
Common neurometabolite alterations in mTBI		
Neurometabolite	Role in/Marker of	Alteration in TBI
NAA	Neuronal/axonal integrity	Reduced
Cr	Cellular energy metabolism	Constant
Cho	Membrane synthesis/repair	Increased
Lac	Anaerobic glycolysis	Increased
Glx	Excitatory neurotransmitters	Increased
Ins	Inflammation (glial cells)	Increased

Abbreviations: Cho, choline; Cr, creatine; Glx, glutamate/glutamine; Ins, myoinositol; Lac, lactate; mTBI, mild traumatic brain injury; NAA, N-acetyl aspartate; TBI, traumatic brain injury.

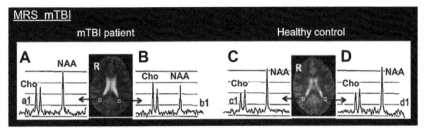

Fig. 4. Comparison of proton magnetic resonance spectra from a young patient with mTBI (*A, B*) and a healthy control subject (*C, D*) showing significant alteration of NAA and Cho in b1 compared with spectra a1, c1, and d1. The b1 voxel is located near injury seen on patient's T2 MRI in the left splenium. (*Adapted from* Govind V, Gold S, Kaliannan K, et al. Whole-brain proton MR spectroscopic imaging of mild-to-moderate traumatic brain injury and correlation with neuropsychological deficits. J Neurotrauma 2010;27(3):483–96; and *Reprinted from* Toledo E, Lebel A, Becerra L, et al. The young brain and concussion: imaging as a biomarker for diagnosis and prognosis. Neurosci Biobehav Rev 2012;36(6):1510–31; with permission.)

widespread research and clinical use because it does not require exposure to any radioactive substance, as do other functional techniques, and because it has a temporal resolution limited only by brain hemodynamics and a spatial resolution comparable to that of conventional MRI.[90]

Evidence is mounting that fMRI is sensitive to changes in neural function following TBI and holds promise as a tool for understanding mTBI and investigating recovery of function. fMRI studies are providing insight into the neural basis of cognitive and behavioral dysfunction following TBI (eg, **Fig. 5**). Although fMRI studies of mTBI are

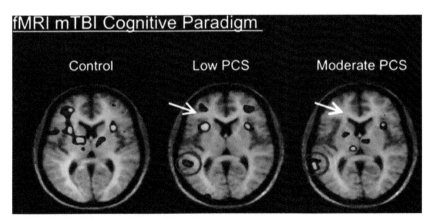

Fig. 5. Functional MRI comparing activation patterns during a verbal working memory task in healthy controls, patients with mTBI and low postconcussive symptoms (PCS), and those with moderate PCS. Additional activation in the posterior brain regions (*red circles*) and less activation in the frontal regions (*white arrows*) is seen in patients with low and moderate PCS compared with control subjects. (*From* Chen JK, Johnston KM, Collie A, et al. A validation of the post concussion symptom scale in the assessment of complex concussion using cognitive testing and functional MRI. J Neurol Neurosurg Psychiatry 2007;78(11):1231–8; with permission.)

scant, the studies that have been done have shown weaker BOLD changes in the dorsolateral prefrontal cortex, a crucial area for monitoring information in working memory.[91]

Studies in concussed athletes showed that they had significantly higher activation in the parietal cortex, right dorsolateral prefrontal cortex, and right hippocampus during performance of visual and spatial memory tasks compared with healthy controls.[92] The response to higher processing tasks in TBI suggested that these subjects did not have actual deficits in working memory ability but that they lost ability to recruit additional neural resources during these tasks.[93] The severity of postconcussive symptoms in concussed subjects was correlated with activation of the posterior parietal cortex. Additionally, activation of an area of the medial premotor cortex (Brodmann area 6) is correlated with longer recovery times, as measured by return to play. The latter findings are from a study that compared 28 concussed high school athletes with 13 age-matched controls while they completed the N-back task, a commonly used test of working memory. An additional important finding related to mood status or affect was noted. The presence of depressive symptoms in concussed athletes was singly related to fMRI activation on working memory tasks. Concussed nondepressed athletes performed comparably with healthy control subjects. These findings are contrary to those found in the acute postconcussive phase and suggest that in relatively young athletes, 2 to 6 concussions may not lead to a lifetime of cognitive deficits. This observation illustrates the plasticity of cognitive abilities in younger adults following concussion.[94]

A newer form of fMRI, called resting-state fMRI (RS-fMRI), is based on the analysis of spontaneous low-frequency fluctuations in the BOLD signal in the absence of any external task (eg, **Fig. 6**). Thirty-five patients with acute mTBI and 35 healthy controls matched for age, gender, handedness, and education underwent RS-fMRI.[95] A decrease in functional connectivity was noted in the motor striatal network in the mTBI group. A cluster of increased functional connectivity in the right frontoparietal network was also noted in the mTBI group, an abnormal finding that might reflect increased awareness to external environment and explain excessive cognitive fatigue reported by patients with mTBI. This increased connectivity also may underlie the physical postconcussive symptoms of headache, photophobia, and sonophobia. Whole-brain functional connectivity is altered within 4 weeks after mTBI, suggesting that changes in functional networks underlie the cognitive deficits and postconcussive complaints reported by this patient population. A recent study showed abnormal thalamic resting-state networks that point to subtle thalamic injury in patients with symptomatic mTBI, suggesting thalamocortical connectivity abnormalities, which may help to explain the complex persistent postconcussive syndrome.[96]

Future fMRI studies should address psychosocial factors, including psychiatric symptoms, such as posttraumatic stress disorder, as well as other potential confounding variables, such as conversion disorder and factitious disorders related to head injury. Genetic variation is another highly probable source of individual differences in mTBI and recovery profiles, and pharmacogenomics combined with fMRI is likely to be incorporated into the development of personalized medicine approaches for mTBI. It is also important to examine (1) the interaction between mTBI and aging and (2) the acute, subacute, and chronic phases of TBI. Task-related activation, deactivation, and RS-fMRI should continue to be investigated for use in the study of changes in functional connectivity, as it may be an important biomarker in research on neurorehabilitative interventions, including behavioral and pharmacologic approaches. A final benefit is likely to arise from the multimodality imaging studies that combine structural, functional, and molecular techniques.[97]

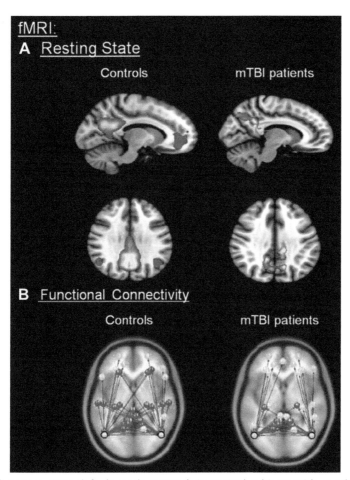

Fig. 6. (A) Resting state default mode network in control subjects with voxels showing significant functional connectivity in red–yellow. For patients with TBI, voxels showing greater connectivity than controls are shown in red–yellow. Note increased functional connectivity in posterior cingulate cortex and precuneus in patients, hypothesized to be a reflection of TBI and adaptive response to cognitive impairment. (B) Functional connectivity maps comparing resting state networks of healthy volunteers and patients with mTBI show differences between shared (red) and non-shared (yellow) connections from left and right parietal ROI. (From [A] Sharp DJ, Beckmann CF, Greenwood R, et al. Default mode network functional and structural connectivity after traumatic brain injury. Brain 2011;134:2233–47, with permission; and [B] Johnson B, Zhang K, Gay M, et al. Alteration of brain default network in subacute phase of injury in concussed individuals: resting-state fMRI study. Neuroimage 2012;59(1):511–8, with permission; and Reprinted from Toledo E, Lebel A, Becerra L, et al. The young brain and concussion: imaging as a biomarker for diagnosis and prognosis. NeurosciBiobehav Rev 2012;36(6):1510–31.)

Perfusion-Weighted Imaging

CT perfusion provides functional information about CBF and can help to identify patients with impaired autoregulation. Continuous scanning of a single slice or contiguous slices can yield time-density curves for each pixel within the image. Cerebral

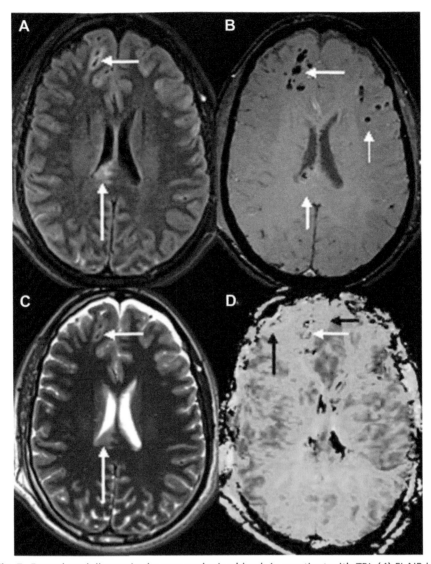

Fig. 7. Frontal medullary vein damage and microbleeds in a patient with TBI. (A) FLAIR image and (C) T2-weighted scan showing 2 of the damaged frontal areas (*short arrow*) and enhanced signal in the splenium of corpus callosum (*long arrow*). (B) SWI showing multiple bleeds in the frontal, lateral, and the splenium of the corpus callosum (*short arrows*). (D) Mean transit time images from the PWI data showing possible delayed arrival times in frontal regions and medial gray matter regions (*black arrows*) representing reduced perfusion to these tissues. Note the dark regions correspond to the bleeds (eg, area denoted by *white arrow*), and because of the long echo times used for PWI, the signal there was too small to be used to determine PWI parameters correctly and hence are set to zero here. (*From* Haacke EM, Raza W, Wu B, et al. The presence of venous damage and microbleeds in traumatic brain injury and the potential future role of angiographic and perfusion magnetic resonance imaging. In: Kriepke CW, Rafols JA, editors. Cerebral blood flow, metabolism, and head trauma: the pathotrajectory of traumatic brain injury. New York: Springer; 2013. p. 75–94; with permission.)

blood volume (CBV), CBF, mean transit time (MTT), and time to peak (TTP) are measured based on the passage of contrast bolus within the brain.[98] Studies have shown that normal brain perfusion or hyperemia is associated with favorable outcomes, whereas oligemia is associated with unfavorable outcomes. In the acute phase of mTBI, disturbed cerebral perfusion is seen in patients with normal noncontrast CT, correlating with the severity of injury and outcome. In patients with decreased GCS scores, a significant decrease of CBF and CBV can be detected in the frontal and occipital gray matter.[99] Xenon-131–enhanced CT assesses the distribution of inhaled Xe^{131} in the bloodstream and tissues and is often cited as the standard for quantitative measurement of CBF. Xenon-131–enhanced CT demonstrates regional hypoperfusion, typically more pronounced in pericontusional tissue.[100]

MR perfusion-weighted imaging (PWI) using arterial spin labeling is a technique that uses an endogenous contrast mechanism in which blood cells flowing into the brain are labeled by the MR signal without need for administration of an external contrast agent, making this method completely noninvasive and repeatable. Regional flow distributions can be assessed independently (eg, **Fig. 7**). In addition, truly quantitative values of CBF can be obtained.[101] Only a few studies have been published, but it has been demonstrated that hemodynamic impairment can occur and persist in patients with mTBI, the extent of which is more severe in the thalamic regions and correlates with neurocognitive dysfunction during the extended course of the disease.[102] In addition, regional hyperperfusion has been reported in the posterior cingulate cortices, thalami, and multiple locations in the frontal cortices.[103] PWI within 1 to 3 hours after injury shows far more severe and widespread perfusion deficits compared with imaging studies that are undertaken 24 hours after head injury.[104]

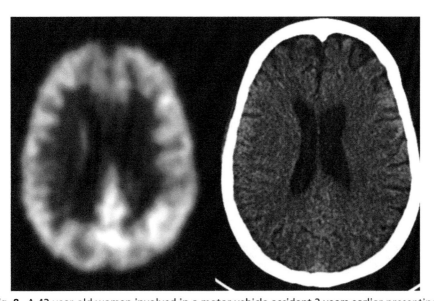

Fig. 8. A 43-year-old woman involved in a motor vehicle accident 2 years earlier presenting with headaches, diplopia, poor balance, and memory impairment. CT (*right*) reveals subtle loss of frontal volume. PET (*left*) reveals mild, patchy frontal cortical hypometabolism with moderate decrements in right polar and medial frontal cortex. Patchy, irregular white matter hypometabolism is also seen.

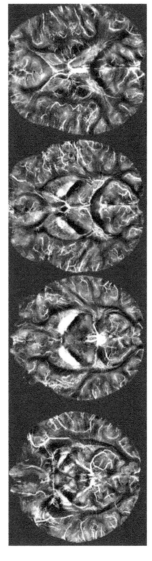

Fig. 9. QSM. Four slices from a 3D GRE multi-echo dataset acquired in a healthy volunteer at 7 T. The QSM maps created are shown as magnitude of tissue magnetic susceptibly with intensity. Vascular blood is thresholded from the QSM values and overlaid onto original QSM maps. (*Courtesy of* Liu C, PhD, and Moseley ME, PhD, Stanford, CA.)

Positron-Emission Tomography

Positron-emission tomography (PET) is a minimally invasive method that requires injection of a radioactive compound, with passive scanning performed at a predetermined interval following the injection. The most commonly used compound is [18F]-2-fluoro-2-deoxy-D-glucose (FDG). This compound provides data on regional brain utilization of glucose, a surrogate for brain metabolism. In sports-related concussion, early dysfunction may be secondary to altered cerebral utilization of glucose as a principal source of metabolic substrate for the production of ATP. The clinical conditions for which PET scans have performed well are those with altered cerebral metabolism. Cost, availability, and restricted use of radioactive materials have prevented more widespread use of this modality. No specific studies have reported the use of PET scanners in investigation or acute management of sports-related concussions. In TBI, clear abnormalities on O^{15} PET combined with FDG demonstrate regional and global alterations of metabolic activity. Diffuse cerebral hypometabolism carries a poorer prognosis for functional outcomes (eg, **Fig. 8**). In mTBI, a few small, chronic-stage disease studies have shown inconsistent findings, but they have shown correlation with cognitive tests.[105]

A recently developed compound, [18F]-fluoroethyl-methyl-amino-2-naphthyl-ethylidene-malononitrile (FDDNP), can highlight pathologic deposits of beta-amyloid and tau protein, and it shows promise as a marker for CTE. A recent small study revealed that FDDNP signals were higher in symptomatic retired National Football League players than they were in controls, in all subcortical regions and the amygdala, areas that commonly produce tau deposits in patients who have suffered TBI. The investigators rightly concluded that the study was limited by the small sample size and lack of autopsy confirmation.[106] Another newer compound, [18F]-THK523, shows promise as being specific for tau alone.[107]

EMERGING TECHNIQUES

The preceding discussion regarding observations made from DTI-based studies of mTBI substantiates that the ability to image the structural integrity of white matter tracts is a key development in the advanced neuroimaging of mTBI. DTI may no longer be the only structural imaging technique for assessing white matter tracts noninvasively in vivo. Similar to diffusion anisotropy, the magnetic susceptibility of white matter has been shown to be orientation dependent or anisotropic.[108] Variations in tissue magnetic susceptibility can be measured voxel-by-voxel to generate susceptibility tensors. Information obtained from susceptibility tensor imaging (STI) appears to be complementary to that obtained from DTI (**Fig. 9**). Thus, probing white matter

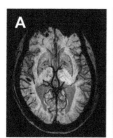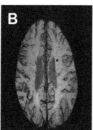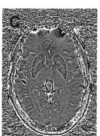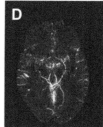

Fig. 10. A patient with motor vehicle accident–related TBI and postconcussive symptoms. (*A, B*) SWI showing microbleeds (hemorrhagic DAI). (*C*) SWI filtered phase and (*D*) SWIM. (*Courtesy of* Haacke EM, PhD, Detroit, MI.)

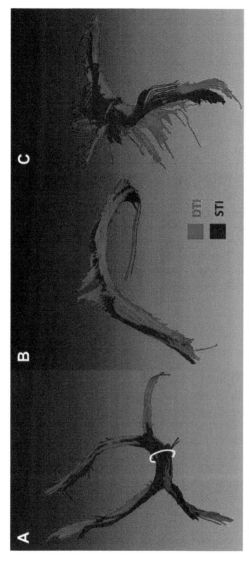

Fig. 11. Comparison of fiber tracts reconstructed using STI and DTI in (A) the anterior commissure, (B) the hippocampal commissure, and (C) the posterior corpus callosum. Yellow circle in (A) represents the middle of the anterior commissure. In general, the 2 methods of fiber tracking yield comparable results for large fiber bundles with STI fibers being generally shorter. In particular, for smaller and more complicated fiber structures, DTI results in longer and smoother pathways than does STI. (*From* Liu C, Li W, Wu B, et al. 3D fiber tractography with susceptibility tensor imaging. Neuroimage 2012;59:1290–8; with permission.)

microstructure simultaneously with susceptibility and diffusion imaging may provide a more complete characterization. Moreover, susceptibility imaging may have certain advantages over diffusion imaging. Resolution of DWI is fairly limited. Susceptibility images, on the other hand, can be readily acquired at much higher spatial resolution and are inherently 3D. As we move from high-field strength (3 T) to ultrahigh field strength ($\geq$7 T) magnets, susceptibility contrast will prove to be advantageous because of increased phase contrast and minimal sensitivity to field inhomogeneity.[108] Quantitative susceptibility mapping (QSM), alternatively referred to as susceptibility-weighted imaging and mapping (SWIM) (**Figs. 10** and **11**), is a novel technique that is showing promise in reducing the inconsistency of standard MRI sequences in cerebral microbleed burden measurements, and may find applications in the advanced neuroimaging of TBI.[109,110]

SUMMARY

TBI has attracted a great deal of social and mainstream media attention in recent years, partly because of our growing experience with war veterans with TBI and concerns regarding professional athletes' short-term risks and long-term morbidity as a result of concussions. The most common form of TBI in both military and civilian populations is mTBI. Most patients with mTBI become asymptomatic within a few days to weeks after injury, but an unfortunate 15% develop persistent disabling symptoms: the so-called "miserable minority."[111] Predicting which patients will develop persistent symptoms and which will recover fully has been a challenge. Even when long-term outcomes are known, conventional neuroimaging fails to distinguish patients with mTBI and persistent symptoms from those who recover, as the images are unremarkable in both cases. Further, in the absence of "organic" causes, many of the persistent symptoms have been branded as "psychogenic," complicating the management of these patients.

As in other subspecialties of neurology, advances in neuroimaging have provided new and improved structural imaging techniques that are being increasingly used in clinical practice for mTBI. At the same time, functional neuroimaging techniques are shedding new light on neurometabolic alterations and disturbances of functional connectivity in the brains of patients with TBI. The specific applications of various structural and functional imaging techniques in the evaluation of TBI are listed in **Table 2**. Some of the advanced structural and functional imaging techniques are not available for "prime time" clinical use, but it would not be overly optimistic to say that they will be applied for diagnostic and prognostic purposes in TBI within a few years.

As advanced neuroimaging unravels fine structural and functional abnormalities in a subset of patients with mTBI, and as efforts are under way to correlate these findings with clinical outcomes, the accuracy and adequacy of the term "mild traumatic brain injury" should be scrutinized. Although the classification of TBI patients as "mild" based on initial GCS score is undoubtedly useful in the acute setting, the terminology is rather inaccurate for those "mild" TBI patients who develop complicated and often very disabling symptoms. For similar reasons, the classification is inadequate in that it encompasses divergent clinical outcomes. The hope is that, in the near future, advanced neuroimaging will identify ways to further stratify the mTBI population into subgroups that are at low risk versus high risk for developing long-term sequelae. This specificity will allow clinicians to specifically target the high-risk patients for early treatment and improve outcomes. These advances are likely to emerge by way of development of biomarkers of injury, staging of reorganization, and reversal of white matter changes following injury, and tracking and characterizing changes in brain

Table 2
Applications of various neuroimaging techniques in evaluation of TBI

Technique/Modality	Principal Application in TBI
Structural	
CT	Intra/extra-axial hemorrhage, skull fracture, cerebral edema, herniation
MRI	
FLAIR	Contusion, nonhemorrhagic DAI, subarachnoid hemorrhage
DWI, ADC	DAI, cerebral edema
STIR	Orbital or calvarial trauma
GRE, SWI	Microhemorrhages (hemorrhagic DAI) from shearing
DTI	White matter integrity and connectivity
VBM	Atrophy, ventriculomegaly
Functional	
fMRI	Neuronal activation during functional tasks inferred from BOLD signal
CT/MR perfusion	Quantitative cerebral perfusion
MR spectroscopy	Neuronal loss, edema, inflammation, hypoxia
FDG-PET	Metabolic changes, task-related metabolism

Abbreviations: ADC, apparent diffusion coefficient; BOLD, blood oxygen level–dependent; CT, computed tomography; DAI, diffuse axonal injury; DTI, diffusion tensor imaging; DWI, diffusion-weighted imaging; FDG-PET, [18F]-2-fluoro-2-deoxy-D-glucose–positron emission tomography; FLAIR, fluid-attenuated inversion recovery; fMRI, functional magnetic resonance imaging; GRE, gradient-recalled echo; MRI, magnetic resonance imaging; STIR, short tau inversion recovery; SWI, susceptibility-weighted imaging; TBI, traumatic brain injury; VBM, voxel-based morphometry.

injury over time. Also, such tools will likely be used in future research to evaluate treatment efficacy.

ACKNOWLEDGMENTS

The authors express their sincere gratitude to Tzipora Sofare, MA, for editing this article, to Kaveer Nandigam, MD, for his help with figures and early drafts, and to Amanda Fisher for her help with obtaining figure permissions and providing administrative assistance.

REFERENCES

1. Goldstein M. Traumatic brain injury: a silent epidemic. Ann Neurol 1990;27:327.
2. Centers for Disease Control and Prevention. Heads up: Concussion. Available at: www.cdc.gov/concussion/headsup/index.html. Accessed May 28, 2013.
3. National Center for Injury Prevention and Control. Report to Congress on mild traumatic brain injury in the United States: steps to prevent a serious public health problem. Atlanta (GA): Centers for Disease Control and Prevention; 2003.
4. Alexander MP. Mild traumatic brain injury: pathophysiology, natural history, and clinical management. Neurology 1995;45:1253–60.
5. Bigler ED. Neuropsychology and clinical neuroscience of persistent post-concussive syndrome. J Int Neuropsychol Soc 2008;14:1–22.
6. Menon DK, Schwab K, Wright DW, et al. Position statement: definition of traumatic brain injury. Arch Phys Med Rehabil 2010;91:1637–40.

7. Teasdale G, Jennett B. Assessment of coma and impaired consciousness. A practical scale. Lancet 1974;2:81–4.
8. Stein SD. Classification of head injury. In: Narayan RK, Wilberger JE, Povlishock JT, editors. Neurotrauma. New York: McGraw-Hill; 1996. p. 31–41.
9. Mild Traumatic Brain Injury Committee of the Head Injury Interdisciplinary Special Interest Group of the American Congress of Rehabilitation Medicine. Definition of mild traumatic brain injury. J Head Trauma Rehabil 1993;8(3):86–7.
10. Carroll LJ, Cassidy JD, Holm L, et al. Methodological issues and research recommendations for mild traumatic brain injury: the WHO Collaborating Centre Task Force on Mild Traumatic Brain Injury. J Rehabil Med 2004;(Suppl 43): 113–25.
11. Ruff RM, Iverson GL, Barth JT, et al. Recommendations for diagnosing a mild traumatic brain injury: a National Academy of Neuropsychology education paper. Arch Clin Neuropsychol 2009;24:3–10.
12. Ling GS, Marshall SA, Moore DF. Diagnosis and management of traumatic brain injury. Continuum (Minneap Minn) 2010;16:27–40.
13. Giza CC, Hovda DA. The neurometabolic cascade of concussion. J Athl Train 2001;36:228–35.
14. Hernandez-Ontiveros DG, Tajiri N, Acosta S, et al. Microglia activation as a biomarker for traumatic brain injury. Front Neurol 2013;4:30.
15. Pettus EH, Povlishock JT. Characterization of a distinct set of intra-axonal ultrastructural changes associated with traumatically induced alteration in axolemmal permeability. Brain Res 1996;722:1–11.
16. Barkhoudarian G, Hovda DA, Giza CC. The molecular pathophysiology of concussive brain injury. Clin Sports Med 2011;30:33–48, vii–iii.
17. Medana IM, Esiri MM. Axonal damage: a key predictor of outcome in human CNS diseases. Brain 2003;126:515–30.
18. Kinnunen KM, Greenwood R, Powell JH, et al. White matter damage and cognitive impairment after traumatic brain injury. Brain 2011;134:449–63.
19. World Health Organization. International classification of diseases and related health problems, 10th revision. Geneva (Switzerland): WHO; 2012.
20. Martland J. Punch drunk. JAMA 1928;91:1103–7.
21. Guskiewicz KM, Marshall SW, Bailes J, et al. Association between recurrent concussion and late-life cognitive impairment in retired professional football players. Neurosurgery 2005;57:719–26.
22. McKee AC, Cantu RC, Nowinski CJ, et al. Chronic traumatic encephalopathy in athletes: progressive tauopathy after repetitive head injury. J Neuropathol Exp Neurol 2009;68:709–35.
23. Gallagher CN, Hutchinson PJ, Pickard JD. Neuroimaging in trauma. Curr Opin Neurol 2007;20:403–9.
24. Le TH, Gean AD. Neuroimaging of traumatic brain injury. Mt Sinai J Med 2009; 76:145–62.
25. National Institute for Clinical Excellence. Head injury: triage, assessment, investigation and early management of head injury in infants, children, and adults: Quick reference guide. 2007. Available at: www.nice.org.uk/nicemedia/live/11836/36257/36257.pdf. Accessed May 28, 2013.
26. Stiell IG, Wells GA, Vandemheen K, et al. The Canadian CT Head Rule for patients with minor head injury. Lancet 2001;357:1391–6.
27. Jagoda AS, Bazarian JJ, Bruns JJ Jr, et al. Clinical policy: neuroimaging and decision making in adult mild traumatic brain injury in the acute setting. Ann Emerg Med 2008;52:714–48.

28. Haydel MJ, Preston CA, Mills TJ, et al. Indications for computed tomography in patients with minor head injury. N Engl J Med 2000;343:100–5.
29. Stiell IG, Clement CM, Rowe BH, et al. Comparison of the Canadian CT Head Rule and the New Orleans Criteria in patients with minor head injury. JAMA 2005;294:1511–8.
30. Smits M, Dippel DW, de Haan GG, et al. External validation of the Canadian CT Head Rule and the New Orleans Criteria for CT scanning in patients with minor head injury. JAMA 2005;294:1519–25.
31. Melnick ER, Szlezak CM, Bentley SK, et al. CT overuse for mild traumatic brain injury. Jt Comm J Qual Patient Saf 2012;38:483–9.
32. American College of Radiology. ACR Appropriateness Criteria–Head trauma. 1996. Available at: www.acr.org/~/media/ACR/documents/appcriteria/diagnostic/headtrauma.pdf. Accessed May 28, 2013.
33. Haydel MJ, Shembekar AD. Prediction of intracranial injury in children aged five years and older with loss of consciousness after minor head injury due to nontrivial mechanisms. Ann Emerg Med 2003;42:507–14.
34. Simon B, Letourneau P, Vitorino E, et al. Pediatric minor head trauma: indications for computed tomographic scanning revisited. J Trauma 2001;51:231–7.
35. Fearnside M, McDougall P. Moderate head injury: a system of neurotrauma care. Aust N Z J Surg 1998;68:58–64.
36. Ginde AA, Foianini A, Renner DM, et al. Availability and quality of computed tomography and magnetic resonance imaging equipment in US emergency departments. Acad Emerg Med 2008;15:780–3.
37. Almenawer SA, Bogza I, Yarascavitch B, et al. The value of scheduled repeat cranial computed tomography after mild head injury: single-center series and meta-analysis. Neurosurgery 2013;72:56–62 [discussion: 3–4].
38. Washington CW, Grubb RL Jr. Are routine repeat imaging and intensive care unit admission necessary in mild traumatic brain injury? J Neurosurg 2012;116:549–57.
39. Stippler M, Smith C, McLean AR, et al. Utility of routine follow-up head CT scanning after mild traumatic brain injury: a systematic review of the literature. Emerg Med J 2012;29:528–32.
40. Enterline DS, Kapoor G. A practical approach to CT angiography of the neck and brain. Tech Vasc Interv Radiol 2006;9:192–204.
41. Delgado Almandoz JE, Schaefer PW, Kelly HR, et al. Multidetector CT angiography in the evaluation of acute blunt head and neck trauma: a proposed acute craniocervical trauma scoring system. Radiology 2010;254:236–44.
42. Brenner DJ, Hall EJ. Computed tomography—an increasing source of radiation exposure. N Engl J Med 2007;357:2277–84.
43. Wiest PW, Locken JA, Heintz PH, et al. CT scanning: a major source of radiation exposure. Semin Ultrasound CT MR 2002;23:402–10.
44. Smith-Bindman R, Lipson J, Marcus R, et al. Radiation dose associated with common computed tomography examinations and the associated lifetime attributable risk of cancer. Arch Intern Med 2009;169:2078–86.
45. King MA, Kanal KM, Relyea-Chew A, et al. Radiation exposure from pediatric head CT: a bi-institutional study. Pediatr Radiol 2009;39:1059–65.
46. Brody AS, Frush DP, Huda W, et al. Radiation risk to children from computed tomography. Pediatrics 2007;120:677–82.
47. Frush DP, Donnelly LF, Rosen NS. Computed tomography and radiation risks: what pediatric health care providers should know. Pediatrics 2003;112:951–7.

48. Shah NB, Platt SL. ALARA: is there a cause for alarm? Reducing radiation risks from computed tomography scanning in children. Curr Opin Pediatr 2008;20: 243–7.
49. McCullough BJ, Jarvik JG. Diagnosis of concussion: the role of imaging now and in the future. Phys Med Rehabil Clin N Am 2011;22:635–52, viii.
50. Duckworth JL, Stevens RD. Imaging brain trauma. Curr Opin Crit Care 2010;16: 92–7.
51. Gean AD, Fischbein NJ. Head trauma. Neuroimaging Clin N Am 2010;20: 527–56.
52. Delfaut EM, Beltran J, Johnson G, et al. Fat suppression in MR imaging: techniques and pitfalls. Radiographics 1999;19:373–82.
53. Bagley LJ, McGowan JC, Grossman RI, et al. Magnetization transfer imaging of traumatic brain injury. J Magn Reson Imaging 2000;11:1–8.
54. Sinson G, Bagley LJ, Cecil KM, et al. Magnetization transfer imaging and proton MR spectroscopy in the evaluation of axonal injury: correlation with clinical outcome after traumatic brain injury. AJNR Am J Neuroradiol 2001;22:143–51.
55. McGowan JC, Yang JH, Plotkin RC, et al. Magnetization transfer imaging in the detection of injury associated with mild head trauma. AJNR Am J Neuroradiol 2000;21:875–80.
56. Smith DH, Meaney DF, Shull WH. Diffuse axonal injury in head trauma. J Head Trauma Rehabil 2003;18:307–16.
57. Tong KA, Ashwal S, Holshouser BA, et al. Hemorrhagic shearing lesions in children and adolescents with posttraumatic diffuse axonal injury: improved detection and initial results. Radiology 2003;227:332–9.
58. Greenberg SM, Vernooij MW, Cordonnier C, et al. Cerebral microbleeds: a guide to detection and interpretation. Lancet Neurol 2009;8:165–74.
59. Haacke EM, Mittal S, Wu Z, et al. Susceptibility-weighted imaging: technical aspects and clinical applications, part 1. AJNR Am J Neuroradiol 2009;30: 19–30.
60. Mittal S, Wu Z, Neelavalli J, et al. Susceptibility-weighted imaging: technical aspects and clinical applications, part 2. AJNR Am J Neuroradiol 2009;30:232–52.
61. Beauchamp MH, Beare R, Ditchfield M, et al. Susceptibility-weighted imaging and its relationship to outcome after pediatric traumatic brain injury. Cortex 2013;49:591–8.
62. Babikian T, Freier MC, Tong KA, et al. Susceptibility-weighted imaging: neuropsychologic outcome and pediatric head injury. Pediatr Neurol 2005;33:184–94.
63. Colbert CA, Holshouser BA, Aaen GS, et al. Value of cerebral microhemorrhages detected with susceptibility-weighted MR imaging for prediction of long-term outcome in children with nonaccidental trauma. Radiology 2010;256: 898–905.
64. Hasiloglu ZI, Albayram S, Selcuk H, et al. Cerebral microhemorrhages detected by susceptibility-weighted imaging in amateur boxers. AJNR Am J Neuroradiol 2011;32:99–102.
65. Galloway NR, Tong KA, Ashwal S, et al. Diffusion-weighted imaging improves outcome prediction in pediatric traumatic brain injury. J Neurotrauma 2008;25: 1153–62.
66. Schaefer PW, Huisman TA, Sorensen AG, et al. Diffusion-weighted MR imaging in closed head injury: high correlation with initial Glasgow Coma Scale score and score on modified Rankin scale at discharge. Radiology 2004;233:58–66.
67. Suh DY, Davis PC, Hopkins KL, et al. Nonaccidental pediatric head injury: diffusion-weighted imaging findings. Neurosurgery 2001;49:309–18.

68. Jellison BJ, Field AS, Medow J, et al. Diffusion tensor imaging of cerebral white matter: a pictorial review of physics, fiber tract anatomy, and tumor imaging patterns. AJNR Am J Neuroradiol 2004;25:356–69.

69. Zappala G, Thiebaut de Schotten M, Eslinger PJ. Traumatic brain injury and the frontal lobes: what can we gain with diffusion tensor imaging? Cortex 2012;48: 156–65.

70. Aoki Y, Inokuchi R, Gunshin M, et al. Diffusion tensor imaging studies of mild traumatic brain injury: a meta-analysis. J Neurol Neurosurg Psychiatry 2012; 83:870–6.

71. Wilde EA, McCauley SR, Hunter JV, et al. Diffusion tensor imaging of acute mild traumatic brain injury in adolescents. Neurology 2008;70:948–55.

72. Cubon VA, Putukian M, Boyer C, et al. A diffusion tensor imaging study on the white matter skeleton in individuals with sports-related concussion. J Neurotrauma 2011;28:189–201.

73. Smits M, Houston GC, Dippel DW, et al. Microstructural brain injury in post-concussion syndrome after minor head injury. Neuroradiology 2011;53: 553–63.

74. Niogi SN, Mukherjee P, Ghajar J, et al. Extent of microstructural white matter injury in postconcussive syndrome correlates with impaired cognitive reaction time: a 3T diffusion tensor imaging study of mild traumatic brain injury. AJNR Am J Neuroradiol 2008;29:967–73.

75. Mayer AR, Ling J, Mannell MV, et al. A prospective diffusion tensor imaging study in mild traumatic brain injury. Neurology 2010;74:643–50.

76. Jorge RE, Acion L, White T, et al. White matter abnormalities in veterans with mild traumatic brain injury. Am J Psychiatry 2012;169:1284–91.

77. Gale SD, Baxter L, Roundy N, et al. Traumatic brain injury and grey matter concentration: a preliminary voxel-based morphometry study. J Neurol Neurosurg Psychiatry 2005;76:984–8.

78. Ashburner J, Friston KJ. Voxel-based morphometry—the methods. Neuroimage 2000;11:805–21.

79. MacKenzie JD, Siddiqi F, Babb JS, et al. Brain atrophy in mild or moderate traumatic brain injury: a longitudinal quantitative analysis. AJNR Am J Neuroradiol 2002;23:1509–15.

80. Cohen BA, Inglese M, Rusinek H, et al. Proton MR spectroscopy and MRI-volumetry in mild traumatic brain injury. AJNR Am J Neuroradiol 2007;28: 907–13.

81. Ross DE. Review of longitudinal studies of MRI brain volumetry in patients with traumatic brain injury. Brain Inj 2011;25:1271–8.

82. Zhou Y, Kierans A, Kenul D, et al. Mild traumatic brain injury: longitudinal regional brain volume changes. Radiology 2013;267:880–90.

83. Gasparovic C, Yeo R, Mannell M, et al. Neurometabolite concentrations in gray and white matter in mild traumatic brain injury: an 1H-magnetic resonance spectroscopy study. J Neurotrauma 2009;26:1635–43.

84. Holshouser BA, Tong KA, Ashwal S. Proton MR spectroscopic imaging depicts diffuse axonal injury in children with traumatic brain injury. AJNR Am J Neuroradiol 2005;26:1276–85.

85. Brooks WM, Friedman SD, Gasparovic C. Magnetic resonance spectroscopy in traumatic brain injury. J Head Trauma Rehabil 2001;16:149–64.

86. Henry LC, Tremblay S, Boulanger Y, et al. Neurometabolic changes in the acute phase after sports concussions correlate with symptom severity. J Neurotrauma 2010;27:65–76.

87. Vagnozzi R, Signoretti S, Tavazzi B, et al. Temporal window of metabolic brain vulnerability to concussion: a pilot 1H-magnetic resonance spectroscopic study in concussed athletes—part III. Neurosurgery 2008;62:1286–95.

88. Garnett MR, Blamire AM, Corkill RG, et al. Early proton magnetic resonance spectroscopy in normal-appearing brain correlates with outcome in patients following traumatic brain injury. Brain 2000;123(Pt 10):2046–54.

89. Ptito A, Chen JK, Johnston KM. Contributions of functional magnetic resonance imaging (fMRI) to sport concussion evaluation. NeuroRehabilitation 2007;22: 217–27.

90. McDonald BC, Saykin AJ, McAllister TW. Functional MRI of mild traumatic brain injury (mTBI): progress and perspectives from the first decade of studies. Brain Imaging Behav 2012;6:193–207.

91. Chen H, Yao D, Liu Z. A study on asymmetry of spatial visual field by analysis of the fMRI BOLD response. Brain Topogr 2004;17:39–46.

92. Zhang K, Johnson B, Pennell D, et al. Are functional deficits in concussed individuals consistent with white matter structural alterations: combined fMRI & DTI study. Exp Brain Res 2010;204:57–70.

93. Lovell MR, Pardini JE, Welling J, et al. Functional brain abnormalities are related to clinical recovery and time to return-to-play in athletes. Neurosurgery 2007;61: 352–9.

94. Terry DP, Faraco CC, Smith D, et al. Lack of long-term fMRI differences after multiple sports-related concussions. Brain Inj 2012;26:1684–96.

95. Shumskaya E, Andriessen TM, Norris DG, et al. Abnormal whole-brain functional networks in homogeneous acute mild traumatic brain injury. Neurology 2012;79: 175–82.

96. Tang L, Ge Y, Sodickson DK, et al. Thalamic resting-state functional networks: disruption in patients with mild traumatic brain injury. Radiology 2011;260: 831–40.

97. Rosenbaum SB, Lipton ML. Embracing chaos: the scope and importance of clinical and pathological heterogeneity in mTBI. Brain Imaging Behav 2012;6: 255–82.

98. Wintermark M, van Melle G, Schnyder P, et al. Admission perfusion CT: prognostic value in patients with severe head trauma. Radiology 2004;232:211–20.

99. Metting Z, Rodiger LA, Stewart RE, et al. Perfusion computed tomography in the acute phase of mild head injury: regional dysfunction and prognostic value. Ann Neurol 2009;66:809–16.

100. Depreitere B, Aviv R, Symons S, et al. Study of perfusion in and around cerebral contusions by means of computed tomography. Acta Neurochir Suppl 2008; 102:259–62.

101. Warmuth C, Gunther M, Zimmer C. Quantification of blood flow in brain tumors: comparison of arterial spin labeling and dynamic susceptibility-weighted contrast-enhanced MR imaging. Radiology 2003;228:523–32.

102. Ge Y, Patel MB, Chen Q, et al. Assessment of thalamic perfusion in patients with mild traumatic brain injury by true FISP arterial spin labelling MR imaging at 3T. Brain Inj 2009;23:666–74.

103. Kim J, Whyte J, Patel S, et al. Resting cerebral blood flow alterations in chronic traumatic brain injury: an arterial spin labeling perfusion fMRI study. J Neurotrauma 2010;27:1399–411.

104. Pasco A, Lemaire L, Franconi F, et al. Perfusional deficit and the dynamics of cerebral edemas in experimental traumatic brain injury using perfusion and diffusion-weighted magnetic resonance imaging. J Neurotrauma 2007;24:1321–30.

105. Lin AP, Liao HJ, Merugumala SK, et al. Metabolic imaging of mild traumatic brain injury. Brain Imaging Behav 2012;6:208–23.

106. Small GW, Kepe V, Siddarth P, et al. PET scanning of brain tau in retired national football league players: preliminary findings. Am J Geriatr Psychiatry 2013;21: 138–44.

107. Fodero-Tavoletti MT, Okamura N, Furumoto S, et al. 18F-THK523: a novel in vivo tau imaging ligand for Alzheimer's disease. Brain 2011;134:1089–100.

108. Liu C, Murphy NE, Li W. Probing white-matter microstructure with higher-order diffusion tensors and susceptibility tensor MRI. Front Integr Neurosci 2013;7:11.

109. Li X, Vikram DS, Lim IA, et al. Mapping magnetic susceptibility anisotropies of white matter in vivo in the human brain at 7 T. Neuroimage 2012;62:314–30.

110. Liu T, Surapaneni K, Lou M, et al. Cerebral microbleeds: burden assessment by using quantitative susceptibility mapping. Radiology 2012;262:269–78.

111. Ruff R. Two decades of advances in understanding of mild traumatic brain injury. J Head Trauma Rehabil 2005;20:5–18.

Neuroimaging of Dementia

John A. Bertelson, MD[a],*, Bela Ajtai, MD, PhD[b]

KEYWORDS

- Magnetic resonance imaging (MRI) • Alzheimer disease (AD)
- Positron emission tomography (PET) • Frontotemporal lobar degeneration (FTLD)
- Lewy body dementia (LBD) • Prion disease • Multiple sclerosis (MS)
- Vascular cognitive impairment

KEY POINTS

- Routine use of structural neuroimaging with computed tomography (CT) or MRI is recommended in the evaluation of patients with dementia.
- The latest criteria for the diagnosis of AD incorporate imaging biomarkers to support a clinical diagnosis. Imaging biomarkers for AD include PET and volumetric MRI.
- Florbetapir, an amyloid-binding PET tracer, was recently approved by the US Food and Drug Administration for use in the assessment of patients with cognitive impairment. Although a positive scan is nonspecific and of limited clinical usefulness, a negative scan may be clinically relevant and suggests the presence of a non-AD cause of cognitive decline.
- The best conventional MRI modality for prion disorders is diffusion-weighted imaging (DWI). The hyperintense DWI signal is caused by restricted diffusion in the vacuolar (spongiform) areas. The pulvinar sign is part of the World Health Organization diagnostic criteria for variant Creutzfeldt-Jakob disease.
- Cognitive deficits in multiple sclerosis (MS) can be attributed not only to visible white matter lesions but also to affected gray matter and normal-appearing brain tissue.
- In MS (or any immunocompromised host), the appearance of patchy, confluent T2 hyperintense signal that extends to the subcortical U-fibers is worrisome for the development of progressive multifocal leukoencephalopathy.
- Neurosarcoidosis or central nervous system (CNS) lupus may be difficult to differentiate from MS on MRI. In neurosarcoidosis, the pituitary stalk and hypothalamus may be involved. Leptomeningeal enhancement, when present, is characteristic of neurosarcoidosis. Lesions in CNS lupus tend to be subcortical, round and patchy (not linear), and spare the callosum.
- MRI is the preferred imaging modality to characterize the pathologic correlates to vascular cognitive impairment, which can be caused by large-vessel infarction, lacunar infarct(s), chronic microvascular ischemia, watershed ischemia, or hemorrhage.

Funding Sources: Dr Bertelson, Seton Brain and Spine Institute; Dr Ajtai, Dent Neurologic Institute.
Conflict of Interest: None.
[a] Seton Brain and Spine Institute, 1600 West 38th Street, Suite 308, Austin, TX 78731, USA;
[b] Dent Neurologic Institute, 3980A Sheridan Drive, Amherst, NY 14226, USA
* Corresponding author.
E-mail address: jabertelson@yahoo.com

INTRODUCTION

Dementia is a common cause of morbidity and mortality worldwide, particularly in the elderly population. The worldwide prevalence of dementia in 2010 was estimated to be more than 35 million, with a projected prevalence in 2050 of more than 115 million.[1] In the United States, 13% of people 65 years and older, and almost 50% of those 85 years and older, have Alzheimer disease (AD).[2] The prevalence of AD in the United States is expected to increase from 5.4 million in 2012 to as much as 16 million in 2050.[2] Although dementia remains a clinical diagnosis, neuroimaging is an increasingly valuable clinical and research tool in the assessment of patients with cognitive symptoms. The introduction of CT in the 1970s allowed for the first time routine visualization of cerebral anatomy in vivo, to assess for structural lesions that could mimic degenerative forms of dementia. MRI, PET, and other imaging modalities allow for improved visualization of the pathophysiologic processes associated with dementia and are routinely used in clinical practice.

IMAGING GUIDELINES

The indications for utilization of neuroimaging in the routine evaluation of dementia have evolved over the past several decades (**Table 1**). In the 1990s, guidelines published by American and Canadian organizations recommended that neuroimaging be considered in the evaluation of patients with dementia, but routine use of CT or MRI was not recommended for all patients.[3,4] However, initial and subsequently revised guidelines by the European Federation of Neurological Societies, and revised guidelines by the American Academy of Neurology recommended the use of structural neuroimaging (either CT or MRI) in the routine evaluation of patients with dementia.[5–7]

Table 1
Evolution of guidelines for neuroimaging in patients with dementia

Entity	Year	Recommendations
AAN[a]	1994	Neuroimaging is not routinely recommended (option[b])
CCCD[c]	1999	Neuroimaging (head CT) is recommended in select clinical situations, such as age <60 y, rapid progression, or gait disturbance (level B[d])
AAN[a]	2001	Structural neuroimaging (noncontrast CT or MRI) is appropriate in the routine initial evaluation of patients with dementia (guideline[e])
EFNS[f]	2007	Structural imaging is recommended in every patients suspected of dementia: • Noncontrast CT can identify surgically treatable lesions and vascular disease (level A[g]). • To increase specificity, MRI should be used (level A[g]).
EFNS[f]	2012	Structural imaging (CT or MRI) is recommended in the routine evaluation of every patient with dementia, to exclude secondary causes of dementia (level A[g])

[a] American Academy of Neurology.
[b] Practice option: unclear clinical certainty (inconclusive or conflicting evidence or opinion).
[c] Canadian Consensus Conference on Dementia.
[d] Level B: based on fair evidence.
[e] Practice guideline: recommendation that reflects moderate clinical certainty, usually class II evidence or strong consensus of class III evidence.
[f] European Federation of Neurological Societies.
[g] Level A: established as effective, based on at least 1 convincing class I study or at least 2 convincing class II studies.

Historically, the primary indication for neuroimaging has been to rule out reversible processes; it has been estimated that up to 5% of patients with dementia without focal signs or symptoms may have a potentially reversible lesion identifiable on routine neuroimaging.[8] Although there are limited data on the subject, at least one North American reference suggests that neurologists may strongly adhere to these recommendations, reporting that 99% of the patients with dementia in a Veterans Administration practice received either a CT or MRI as part of their evaluation.[9]

ROUTINE IMAGING MODALITIES

In patients presenting with dementia, structural imaging modalities such as noncontrast CT or MRI can readily identify clinically significant mass lesions, such as subdural hematomas, neoplasms, and hydrocephalus, which are potentially amenable to surgical intervention (**Fig. 1**). CT scans are well suited to visualize soft tissue such as brain parenchyma, but bony and similar structures can also be clearly assessed using different windowing settings. In patients with dementia, most lesions amenable to surgical intervention can be identified with CT. A total CT scan time in the order of seconds is particularly valuable in the population with dementia, given potential intolerance of the prolonged immobilization required for MRI. Although traditional CT brain protocols have provided only axial images, multiplanar reconstructions including coronal and sagittal images are becoming more widely available. Limitations to CT include exposure to ionizing radiation, diminished visualization of structures within the posterior fossa, and artifact from implanted metallic devices (**Fig. 2**).

With its superior resolution and standard multiplanar capability, MRI is the preferred imaging modality in the evaluation of patients with dementia. In contrast to standard CT protocols, MRI of the brain routinely includes sagittal, coronal, and axial sequences (**Fig. 3**). In addition, standard MRI protocols include sequences that are sensitive to edema (fluid-attenuated inversion recovery [FLAIR] and T2-weighted), acute ischemia (diffusion-weighted imaging [DWI]), blood products (gradient echo or susceptibility-weighted imaging [SWI]), and other pathologic processes. Limitations to MRI include

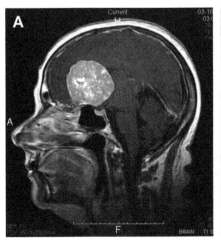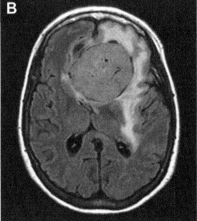

Fig. 1. A 65-year-old woman presenting with memory loss and bradyphrenia. Imaging findings are characteristic of meningioma. (A) T1-weighted sagittal, contrast-enhanced MRI and (B) fluid-attenuated inversion recovery axial MRI.

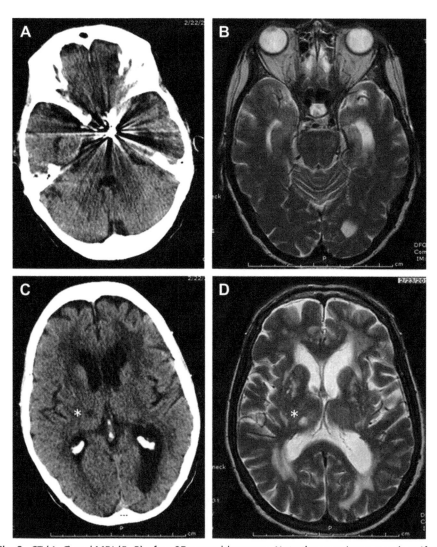

Fig. 2. CT (*A, C*) and MRI (*B, D*) of an 85-year-old woman. Note the prominent streak artifact on CT (*A*) caused by coiled aneurysm with minimal degradation of the corresponding MR image (*B*). Both series show mild ventriculomegaly, prominent periventricular white matter disease (likely ischemic), and a right thalamic lacunar infarct (*asterisk*).

longer scan times, greater potential for motion artifact, and contraindications in patients with certain implanted hardware, such as most pacemakers. In appropriate clinical scenarios, in particular if neoplasm, intracranial infection, or demyelination are suspected, contrast-enhanced MRI sequences should be strongly considered. Although not universally used in clinical practice to assess patients with dementia, additional MRI techniques have shown promise in further elucidating the pathophysiology of AD and other dementias (**Box 1**).

Nuclear medicine protocols with clinical relevance to dementia imaging include PET and single-photon emission CT (SPECT). The most commonly used PET ligand in

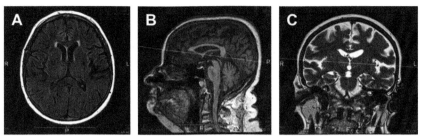

Fig. 3. Select MRI sequences used in the assessment of patients with dementia. (*A*) Axial FLAIR, (*B*) sagittal T1-weighted, and (*C*) coronal T2-weighted images.

dementia is 2-deoxy-2-[18F]fluoro-D-glucose ([^{18}F]FDG), which serves as a marker for regional brain metabolism (**Fig. 4**). [^{18}F]FDG, a glucose analogue, is transported into the neuron proportional to the degree of cellular metabolic activity. In 2004, [^{18}F] FDG-PET became the first nuclear medicine modality to be reimbursed by Centers for Medicare and Medicaid Services (CMS) for the evaluation of patients with dementia. Certain insurers, including CMS, generally cover [^{18}F]FDG-PET studies only to clarify a diagnosis between AD and frontotemporal lobar dementia (FTLD), assuming that other criteria are also met. In contrast, SPECT imaging is not generally reimbursed by CMS for the assessment of dementia, and in the United States is used less commonly than PET in routine clinical assessment of patients with dementia.

ALZHEIMER DISEASE

AD is the most common cause of dementia in the United States. In addition to a strong association with advancing age, risk factors associated with AD include female gender, genetic factors such as apolipoprotein E status, hypertension, and diabetes mellitus. The characteristic pathologic findings associated with AD include β-amyloid plaques, neurofibrillary tangles, and atrophy. The current consensus is that the first step in the AD cascade is the production of β-amyloid (in particular Aβ-42) by β-secretase and γ-secretase cleavage of the amyloid precursor protein. There is subsequent deposition of insoluble β-amyloid, with the development of neuritic plaques. Hyperphosphorylation of tau protein and development of neurofibrillary tangles follow, and atrophy and other imaging hallmarks of AD occur (**Fig. 5**).[10] The cognitive symptoms associated with AD occur late in the AD cascade. Noninvasive confirmation of AD such as through neuroimaging will likely become increasingly important as disease-modifying agents specific to AD become available.

Box 1
Additional MRI protocols with applications for dementia evaluation
Magnetic resonance spectroscopy
Diffusion tensor imaging
Magnetization transfer imaging
Functional MRI
Magnetic resonance perfusion
Cerebrospinal fluid flow studies

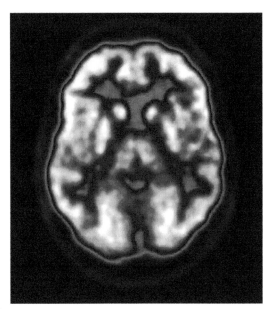

Fig. 4. Normal [^{18}F]FDG-PET in the axial plane.

Recently, the diagnostic criteria for dementia of the Alzheimer type have been revised to incorporate imaging and laboratory biomarkers, factors associated with the pathophysiologic process of AD.[11] There are 2 categories of AD biomarkers, those pertaining to β-amyloid deposition and others that reflect neuronal degeneration or injury. β-Amyloid neuroimaging biomarkers include amyloid binding with specific PET tracers. Neuroimaging biomarkers for neuronal degeneration include regional hypometabolism, visualized on [^{18}F]FDG-PET, and atrophy, best visualized on MRI.

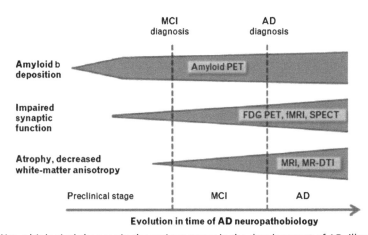

Fig. 5. Neurobiological changes in the various stages in the development of AD, illustrated by specific imaging techniques. A larger area in red indicates a greater degree of the neurobiological disorder (ie, Aβ deposition or atrophy). (*Adapted with permission from* Lippincott Williams and Wilkins/Wolters Kluwer Health: Curr Opin Neurol, Masdeu J, et al, The neurobiology of Alzheimer disease defined by neuroimaging, 2012.)

Many recent advances in AD imaging research have resulted from the Alzheimer's Disease Neuroimaging Initiative (ADNI), which began enrollment in 2004 and was initially scheduled to be completed in 2009. The primary goal of ADNI was to develop clinical, imaging, genetic, and biochemical markers for the early detection and monitoring of AD. Funding for ADNI has been extended, and the active protocol in North America is known as ADNI-2, which includes MRI, [^{18}F]FDG-PET, and amyloid PET imaging. There are also now ADNI sites in Europe, Australia, and Asia, with others under development.[12]

Imaging Modalities in AD

MRI is the preferred imaging modality for the routine assessment of patients with dementia of the Alzheimer type. The most common MRI finding in patients with AD is atrophy, which can be focal, multifocal, or generalized. Atrophy of the medial temporal lobe and other select regions has been reported not only in patients with dementia but also in mild cognitive impairment (MCI) and even asymptomatic individuals with genetic risk factors for AD.[13–15] Patients with less common forms of AD, for example posterior cortical atrophy (**Fig. 6**), may show patterns of atrophy reflective of their particular subtype.

Measurements of cortical thickness have been proposed as a promising MRI biomarker of atrophy, because patients with AD have been noted to have selective areas of cortical thinning. One such metric, calculated from averaging cortical thickness in multiple regions of interest, including the medial temporal lobe, has been used to predict time to development of dementia in patients with baseline normal cognitive function.[16] A similar study shows a trend toward more AD-like cerebrospinal fluid (CSF) (abnormally low CSF β-amyloid) and a greater risk of cognitive and neuropsychological decline over 3 years in patients with greater baseline atrophy.[17] Ventricular volume measurements, as a marker of atrophy, have also been investigated. Patients with AD have been shown to have larger ventricular volumes than patients with MCI and normal controls.[18] In addition, ventricular volume measurements may predict which patients with MCI may progress to dementia compared with those who remain clinically stable.[18]

A fully automated and commercially available process (NeuroQuant, CorTechs Labs, La Jolla, CA) has been developed, which performs age-matched and gender-matched volumetric analysis of the hippocampi, inferior lateral ventricles, and other key structures (**Fig. 7**). A typical AD pattern is a significant reduction in hippocampal volume, with corresponding enlargement of the adjacent inferior portion of the lateral ventricle (**Fig. 8**). This process has been used to show that patients with greater hippocampal atrophy at baseline progress to dementia more rapidly than those with less baseline atrophy.[19] Other tools for volumetric analysis include FreeSurfer (http://surfer.nmr.mgh.harvard.edu) and Functional MR Imaging of the Brain Software Library (http://www.fmrib.ox.ac.uk/fsl).

It is increasingly recognized that AD pathology is not restricted to cortically-based plaques and tangles; white matter derangements can also occur and can be assessed with MRI. For example, diffusion tensor imaging (DTI) can characterize white matter integrity through measurements of fractional anisotropy (FA). A meta-analysis of DTI studies[20] identified widespread reduced FA in patients with AD and MCI, compared with normal controls. Neuropsychiatric symptoms including agitation and apathy have been associated with reduced FA in the anterior cingulum and other regions in patients with MCI and AD.[21,22]

Another advanced MRI technique with potential usefulness in AD is magnetic resonance spectroscopy (MRS). Patients with AD show a reduction in the *N*-acetyl

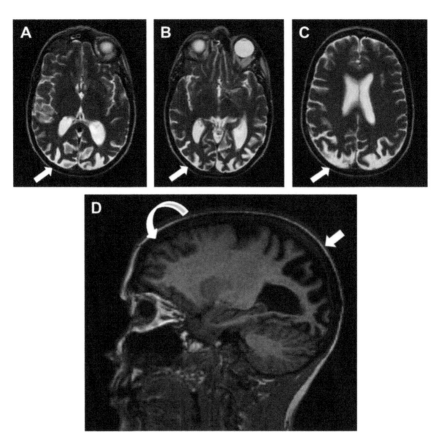

Fig. 6. MRI of a 69-year-old woman with the posterior cortical atrophy variant of AD. (*A–C*) Axial T2-weighted and (*D*) parasagittal T1-weighted sequences. Note the sulcal prominence representing atrophy in the parietal and occipital regions (*straight arrows*), compared with the normal frontal (*curved arrow*) and temporal lobes.

aspartate (NAA)/creatine (Cr) ratio, reflecting diminished neuronal density, in regions such as the posterior cingulate gyrus (**Fig. 9**).[23]

After CT and MRI, the imaging modality most commonly used in the clinical assessment of AD is [18F]FDG-PET. Typical findings in AD are hypometabolism in the parietotemporal region and posterior cingulate cortex (**Fig. 10**), although abnormalities can sometimes be appreciated in the medial temporal lobes. As AD progresses, hypometabolism becomes more extensive, with involvement of the prefrontal cortex and other cortical regions. However, certain regions, including the cerebellum, primary visual cortex, and primary motor cortex, are relatively spared throughout the course of the disease.[24] Primarily because reimbursement is limited to cases indeterminate between AD and FTLD, [18F]FDG-PET is only used in select clinical assessments.

Recently, considerable interest has been generated regarding novel PET tracers that bind to intracerebral β-amyloid. The first such tracer to be developed was the Pittsburgh compound B (PiB),[25] which has been shown to have a high affinity for amyloid. More than 90% of patients with AD, 60% of patients with MCI, and 30% of normal elderly individuals show abnormal PiB binding (**Fig. 11**).[26] Although data suggest that amyloid deposition generally occurs before the onset of cognitive impairment

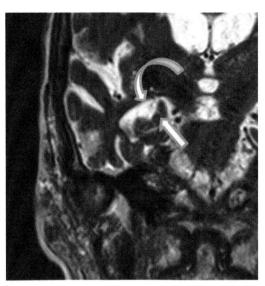

Fig. 7. Coronal T2-weighted MRI showing cross section of the right hippocampus (*straight arrow*) and inferior lateral ventricle (*curved arrow*).

associated with AD, it remains to be determined whether or not significant amyloid deposition can represent a benign process in some elderly individuals, without the inevitable development of dementia.

A significant limitation of PiB imaging is the short half-life of the PiB tracer (about 20 minutes), which essentially restricts its use to centers with immediate access to a cyclotron. More recently, amyloid-binding PET tracers with longer half-lives have been developed. One such agent, florbetapir (Amyvid, Lilly USA, Indianapolis, IN) with a half-life of almost 2 hours, was approved by the US Food and Drug Administration in 2012 (**Table 2**). Studies have confirmed that florbetapir-PET scans accurately

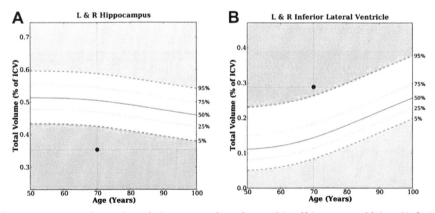

Fig. 8. Brain MRI volumetric analysis. Presented are the combined hippocampal (*A*) and inferior lateral ventricle volumes (*B*), as % of total intracranial volume (ICV). There is significant reduction in the hippocampal volume (<5th percentile), with corresponding enlargement of the adjacent inferior lateral ventricles (>95th percentile). This pattern suggests hippocampal atrophy, such as can be seen with AD. (*Courtesy of* Coltechs Labs, Inc., La Jolla, CA; with permission.)

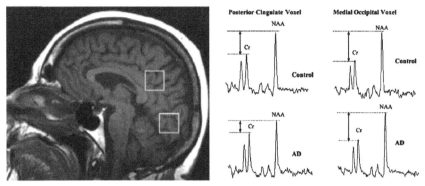

Fig. 9. Proton MRS regional differences in control versus patient with AD. Note that although the NAA/Cr ratios in the medial occipital regions are relatively constant between the normal control and patient with AD, the NAA/Cr ratio in the posterior cingulate is significantly diminished in the patient with AD. (*From* Kantarci K, Jack C. Predicting progression of Alzheimer's disease with magnetic resonance. In: Broderick PA, Rahni DN, Kolodny EH, editors. Bioimaging in neurodegeneration. Totowa (NJ): Humana Press, 2005; with kind permission of Springer Science+Business Media.)

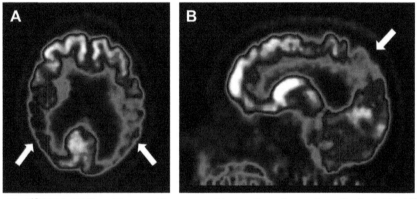

Fig. 10. [^{18}F]FDG-PET in a 61-year-old woman with AD. Note the profoundly diminished [^{18}F] FDG uptake in the temporoparietal and parietal regions bilaterally (*arrows*), seen on (*A*) axial and (*B*) parasagittal images.

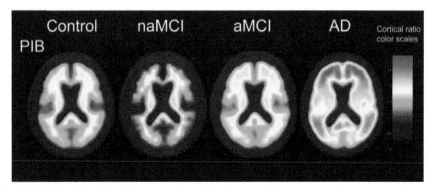

Fig. 11. PiB binding in healthy controls and patients with nonamnestic MCI, amnestic MCI, and AD. The higher cortical ratio color scale corresponds to greater PiB binding. (*From* Lowe VJ, Kemp BJ, Jack CR Jr, et al. Comparison of ^{18}F-FDG and PiB PET in Cognitive Impairment. J Nucl Med 2009;50(6):883; with permission. © by the Society of Nuclear Medicine and Molecular Imaging, Inc.)

Table 2	
Florbetapir-PET imaging in dementia	
Indications for florbetapir-PET scans	
Patients with cognitive impairment being evaluated for AD and other causes of cognitive decline	
To estimate β-amyloid neuritic plaque density	
Adjunct to other diagnostic evaluations	
Positive scan	**Negative scan**
Indicates moderate to frequent β-amyloid neuritic plaques	Indicates sparse to no β-amyloid neuritic plaques
Does not implicate AD as the cause of cognitive decline. Although consistent with AD, a positive scan may also be present in patients with other neurologic conditions and older persons with normal cognition	Inconsistent with a diagnosis of AD and suggests an alternative cause for the cognitive decline

Data from Amyvid package insert, Eli Lilly and Company, Inc., Indianapolis, IN. 2012.

and reliably estimate β-amyloid neuritic plaque density.[27] Given that β-amyloid is relatively nonspecific and is seen not only in patients with AD but also in normal elderly and various non-AD disorders (such as Lewy body disease), a positive scan is of limited clinical usefulness. However, a negative florbetapir scan has clinical value because it is inconsistent with AD and suggests the presence of a dementing disorder other than AD. As of April 2013, a decision from CMS regarding reimbursement for florbetapir-PET had not been announced. High cost and low specificity of florbetapir and other amyloid-binding PET tracers will likely limit their clinical use. For now, amyloid imaging has a valuable role in clinical trials of antiamyloid therapies.[28]

FRONTOTEMPORAL LOBAR DEGENERATION

The term FTLD refers to a heterogeneous group of disorders characterized by degeneration predominantly of the frontal or temporal lobes, with symptoms involving behavior, language, or motor function. An earlier term for this disease spectrum, Pick disease, is no longer routinely used, because many patients with FTLD do not show the characteristic Pick bodies on autopsy. At least three different pathologic substrates are associated with FTLD: tau, transactive response DNA-binding protein 43 (TDP-43), and fused in sarcoma (FUS).[29]

Behavioral variant frontotemporal lobar degeneration (bv-FTLD) is characterized by initial symptoms of prominent personality changes, which can include impulsivity, apathy, and disinhibition. The language variant of FTLD, primary progressive aphasia (PPA), is characterized by language-based symptoms at presentation. The PPA subtypes include the nonfluent/agrammatic, semantic, and logopenic forms.[30] The FTLD variants and subtypes can be distinguished by their clinical, and sometimes imaging, characteristics. For example, different patterns of atrophy may be seen on routine MRI (**Fig. 12**). However, the sensitivity of routine structural MRI for FTLD is highly variable (10%–100%), related to the FTLD subtype, experience of the interpreting physician, and use of objective rating scales.[31,32] Although not routinely used in clinical practice, MRI volumetry protocols have been used to accurately distinguish between AD and FTLD,[33] and also between various FTLD subtypes.[34,35] Sometimes, MRI can reveal focal frontal or temporal atrophy in presymptomatic patients (**Fig. 13**).

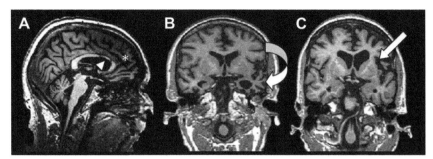

Fig. 12. MRI of different types of FTLD. (*A*) Sagittal T1-weighted image of patient with bv-FTD. Note the thinning of the anterior corpus callosum (*arrowhead*) and relative atrophy of the midline frontal lobe (*asterisk*). (*B*) Coronal T1-weighted image of patient with semantic dementia showing left temporal atrophy (*curved arrow*). (*C*) Coronal T1-weighted image of patient with nonfluent FTD, with left insular atrophy (*arrow*). (*From* Tartaglia M, Rosen H, Miller B. Neuroimaging in Dementia. Neurotherapeutics 2011;8(1):84; with permission.)

Routine MRI imaging can occasionally be helpful in identifying findings other than atrophy in patients with FTLD, such as T2 hyperintensity in the corticospinal tracts of patients with FTLD-amyotrophic lateral sclerosis. Several additional MRI modalities have been studied in patients with FTLD, including arterial spin labeling, functional

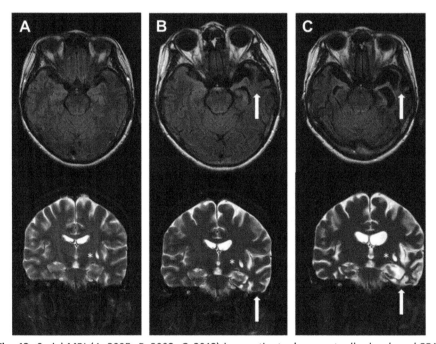

Fig. 13. Serial MRI (*A*, 2005; *B*, 2008; *C*, 2013) in a patient who eventually developed PPA. The onset of dysnomia was in 2011 at 68 years of age. The initial images were obtained because of a history of headache, when language was reportedly normal. Note the progressive atrophy primarily involving the left temporal lobe (*arrows*). There is also evidence of a milder degree of generalized atrophy, with progressive enlargement of the right temporal horn (axial images) and body of the lateral ventricles (axial and coronal images). Incidentally noted is a prominent perivascular space medial to the left insula (*asterisk*).

MRI, perfusion-weighted, diffusion-weighted, and MRS. Multimodal MRI protocols such as those that incorporate DWI, perfusion, and structural imaging[36] are particularly promising.

Imaging with PET is a commercially available option in the United States when structural imaging and the clinical evaluation are indeterminate in distinguishing between FTLD and AD. Characteristic [^{18}F]FDG-PET abnormalities in FTLD include frontal, temporal, or frontotemporal hypometabolism (**Fig. 14**). When compared with MRI, the sensitivity and specificity of SPECT/PET for FTLD is increased from 63.5% and 70.4% to 90.5% and 74.6%, respectively.[37] Other sources confirm the greater sensitivities for FTLD using combined structural (MRI) and functional (PET/SPECT) imaging compared with MRI alone.[38]

DIFFUSE LEWY BODY DEMENTIA

Dementia with Lewy bodies (DLB) is the second most common neurodegenerative cause of dementia after AD[39] and up to 40% of patients with AD harbor comorbid Lewy body pathology as well. The pathologic hallmark of DLB is the Lewy body, an eosinophilic cytoplasmic inclusion mostly composed of α-synuclein. Lewy bodies are found in the substantia nigra, locus ceruleus, dorsal raphe, substantia innominata, dorsal motor nucleus of the vagus nerve, and neocortex. Clinical signs of DLB include visual hallucinations, extrapyramidal features, fluctuating level of alertness, and sensitivity to neuroleptics. Visuospatial and executive dysfunction are often prominent.

Conventional MRI does not show specific abnormalities in Lewy body disease. Cerebral volume loss may be seen. Hippocampal atrophy can be present, but not to the same degree as in AD.[40] Relatively preserved medial temporal lobe volume argues for DLB and against AD. SPECT and PET can be helpful to support the diagnosis. The most common finding with these techniques is occipital lobe hypoperfusion (SPECT) and hypometabolism (PET), involving primary visual and visual association cortices.[41,42] Involvement of these regions is believed to be the basis of the visual hallucinations. Additional findings on SPECT may include frontal and striatal hyperperfusion and parietal/temporal hypoperfusion (**Fig. 15**). The sensitivity of SPECT in DLB is about 65%, and its specificity in distinguishing from AD and normal controls is around 87%.[43–45] Occipital hypometabolism on PET has been found to distinguish DLB from AD, with a 92% sensitivity and specificity.[46] Relative sparing

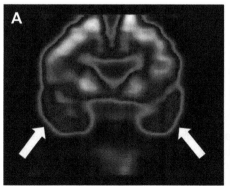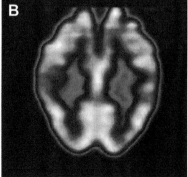

Fig. 14. PET in a patient with frontotemporal dementia. Note the prominent hypometabolism of the temporal lobes bilaterally (*arrows*) in the coronal image (*A*), with normal-appearing frontal and parietal lobes (axial image, *B*).

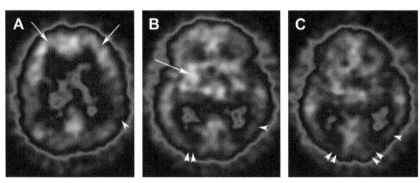

Fig. 15. Neurolite-SPECT scan of a patient with Lewy body dementia. (*A*) Frontal hyperperfusion (*arrows*) and parietal hypoperfusion (*arrowhead*). (*B*) Striatal hyperperfusion, right>left (*arrow*), posterolateral temporal hypoperfusion (*arrowhead*), occipital hypoperfusion (*double arrowhead*). (*C*) Posterolateral temporal hypoperfusion (*arrowhead*), occipital hypoperfusion (*double arrowhead*).

of the midsegment and posterior segment of the cingulate gyrus (lack of hypoperfusion and hypometabolism), when present on SPECT and PET, has been found to be 100% specific to DLB.[47]

An interesting field in SPECT imaging for DLB is dopamine transporter (DAT) imaging, using ligands that bind to the DAT. Decreased striatal DAT uptake is a suggestive imaging finding in DLB. It has been also found useful to distinguish DLB from AD and normal controls.[48] The sensitivity and specificity of the technique to differentiate DLB from Parkinson disease (PD) with or without dementia is controversial.[49,50] For a comprehensive review of imaging in DLB, see the summary by Tateno and coworkers.[51]

PROGRESSIVE SUPRANUCLEAR PALSY

Progressive supranuclear palsy (PSP) is a neurodegenerative disorder, characterized by predominantly axial rigidity, balance impairment with frequent falling, vertical gaze paresis, and, in most cases, subcortical-type dementia. Structural imaging features of PSP include thinning of the cranial midbrain tectum and a concave aspect of the third ventricular floor (**Fig. 16**). Atrophy may also involve the frontal and temporal lobes. Subtle T2 hyperintensity may be present in the periaqueductal area.

The finding of reduced anteroposterior midbrain diameter (routinely measurable on axial images), especially if less than 14 mm, favors PSP over PD. A more complex measurement that has been proposed to differentiate PSP from PD, as well as the parkinsonian variant of multiple system atrophy (MSA-p) is the MR parkinsonism index. It is expressed by the formula:

$$[(P/M) \times (MCP/SCP)]$$

where P/M is the ratio of the pons area to midbrain area on midsagittal images and MCP/SCP is the middle cerebellar peduncle width (on a parasagittal image) divided by that of the superior cerebellar peduncle on a coronal image. This MR parkinsonism index value was found to be significantly larger in the PSP patient group than in the PD, MSA-p, or normal control groups, without overlap. Hence, sensitivity and specificity values of 100% have been shown using this method in the pairwise differentiation of PSP from PD, MSA-p, and controls.[52]

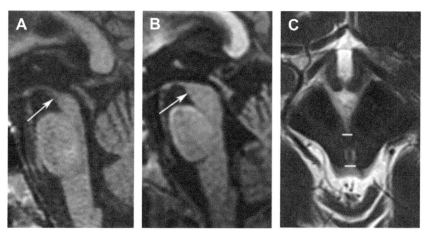

Fig. 16. Progressive supranuclear palsy. (*A*) Thin-slice T1-weighted images. Arrow indicates the thinning of the cranial midbrain. Dorsally, note the concave aspect of the third ventricular floor. (*B*) Normal control. (*C*) T2-weighted image showing reduced anteroposterior diameter of the midbrain (*between horizontal bars*).

HUNTINGTON DISEASE

The typical MRI finding in Huntington disease (HD) is atrophy of the caudate nucleus (**Fig. 17**). Atrophy of the putamen and frontal lobes is also frequently seen. With disease progression, diffuse cortical, thalamic, and limbic atrophy may also appear. Putaminal signal changes may be present, which can be hyperintense or hypointense on T2-weighted images. The T2 hyperintense signal change is attributed to more marked neuronal loss and gliosis. T2 hypointense signal change is less frequent and may correlate with putaminal iron deposition.

MSA-P

In this neurodegenerative disorder, extrapyramidal/parkinsonian features with impaired balance (but generally no resting tremor), dysautonomia, and, at times, pyramidal signs

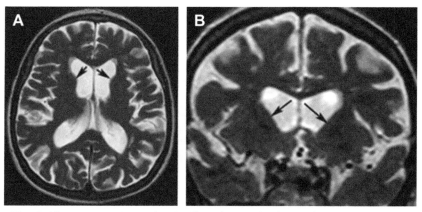

Fig. 17. HD. The arrows point to the significantly atrophic head of the caudate nucleus on axial (*A*) and coronal (*B*) T2-weighted images.

are present. Cognitive testing often reveals executive dysfunction. T2 and FLAIR MRI sequences may show significant hypointensity in the posterior and lateral putamen (potentially because of the magnetic susceptibility effects of accumulated iron, manganese, neuromelanin, and hematin). A thin line of T2 hyperintense signal change along the lateral aspect of the putamen may also be present, presumably caused by neuronal loss and gliosis (**Fig. 18**). Another typical imaging finding, when present, is cruciform T2 hyperintense signal in the pons, referred to as the hot-cross-bun sign. In a patient with levodopa-resistant parkinsonism, these findings strongly support the diagnosis of MSA-p.

NORMAL PRESSURE HYDROCEPHALUS

Normal pressure hydrocephalus (NPH) is an uncommon cause of dementia in the middle-aged and elderly, with an estimated prevalence of 0.41% to 2.94%.[53] NPH can be secondary to a history of precipitating events such as intracerebral hemorrhage, meningitis, or brain trauma; other forms of NPH are considered idiopathic and may account for one-third of the total cases.[54] The cause of NPH is unknown but may be related to impaired CSF absorption at the level of the arachnoid villi.

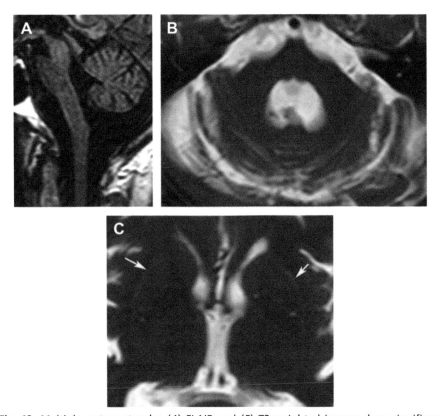

Fig. 18. Multiple system atrophy. (*A*) FLAIR and (*B*) T2-weighted images show significant brainstem and cerebellar volume loss. (*C*) Thin, linear T2 hyperintense signal change (*arrows*) along the lateral aspect of the putamen on an axial T2-weighted image, presumably caused by neuronal loss and gliosis.

The classic clinical triad of dementia, gait apraxia, and urinary incontinence is often not present; a recently proposed diagnostic criterion for probable idiopathic NPH requires only the presence of the characteristic gait disorder, plus at least one of dementia or urinary incontinence.[55] As a type of communicating hydrocephalus, requisite imaging findings for NPH include ventriculomegaly without macroscopic evidence of obstruction of CSF (**Table 3**). In addition, some patients with idiopathic NPH show patchy sulcal prominence, with other sulci either appearing normal or effaced (**Fig. 19**).[54]

PRION DISEASES

Prion diseases are rare causes of rapidly progressing dementia. Sporadic Creutzfeldt-Jakob disease (sCJD) and variant Creutzfeldt-Jakob disease (vCJD) are the most studied entities. Pathologically, the disease is characterized by neuronal loss, prion deposition, vacuolation, and some astrogliosis. The fluid-filled vacuoles, less accurately referred to as spongiform changes, are significant in causing characteristic MRI changes.

The most useful conventional MRI techniques to evaluate sCJD are FLAIR and DWI sequences. With these techniques, the involved regions show hyperintense signal, which is more conspicuous on DWI. Potentially involved structures include the caudate nucleus and putamen (usually in a symmetric fashion), thalamus, or the various segments of the neocortex (cortical ribbon hyperintensity), either symmetric or asymmetric (**Fig. 20**). Frontotemporal, temporoparietal, lateral, and medial occipital and anterior cingulate cortical involvement can be encountered in various patterns, which can change during the disease course. A large multicenter study of sCJD suggested that a characteristic pattern of involvement may occur, depending on the molecular subtype.[56] Isolated involvement of the limbic regions, without other brain regions, is not believed to happen in CJD, and involvement of the precentral gyrus is also rare. Also, the phenomenon of the hyperintensity being more prominent on DWI than on FLAIR sequence is an imaging feature highly in favor of sCJD as opposed to other rapidly progressive dementias.[57] The cause for the DWI hyperintensity is believed to be restriction of diffusion.[58–60] It has been suggested that the spongiform changes should rather be referred to as vacuolation and the fluid-filled vacuoles likely cause restriction of water movement.[57]

Table 3
Imaging findings associated with idiopathic NPH

Required	Optional
1. Ventriculomegaly out of proportion to atrophy or congenital enlargement	1. Preclinical imaging study showing smaller ventricular size
2. No macroscopic obstruction to CSF flow	2. Radionucleotide cisternogram showing delayed clearance of tracer over the cerebral convexities after 48–72 h
3. At least 1 of the following:	3. Cine MRI or similar study showing increased ventricular flow rate
a. Enlarged temporal horns out of proportion to hippocampal atrophy	4. Negative SPECT-acetazolamide challenge (decreased periventricular perfusion unaltered by acetazolamide)
b. Callosal angle of 40° or more	
c. Periventricular signal change not attributable to chronic microvascular ischemia or other signs of abnormal brain water content	
d. Aqueductal or fourth ventricular flow void	

Adapted from Relkin N, Marmarou A, Klinge P, et al. Diagnosing idiopathic normal-pressure hydrocephalus. Neurosurgery 2005;57:S2–6.

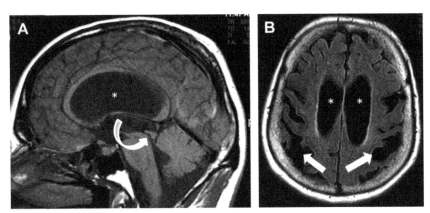

Fig. 19. Imaging characteristics of NPH. (*A*) A 61-year-old man with ventriculomegaly (*asterisk*) and grossly patent cerebral aqueduct (*curved arrow*). (*B*) A 69-year-old man with enlarged lateral ventricles (*asterisk*) and multifocal sulcal dilation (*straight arrows*).

DWI (and FLAIR) signal abnormalities are not diagnostic by themselves and may change depending on the stage of the disease.[61] Disappearance of the DWI hyperintensity in late stages has been described.[62] MRI changes identical to those in sCJD have been reported in extrapontine myelinolysis, hyperglycemia, and uncontrolled seizures, and, therefore, clinical correlation is essential.[57]

With proton MRS, the characteristic findings in sCJD include reduced NAA levels and NAA/Cr ratios and increased myoinositol levels.[63] In one study,[64] the combination of thalamic DWI hyperintensity and reduced NAA/Cr ratio correctly classified 93% of the patients as having prion disease.

vCJD (causally linked to bovine spongiform encephalopathy) presents with a different appearance on conventional MRI. The imaging finding, referred to as pulvinar sign (hyperintensity involving the posterior thalami (pulvinar)), in a symmetric fashion is characteristic for vCJD. Additional commonly involved regions include the dorsomedial thalamic nuclei, head of the caudate nucleus, and periaqueductal gray matter. The combination of pulvinar and dorsomedial thalamic hyperintensity is also referred to as the hockey-stick sign (**Fig. 21**).[65] Because of its high diagnostic value, the pulvinar sign is part of the World Health Organization diagnostic criteria for vCJD.[66] With

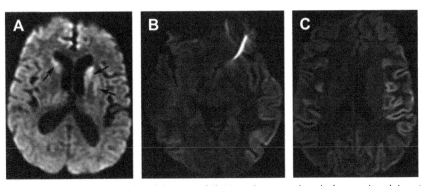

Fig. 20. sCJD. Diffusion-weighted images. (*A*) Hyperintense signal change involving the head of the caudate nucleus bilaterally and the left putamen (*arrows*). (*B, C*) Cortical ribbon hyperintensity involving various segments of the neocortex, in an asymmetric fashion.

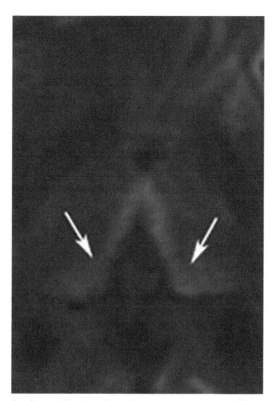

Fig. 21. vCJD. The hockey-stick sign: hyperintense signal on diffusion-weighted image, involving the pulvinar and medial thalamus bilaterally.

proton MRS studies in vCJD, the pulvinar shows significantly decreased NAA and increased myoinositol levels and the magnitude of increase suggests potential for even earlier diagnosis.[67]

PET scanning is not being used routinely in the evaluation of prion diseases. In a landmark study, the observed pattern of hypometabolism was different from the distribution of the lesions on MRI: hypometabolism was present predominantly in the cerebellum and the cerebral cortex (frontal, occipital, parietal) rather than the thalamus or striatum.[68] Showing occipital lobe hypometabolism can be useful in identifying patients with mostly visual complaints, the so-called Heidenhain variant.[69]

Prion disease–related changes have been studied with SPECT scanning as well. In 1 study, 89% of the patients showed perfusion pattern change involving the cerebellum, occipital lobes, even a whole hemisphere.[70] Focal hypoperfusion has been detected in the basal ganglia,[71] the thalamus,[72] and frontotemporal areas.[73] The perfusion pattern change in prion disorders is different from other dementias, and the changes occur earlier than on MRI.[73,74]

MULTIPLE SCLEROSIS

Cognitive deficits and dementia are well-known sequelae of multiple sclerosis (MS).[75] Studies have shown that up to 70% of patients with MS have some degree of cognitive dysfunction. Cognitive impairment can also present in as many as 53.7% of early-stage patients, with no correlation with physical disability.[76] The cognitive domains most frequently affected include attention, executive functioning, information-processing speed and efficiency, and episodic and working memory.

The earliest studies on MRI findings and cognitive deficits in MS focused on parameters measurable by conventional MRI techniques (T2 and T1 lesion load, ventricular/brain ratio, third ventricle width, and size of the corpus callosum). The results regarding the correlation between T2 lesion burden and cognitive impairment are conflicting.[77,78] Attempts to correlate lesion location with specific cognitive deficits also yielded mixed results. A generally accepted hypothesis holds that the main mechanism of cognitive deficits related to damage white matter is disconnection. Disruption of frontoparietal subcortical networks was found to be associated with impairment of complex attention and working memory.[79] Cognitively impaired patients tend to have higher lesion frequency in commissural fiber tracts.[80] DTI studies found diffusivity changes in the corpus callosum that correlated with visual and verbal memory tests.[81] Although disconnection is a proven mechanism of cognitive deficits, linking a certain cognitive deficit to a precise lesion location is more challenging. Diffusion tensor MRI tractography studies helped to identify cognitively relevant white matter tracts. These tracts included the cingulum (lesion of which was found to predict global cognitive performance); the uncinate fasciculus (implicated in visual processing speed, sustained attention, and visuospatial and verbal memory); the superior cerebellar peduncle (which was predictive of global cognitive performance, visual processing speed, sustained attention, verbal learning/memory, and verbal fluency); and the middle cerebellar peduncle.[82] In an earlier series,[83] strong association was found between frontal lobe MS disease and executive deficits. However, this finding was not confirmed in a later study,[84] in which the specific contribution of frontal lobe lesions to executive dysfunction in the setting of widespread lesions could not be ascertained.

The discrepancies between white matter lesion burden and cognitive deficits can be explained by considering that MS represents a considerably more diffuse process, which also involves gray matter[85–88] and otherwise normal-appearing parenchyma. Gray matter lesions are difficult to visualize by conventional T2-weighted images. FLAIR sequences visualize cortical and juxtacortical lesions better, because of the suppression of the signal from the adjacent CSF.[89] A more sensitive technique for imaging cortical lesions is the double inversion recovery sequence,[90] but even this detects only a small percentage of intracortical lesions.[91] Using higher magnetic field strength also increases the sensitivity to detect cortical lesions.

Other emerging techniques in gray matter imaging are magnetization transfer imaging (MTI) and DTI. MS lesions are associated with an altered magnetization transfer ratio (MTR) in the gray matter early in the disease.[92] Cognitively impaired patients with MS have more pronounced reduction in neocortical volume and cortical MTR than cognitively intact patients.[93] With DTI, correlation was found between gray matter mean diffusivity changes and cognitive impairment in patients with relapsing remitting MS.[94]

Normal-appearing white matter (NAWM) and normal-appearing gray matter are regions where conventional MRI techniques fail to reveal lesions, yet histopathology and advanced imaging techniques show the presence of pathologic process. In MS, the NAWM may show microscopic demyelination[95] or axonal transection leading to secondary, Wallerian-like degeneration.[96] MRS studies showed increased myoinositol (a glial and inflammatory marker) in the NAWM, suggestive of an inflammatory process.[97] In a more recent extensive work, using MTI and DTI in correlation with pathologic studies on postmortem multiple sclerosis brains, various pathomechanisms underlying the MTR and DTI abnormalities in the NAWM were suggested, which depended on the distance from the visible white matter lesions.[98] Several studies support the role of disease in the NAWM in cognitive deficits in MS.[94,97,99–102] Changes in the NAWM included fractional isotropy changes on DTI and altered MTR, and these correlated with cognitive impairment.

Proton MRS has also been performed in cognitively impaired patients. Typical findings are reduced NAA and thereby decreased NAA/Cr ratio (indicating decreased neuronal and axonal integrity and viability) and increased myoinositol level (a marker of inflammation and gliosis). Globally, lower NAA/Cr ratio was found to distinguish between cognitively impaired and intact patients with MS.[103] Reduction of the regional NAA/Cr ratio in the frontal cingulate gyrus correlated with distinct memory functions.[104]

Another imaging tool for evaluation of cognitively impaired patients with MS is volumetric analysis. Consistent indicators of cognitive dysfunction are corpus callosum atrophy,[105–107] third ventricle width,[108,109] and thalamic atrophy.[110] Volumetric analysis of deep gray matter structures found correlation with free recall or new learning, and mesial temporal lobe volumetric measures predicted recognition memory performance.[111] Left frontal atrophy was associated with impaired performance on auditory/verbal memory testing, and right frontal atrophy was associated with impairment in visual episodic and working memory.[112] See **Fig. 22** for the MRI appearance in a cognitively impaired patient with advanced MS.

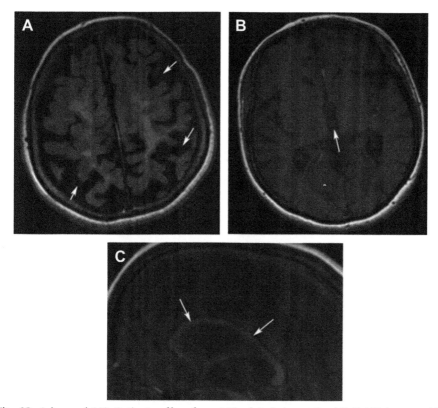

Fig. 22. Advanced MS. Patient suffers from MS-related dementia. (*A*) FLAIR image with confluent hyperintense demyelinating lesions. Note the severe cortical atrophy as shown by sulcal enlargement (*arrows*). (*B*) T1-weighted image shows severe third ventricle enlargement (*arrow*), caused by thalamic atrophy. (*C*) T1-weighted image reveals severe thinning of the corpus callosum.

PROGRESSIVE MULTIFOCAL LEUKOENCEPHALOPATHY

Progressive multifocal leukoencephalopathy (PML) is an infectious demyelinating disease, affecting immunocompromised hosts. It typically involves the white matter, mostly in the frontal, parietal, and occipital lobes. The lesions are usually multifocal, and on MRI appear T1 hypointense and T2/FLAIR hyperintense. Their initially round or oval morphology may later become confluent. The tendency to involve the subcortical white matter, including the U-fibers, is characteristic (**Fig. 23**). In later stages, involvement of the deep gray matter, corpus callosum, and posterior fossa may be

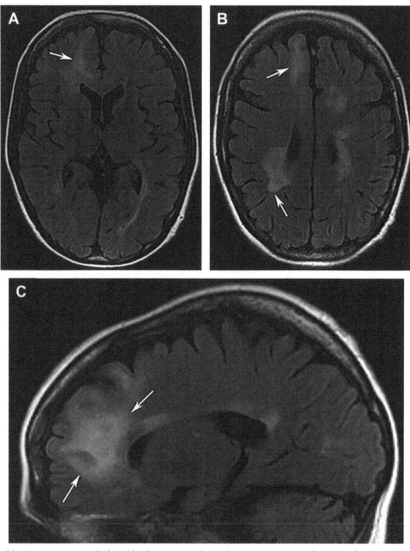

Fig. 23. Progressive multifocal leukoencephalopathy. FLAIR images show confluent T2 hyperintense signal change (*arrows*) extending to the frontal (*A*) and frontal/parietal (*B*) subcortical white matter, including the U-fibers. (*C*) Sagittal image reveals extensive, confluent T2 hyperintense signal in the frontal deep and subcortical white matter (*arrows*).

seen as well. The lesions generally do not show gadolinium enhancement, but faint enhancement may sometimes occur. With DWI sequences, restricted diffusion was described at the spreading, outer margins of the PML lesions, with low signal on the apparent diffusion coefficient map.[113]

HUMAN IMMUNODEFICIENCY VIRUS–ASSOCIATED COGNITIVE DISORDERS

This group of disorders develops as a result of direct involvement of the central nervous system (CNS) by the human immunodeficiency virus (HIV). The classification identifies asymptomatic neurocognitive impairment, mild neurocognitive disorder, and HIV-associated dementia, representing stages of a progressive cognitive decline. Pathologically, the primary targets are macrophages, resulting in microglial nodule formation with the presence of multinucleated giant cells. Demyelination and vacuole formation are also observed.

The imaging features in HIV-associated cognitive disorders are not specific. Demyelination is seen as T2 hyperintense signal changes, best appreciated on FLAIR images. These changes usually start in the periventricular region and centrum semiovale, and later become more diffuse and confluent. The basal ganglia and thalamus may also be involved. Along with these changes, cerebral atrophy develops, with progressive enlargement of the ventricles and sulcal spaces.

CNS LUPUS

Neuropsychiatric symptoms (ranging from subtle cognitive deficits to seizures, psychosis, and dementia) are potential complications of systemic lupus erythematosus (SLE). A variety of underlying diseases have been suggested.[114] Given the wide array of potential pathologic processes in lupus, the neurologic consequences and imaging finding also vary. Thrombotic ischemic strokes, either caused by small-vessel or large-vessel vasculitis may be seen in the deep as well as subcortical white matter. Libman-Sacks endocarditis may lead to embolic infarcts. CNS lupus may present with small, nonspecific T2 hyperintense white matter lesions, which are difficult to distinguish from MS lesions or other vasculitides. Imaging findings suggestive of lupus include round or patchy lesions in the subcortical white matter regions (**Fig. 24**), often along with cortical and deep gray matter lesions. Linear periventricular lesions or corpus callosum involvement are atypical of CNS SLE and should suggest MS. Acute and subacute lesions may enhance with gadolinium in both diseases. Cortical atrophy and parenchymal calcifications are other possible findings in long-standing lupus. However, structural imaging studies in lupus may also be unremarkable; MRI has been found to be abnormal in only 50% of patients.[115,116] In these instances, advanced imaging techniques may be of value. SPECT often reveals multifocal areas of frontal and parietal hypoperfusion. Dual imaging with MRI and SPECT was found to be more useful than either technique alone.[117] In 1 series, 70% of patients with neuropsychiatric lupus had abnormal findings on SPECT scan, mostly parietal hypoperfusion. In patients with abnormal MRI scans, SPECT was also always abnormal.[118]

In a study using PET,[115] 100% of patients with CNS lupus showed hypometabolism in at least 1 cerebral region, whereas MRI was abnormal in only 50% of patients. Most commonly affected was the parieto-occipital region (96%). The technique was believed to be suitable for disease monitoring as well.

With MRS, a consistent finding in CNS lupus has been reduction of the NAA level.[119] Reduced NAA levels were found in all cases of lupus with major neuropsychiatric symptoms, irrespective of these being past or present.[120] In acute-onset neuropsychiatric

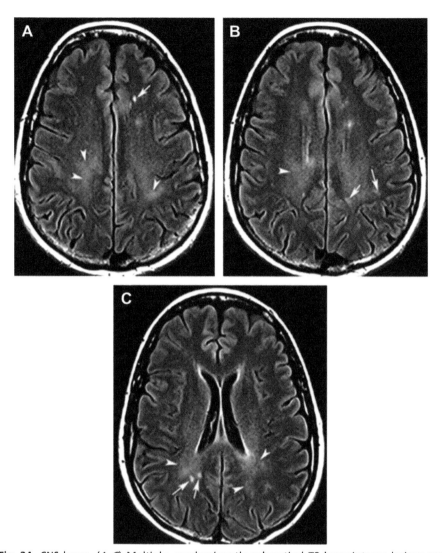

Fig. 24. CNS lupus. (*A–C*) Multiple, predominantly subcortical T2 hyperintense lesions are seen (*arrows*). More faint, confluent T2 hyperintensity is noted in the deeper white matter regions (*arrowheads*).

lupus, the technique is useful for the early detection of metabolic CNS changes and for follow-up after treatment.[121]

NEUROSARCOIDOSIS

About 5% of patients with sarcoidosis develop nervous system complications, including dementia. The granulomatous inflammation may affect the parenchyma, the cranial nerves, and the parenchymal and meningeal (pial) vasculature. In the parenchyma, T2 hyperintense lesions may be present, which are sometimes difficult to distinguish from those of MS or microvascular ischemia. Sometimes, edema

(**Fig. 25**A, B) and larger enhancing lesions are noted, which may be mistaken for metastases. Other characteristically involved structures include the pituitary infundibulum and the hypothalamus. With gadolinium, leptomeningeal enhancement is noted along the penetrating blood vessels, caused by perivascular spreading of the granulomatous process (see **Fig. 25**C, D). The pituitary infundibulum, hypothalamus, and cranial nerves may also show enhancement. Neurosarcoidosis may also lead to cognitive deficits by causing hydrocephalus, either as a result of interference with CSF absorption or obstruction of the ventricular system.

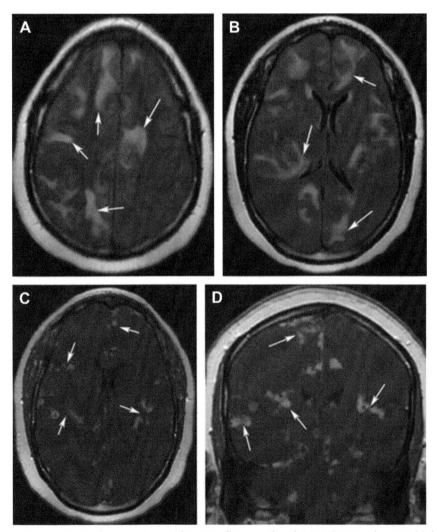

Fig. 25. Neurosarcoidosis. Patient with severe flare-up. (*A, B*) FLAIR images show multiple, confluent T2 hyperintense subcortical and deep white matter lesions (*arrows*). (*C, D*) T1-weighted postcontrast images show partially nodular leptomeningeal enhancement, along the penetrating pial vessels, consistent with an aggressive granulomatous process (*arrows*).

VASCULAR DEMENTIA/VASCULAR COGNITIVE IMPAIRMENT

Formerly known as vascular dementia (VaD), vascular cognitive impairment (VCI) encompasses the spectrum of cognitive syndromes secondary to vascular disease, including MCI and dementia. Superficially, the concept of VCI/VaD seems straightforward (ie, dementia or other cognitive impairment caused by vascular disease). However, in practice, it is often a challenging diagnostic construct, unless there is a clear temporal association with an infarct and cognitive decline. For example, there are numerous diagnostic criteria for VaD.[122] In addition, VaD may occur in conjunction with any number of degenerative dementias; in these situations the term mixed dementia is used. As is reviewed later, there are also a variety of forms of cerebrovascular disease, which can coexist or occur in isolation. Regardless of the diagnostic criteria used, VaD is common in the West, accounting for an estimated 13% to 19% of all cases of dementia.[123] Like AD, VaD is strongly age dependent, with a prevalence of 0.3% in the 65-year to 69-year range, and 5.2% in individuals older than 90 years.[124] MRI is clearly the preferred imaging modality in the assessment of VaD, with greater sensitivity than CT for multiple cerebrovascular diseases, including white matter ischemia and microhemorrhage.

Large-Vessel Disease

Multi-infarct dementia (MID) refers to dementia secondary to multiple large-vessel infarcts (**Fig. 26**), although single, strategically located infarctions can also result in dementia. Dementia more commonly occurs with dominant-hemisphere large-vessel infarcts (such as those involving middle cerebral artery territories) or with bilateral strokes involving the thalami or anterior cerebral artery territories.[125] There is usually significant cortical involvement in MID, in particular of the frontal, temporal, or parietal lobe association cortices. Dementia entirely caused by large-vessel infarction (in the absence of small-vessel disease or AD pathology) seems to be uncommon.[124]

Small-Vessel Disease

There are a variety of pathophysiologic processes that can result in dementia caused by small-vessel disease (**Fig. 27**), including multiple lacunar infarcts, one or more strategically located lacunes, and white matter disease (also referred to as leukoariosis, subcortical arteriosclerotic leukoencephalopathy, Binswanger disease,[126] and so forth). Anatomic regions particularly prone to small-vessel disease include not only the supratentorial subcortical white matter but also the brainstem and

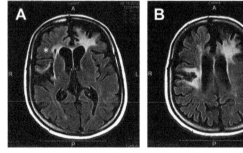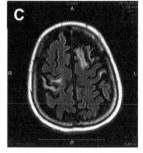

Fig. 26. MID. (*A–C*) Axial FLAIR images showing bilateral cortical/subcortical infarctions, a right frontal lacunar infarct (*asterisk*), and chronic white matter ischemia.

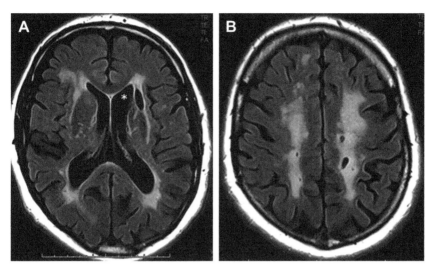

Fig. 27. Patient with dementia and extensive small-vessel ischemic disease. (*A, B*) Axial FLAIR images show lacunar infarctions and confluent white matter changes consistent with chronic microvascular ischemia. Note the mild ex vacuo dilation of the frontal horn of the left lateral ventricle (*asterisk*).

subcortical gray matter structures. Although dementia is well known to occur with fairly extensive small-vessel disease, a recent case series[127] reported multiple thalamic regions associated with dementia caused by single, strategic infarctions, presumably through disruption of the frontal-basal ganglia-thalamus network(s). The white matter changes associated with small-vessel ischemia are most commonly periventricular or subcortical isolated lesions, but with more extensive disease, they can become confluent. Standardized criteria exist to quantify the extent of white matter disease (**Fig. 28**).[128,129]

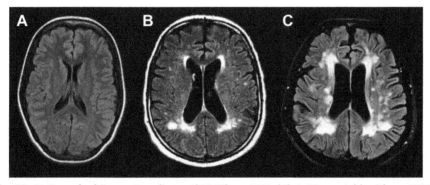

Fig. 28. Rating of white matter disease (WMD) on MRI. (*A*) A 21-year-old with no WMD (Fazekas and Wahlund scores of 0), (*B*) A 51-year-old with moderate WMD (Fazekas score of 2, Wahlund score of 8), (*C*) A 69-year-old with severe WMD (Fazekas score of 3, Wahlund score of 20). (*From* Leonards C, Ipsen N, Malzahn U, et al. White matter lesion severity in mild acute ischemic stroke patients and functional outcome after 1 year. Stroke 2012;43:3046–51; with permission.)

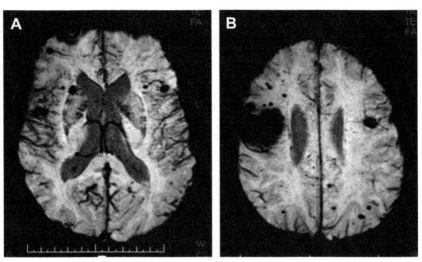

Fig. 29. Cerebral amyloid angiopathy. (*A, B*) Axial SWI show multiple cortical and subcortical hemorrhages.

Other Vascular Diseases

There are several other vascular-spectrum processes that can result in dementia, including hemorrhage (**Fig. 29**), watershed infarcts, hypoxic-ischemic events, and uncommon genetic disorders, such as congenital hypercoagulable states and CADASIL (cerebral autosomal-dominant arteriopathy with subcortical infarcts and leukoencephalopathy) (**Fig. 30**). Additional discussion of imaging of vascular disorders can be found in the article by Nour and Liebeskind elsewhere in this issue.

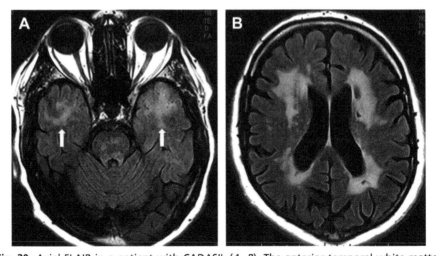

Fig. 30. Axial FLAIR in a patient with CADASIL (*A, B*). The anterior temporal white matter hyperintensities (*arrows*) are suggestive of CADASIL, and are uncommonly seen in other disorders such as MS. Other findings include diffuse leukoariosis and lacunar infarcts. Many patients with CADASIL also show T2 hyperintensities in the basal ganglia and thalamus (*not shown*).

SUMMARY

Significant advances have been made in neuroimaging of dementia over the past decade. MRI, PET, and other imaging technologies often allow for improved visualization of the specific pathophysiologic processes associated with dementia, enabling the clinician to diagnose the various dementing disorders with increased precision and specificity. As disease-modifying agents specific to AD and other disorders become available, amyloid imaging and other novel modalities may become routinely used in clinical practice to assist with diagnosis and monitor response to therapies. However, dementia remains a clinical diagnosis, and even the most advanced imaging techniques should not supersede clinical judgment.

REFERENCES

1. Dementia: a public health priority, World Health Organization 2012. Available at: http://whqlibdoc.who.int/publications/2012/9789241564458_eng.pdf. Accessed March 14, 2013.
2. Alzheimer's Association. 2012 Alzheimer's disease facts and figures. Alzheimers Dement 2012;8(2):131–68.
3. Practice parameter for the diagnosis and management of dementia. Neurology 1994;44:2203–6.
4. Wetmore S, Feighter J, Gass D, et al. Canadian Consensus Conference on Dementia summary of the issues and key recommendations. Can Fam Physician 1999;45:2136–43.
5. Knopman D, DeKosky S, Cummings J, et al. Practice parameter: diagnosis of dementia (an evidence-based review): report of the Quality Standards Subcommittee of the American Academy of Neurology. Neurology 2001;56:1143–54.
6. Waldemar G, Dubois B, Emre M, et al. Recommendations for the diagnosis and management of Alzheimer's disease and other disorders associated with dementia: EFNS guideline. Eur J Neurol 2007;14(1):e1–26.
7. Sorbi S, Hort J, Erkinjuntti T, et al. EFNS-ENS guidelines on the diagnosis and management of disorders associated with dementia. Eur J Neurol 2012;19: 1159–79.
8. Hejl A, Høgh P, Waldemar G. Potentially reversible conditions in 1000 consecutive memory clinic patients. J Neurol Neurosurg Psychiatry 2002;73(4):390–4.
9. Kalkonde Y, Pinto-Patarroyo G, Goldman T, et al. Difference between clinical subspecialties in the outpatient evaluation and treatment of dementia in an academic medical center. Dement Geriatr Cogn Disord 2010;29(1):28–36.
10. Masdeu J, Kreisl W, Berman K. The neurobiology of Alzheimer disease defined by neuroimaging. Curr Opin Neurol 2012;25:410–20.
11. McKhann GM, Knopman DS, Chertkow H, et al. The diagnosis of dementia due to Alzheimer's disease: recommendations from the National Institute on Aging and the Alzheimer's Association workgroup. Alzheimers Dement 2011;7:263–9.
12. Weiner M, Veitch D, Aisen P, et al. The Alzheimer's disease neuroimaging initiative: a review of papers published since its inception. Alzheimers Dement 2012; 8:S1–68.
13. Van de Pol L, Korf E, van der Flier W, et al. Magnetic resonance imaging predictors of cognition in mild cognitive impairment. Arch Neurol 2007;64(7):1023–8.
14. Jack C, Wiste H, Vemuri P, et al. Brain beta-amyloid measures and magnetic resonance imaging atrophy both predict time-to-progression from mild cognitive impairment to Alzheimer's disease. Brain 2010;133:3336–48.

15. Lu P, Thompson P, Leow A. Apolipoprotein E genotype is associated with temporal and hippocampal atrophy rates in healthy elderly adults: a tensor-based morphometry study. J Alzheimers Dis 2011;23(3):433–42.

16. Dickerson B, Stoub T, Shah R, et al. Alzheimer-signature MRI biomarker predicts AD dementia in cognitively normal adults. Neurology 2011;76:1395–402.

17. Dickerson B, Wolk D. MRI cortical thickness biomarker predicts AD-like CSF and cognitive decline in normal adults. Neurology 2012;78:84–90.

18. Nestor S, Rupsingh R, Borrie M, et al. Ventricular enlargement as a possible measure of Alzheimer's disease progression validated using the Alzheimer's disease neuroimaging initiative database. Brain 2008;131:2443–54.

19. Heister D, Brewer J, Madga S, et al. Predicting MCI outcome with clinically available MRI and CSF biomarkers. Neurology 2011;77:1619–28.

20. Sexton C, Kalu U, Filippini N, et al. A meta-analysis of diffusion tensor imaging in mild cognitive impairment and Alzheimer's disease. Neurobiol Aging 2011;32:2322.e5–18.

21. Tighe S, Oishi K, Mori S, et al. Diffusion tensor imaging of neuropsychiatric symptoms in mild cognitive impairment and Alzheimer's dementia. J Neuropsychiatry Clin Neurosci 2012;24(4):484–8.

22. Ota M, Sato N, Nakata Y, et al. Relationship between apathy and diffusion tensor imaging metrics of the brain in Alzheimer's disease. Int J Geriatr Psychiatry 2012;27:722–6.

23. Kantarci K. 1H magnetic resonance spectroscopy in dementia. Br J Radiol 2007;80:S146–52.

24. Berti V, Pupi A, Mosconi L. PET/CT in diagnosis of dementia. Ann N Y Acad Sci 2011;1228:81–92.

25. Klunk W, Engler H, Nordberg A, et al. Imaging brain amyloid in Alzheimer's disease with Pittsburgh compound-B. Ann Neurol 2004;55:306–19.

26. Mosconi L, Berti V, Glodzik L, et al. Pre-clinical detection of Alzheimer's disease using FDG-PET, with or without amyloid imaging. J Alzheimers Dis 2010;20(3):843–54.

27. Yang L, Rieves D, Ganley C. Brain amyloid imaging–FDA approval of florbetapir F18 injection. N Engl J Med 2012;367(10):885–7.

28. Wu L, Rosa-Neto P, Gauthier S. Use of biomarkers in clinical trials of Alzheimer disease. Mol Diagn Ther 2011;15(6):313–25.

29. Tartaglia M. Frontotemporal lobar degeneration: new understanding brings new approaches. Neuroimaging Clin N Am 2012;22:83–97.

30. Gorno-Tempini M, Hillis A, Weintraub S, et al. Classification of primary progressive aphasia and its variants. Neurology 2011;76:1006–14.

31. Kipps C, Davies R, Mitchell J, et al. Clinical significance of lobar atrophy in frontotemporal dementia: application of an MRI visual rating scale. Dement Geriatr Cogn Disord 2007;23:334–42.

32. Suarez J, Tartaglia M, Vitali P, et al. Characterizing radiology reports in patients with frontotemporal dementia. Neurology 2009;73:1073–4.

33. Lehmann M, Douiri A, Kim L, et al. Atrophy patterns in Alzheimer's disease and semantic dementia: a comparison of FreeSurfer and manual volumetric measurements. Neuroimage 2010;49(3):2264–74.

34. Rohrer J, Warren J, Modat M, et al. Patterns of cortical thinning in the language variants of frontotemporal lobar degeneration. Neurology 2009;72(18):1562–9.

35. Whitwell J, Przybelski S, Weigand S, et al. Distinct anatomical subtypes of the behavioural variant of frontotemporal dementia: a cluster analysis study. Brain 2009;132(11):2932–46.

36. Zhang Y, Schuff N, Ching C, et al. Joint assessment of structural, perfusion, and diffusion MRI in Alzheimer's disease and frontotemporal dementia. Int J Alzheimers Dis 2011;2011:546871.

37. Mendez M, Shapira J, McMurtray A, et al. Accuracy of the clinical evaluation for frontotemporal dementia. Arch Neurol 2007;64:830–5.

38. Koedam E, Van der Flier W, Barkhof F, et al. Clinical characteristics of patients with frontotemporal dementia with and without lobar atrophy on MRI. Alzheimer Dis Assoc Disord 2010;24(3):242–7.

39. McKeith I, Mintzer J, Aarsland D, et al. Dementia with Lewy bodies. Lancet Neurol 2004;3:19–28.

40. Hashimoto M, Kitagaki H, Imamura T, et al. Medial temporal and whole-brain atrophy in dementia with Lewy bodies: a volumetric MRI study. Neurology 1998;51:357–62.

41. McKeith IG, Dickson DW, Lowe J, et al. Diagnosis and management of dementia with Lewy bodies: third report of the DLB Consortium. Neurology 2005;65: 1863–72.

42. Albin RL, Minoshima S, D'Amato CJ, et al. Fluoro-deoxyglucose positron emission tomography in diffuse Lewy body disease. Neurology 1996;47:462–6.

43. Lobotesis K, Fenwick JD, Phipps A, et al. Occipital hypoperfusion on SPECT in dementia with Lewy bodies but not AD. Neurology 2001;56:643–9.

44. Varma AR, Talbot PR, Snowden JS, et al. A 99mTc-HMPAO single-photon emission computed tomography study of Lewy body disease. J Neurol 1997;244: 349–59.

45. Pasquier J, Michel BF, Brenot-Rossi I, et al. Value of (99m)Tc-ECD SPET for the diagnosis of dementia with Lewy bodies. Eur J Nucl Med Mol Imaging 2002;29: 1342–8.

46. Ishii K, Imamura T, Sasaki M, et al. Regional cerebral glucose metabolism in dementia with Lewy bodies and Alzheimer's disease. Neurology 1998;51:125–30.

47. Lim SM, Katsifis A, Villemagne VL, et al. The 18F-FDG PET cingulate island sign and comparison to 123I-beta-CIT SPECT for diagnosis of dementia with Lewy bodies. J Nucl Med 2009;50:1638–45.

48. Donnemiller E, Heilmann J, Wenning GK, et al. Brain perfusion scintigraphy with 99mTc-HMPAO or 99mTc-ECD and 123I-beta-CIT single-photon emission tomography in dementia of the Alzheimer-type and diffuse Lewy body disease. Eur J Nucl Med 1997;24:320–5.

49. Ransmayr G, Seppi K, Donnemiller E, et al. Striatal dopamine transporter function in dementia with Lewy bodies and Parkinson's disease. Eur J Nucl Med 2001;28:1523–8.

50. O'Brien JT, Colloby S, Fenwick J, et al. Dopamine transporter loss visualized with FP-CIT SPECT in the differential diagnosis of dementia with Lewy bodies. Arch Neurol 2004;61:919–25.

51. Masaru T, Seiju K, Toshikazu S. Imaging improves diagnosis of dementia with Lewy bodies. Psychiatry Investig 2009;6:233–40.

52. Quattrone A, Nicoletti G, Messina D, et al. MR imaging index for differentiation of progressive supranuclear palsy from Parkinson disease and the Parkinson variant of multiple system atrophy. Radiology 2008;246:214–21.

53. Conn H. Normal pressure hydrocephalus (NPH): more about NPH by a physician who is the patient. Clin Med 2011;11(2):162–5.

54. Kitagaki H, Mori E, Ishii K, et al. CSF spaces in idiopathic normal pressure hydrocephalus: morphology and volumetry. AJNR Am J Neuroradiol 1998;19: 1277–84.

55. Relkin N, Marmarou A, Klinge P, et al. Diagnosing idiopathic normal-pressure hydrocephalus. Neurosurgery 2005;57:S4–16.
56. Meissner B, Kallenberg K, Sanchez-Juan P, et al. MRI lesion profiles in sporadic Creutzfeldt-Jakob disease. Neurology 2009;72:1994–2001.
57. Vitali P, Maccagnano E, Caverzasi E, et al. Diffusion-weighted MRI hyperintensity patterns differentiate CJD from other rapid dementias. Neurology 2011; 76:1711–9.
58. Bahn MM, Kido DK, Lin W, et al. Brain magnetic resonance diffusion abnormalities in Creutzfeldt-Jakob disease. Arch Neurol 1997;54:1411–5.
59. Macfarlane RG, Wroe SJ, Collinge J, et al. Neuroimaging findings in human prion disease. J Neurol Neurosurg Psychiatry 2007;78:664–70.
60. Manners DN, Parchi P, Tonon C, et al. Pathologic correlates of diffusion MRI changes in Creutzfeldt-Jakob disease. Neurology 2009;72:1425–31.
61. Ryutarou U, Tamio K, Takashi K, et al. Serial diffusion-weighted MRI of Creutzfeldt-Jakob disease. AJR Am J Roentgenol 2005;184:560–6.
62. Matoba M, Tonami H, Miyaji H, et al. Creutzfeldt-Jakob disease: serial changes on diffusion-weighted MRI. J Comput Assist Tomogr 2001;25:274–7.
63. Pandya HG, Coley SC, Wilkinson ID, et al. Magnetic resonance spectroscopic abnormalities in sporadic and variant Creutzfeldt-Jakob disease. Clin Radiol 2003;58:148–53.
64. Lodi R, Parchi P, Tonon C, et al. Magnetic resonance diagnostic markers in clinically sporadic prion disease: a combined brain magnetic resonance imaging and spectroscopy study. Brain 2009;132:2669–79.
65. Collie DA, Summers DM, Sellar RJ, et al. Diagnosing variant Creutzfeldt-Jakob disease with the pulvinar sign: MR imaging findings in 86 neuropathologically confirmed cases. AJNR Am J Neuroradiol 2003;24:1560–9.
66. World Health Organization. The revision of the surveillance case definition for variant Creutzfeldt-Jakob disease: report of a WHO Consultation, May 17, 2001, Edinburgh, United Kingdom. World Health Organ Tech Rep Ser. 2004.
67. Cordery RJ, MacManus D, Godbolt A, et al. Short TE quantitative proton magnetic resonance spectroscopy in variant Creutzfeldt-Jakob disease. Eur Radiol 2006;16:1692–8.
68. Engler H, Lundberg PO, Ekbom K, et al. Multitracer study with positron emission tomography in Creutzfeldt-Jakob disease. Eur J Nucl Med Mol Imaging 2003; 30:187.
69. Tsuji Y, Kanamori H, Murakami G, et al. Heidenhain variant of Creutzfeldt-Jakob disease: diffusion-weighted MRI and PET characteristics. J Neuroimaging 2004; 14:63–6.
70. Henkel K, Meller J, Zerr I, et al. Single photon emission computed tomography (SPECT) in 19 patients with Creutzfeldt-Jakob disease. J Neurol 2004;246:490.
71. Lim CC, Tan K, Verma KK, et al. Combined diffusion-weighted and spectroscopic MR imaging in Creutzfeldt-Jakob disease. Magn Reson Imaging 2004; 22:625–9.
72. Hamaguchi T, Kitamoto T, Sato T, et al. Clinical diagnosis of MM2-type sporadic Creutzfeldt-Jakob disease. Neurology 2005;64:643–8.
73. Matsuda M, Tabata K, Hattori T, et al. Brain SPECT with 123I-IMP for the early diagnosis of Creutzfeldt-Jakob disease. J Neurol Sci 2001;183:5–12.
74. Jibiki I, Fukushima T, Kobayashi K, et al. Utility of 123I-IMP SPECT brain scans for the early detection of site-specific abnormalities in Creutzfeldt-Jakob disease (Heidenhain type): a case study. Neuropsychobiology 1994;29:117–9.

75. Chiaravalloti ND, Deluca J. Cognitive impairment in multiple sclerosis. Lancet Neurol 2008;7:1139–51.
76. Achiron A, Barak Y. Cognitive impairment in probable multiple sclerosis. J Neurol Neurosurg Psychiatry 2003;74:443–6.
77. Rao SM, Leo GJ, Haughton VM, et al. Correlation of magnetic resonance imaging with neuropsychological testing in multiple sclerosis. Neurology 1989;39: 161–6.
78. Fultona JC, Grossmana RI, Udupaa J, et al. MR lesion load and cognitive function in patients with relapsing-remitting multiple sclerosis. AJNR Am J Neuroradiol 1999;20:1951–5.
79. Sperling RA, Guttmann CR, Hohol MJ, et al. Regional magnetic resonance imaging lesion burden and cognitive function in multiple sclerosis a longitudinal study. Arch Neurol 2001;58:115–21.
80. Rossi F, Giorgio A, Battaglini M, et al. Relevance of brain lesion location to cognition in relapsing multiple sclerosis. PLoS One 2012;7:e44826.
81. Llufriu S, Blanco Y, Martinez-Heras E, et al. Influence of corpus callosum damage on cognition and physical disability in multiple sclerosis: a multimodal study. PLoS One 2012;7:e37167.
82. Mesaros S, Rocca MA, Kacar K, et al. Diffusion tensor MRI tractography and cognitive impairment in multiple sclerosis. Neurology 2012;78:969–75.
83. Arnett PA, Rao SM, Bernardin L, et al. Relationship between frontal lobe lesions and Wisconsin Card Sorting Test performance in patients with multiple sclerosis. Neurology 1994;44:420–5.
84. Foong J, Rozewicz L, Quaghebeur G, et al. Executive function in multiple sclerosis. The role of frontal lobe pathology. Brain 1997;120:15–26.
85. Kutzelnigg A, Lucchinetti CF, Stadelmann C, et al. Cortical demyelination and diffuse white matter injury in multiple sclerosis. Brain 2005;128:2705–12.
86. Geurts JJ, Barkhof F. Grey matter pathology in multiple sclerosis. Lancet Neurol 2008;7:841–51.
87. Zivadinov R, Minagar A. Evidence for gray matter pathology in multiple sclerosis: a neuroimaging approach. J Neurol Sci 2009;282:1–4.
88. Filippia M, Roccaa MA. MR imaging of gray matter involvement in multiple sclerosis: implications for understanding disease pathophysiology and monitoring treatment efficacy. AJNR Am J Neuroradiol 2010;31:1171–7.
89. Bakshi R, Ariyaratana S, Benedict RH, et al. Fluid-attenuated inversion recovery magnetic resonance imaging detects cortical and juxtacortical multiple sclerosis lesions. Arch Neurol 2001;58:742–8.
90. Geurts JJ, Pouwels PJ, Uitdehaag BM, et al. Intracortical lesions in multiple sclerosis: improved detection with 3D double inversion-recovery MR imaging. Radiology 2005;236:254–60.
91. Calabrese M, De Stefano N, Atzori M, et al. Detection of cortical inflammatory lesions by double inversion recovery magnetic resonance imaging in patients with multiple sclerosis. Arch Neurol 2007;64:1416–22.
92. Ranjeva JP, Audoin B, Au Duong MV, et al. Local tissue damage assessed with statistical mapping analysis of brain magnetization transfer ratio: relationship with functional status of patients in the earliest stage of multiple sclerosis. AJNR Am J Neuroradiol 2005;26:119–27.
93. Amato MP, Portaccio E, Stromillo ML, et al. Cognitive assessment and quantitative magnetic resonance metrics can help to identify benign multiple sclerosis. Neurology 2008;71:632–8.

94. Rovaris M, Iannucci G, Falautano M, et al. Cognitive dysfunction in patients with mildly disabling relapsing-remitting multiple sclerosis: an exploratory study with diffusion tensor MR imaging. J Neurol Sci 2002;195:103–9.

95. Allen IV. Pathology of multiple sclerosis. In: Matthews WB, Compston A, Allen IV, et al, editors. McAlpine's multiple sclerosis. 2nd edition. Edinburgh (United Kingdom): Churchill Livingstone; 1991. p. 341–78.

96. Allen IV, McQuaid S, Mirakhur M, et al. Pathological abnormalities in the normal-appearing white matter in multiple sclerosis. Neurol Sci 2001;22:141–4.

97. Summers M, Swanton J, Fernando K, et al. Cognitive impairment in multiple sclerosis can be predicted by imaging early in the disease. J Neurol Neurosurg Psychiatry 2008;79:955–88.

98. Moll NM, Rietsch AM, Thomas S, et al. Multiple sclerosis normal-appearing white matter: pathology-imaging correlations. Ann Neurol 2011;70:764–73.

99. Cox D, Pelletier D, Genain C, et al. The unique impact of changes in normal appearing brain tissue on cognitive dysfunction in secondary progressive multiple sclerosis patients. Mult Scler 2004;10:626–9.

100. Filippi M, Tortorella C, Rovaris M, et al. Changes in the normal appearing brain tissue and cognitive impairment in multiple sclerosis. J Neurol Neurosurg Psychiatry 2000;68:157–61.

101. Zivadinov R, De Masi R, Nasuelli D, et al. MRI techniques and cognitive impairment in the early phase of relapsing-remitting multiple sclerosis. Neuroradiology 2001;43:272–8.

102. Akbar N, Lobaugh NJ, O'Connor P, et al. Diffusion tensor imaging abnormalities in cognitively impaired MS patients. Can J Neurol Sci 2010;37:608–14.

103. Mathiesen HK, Jonsson A, Tscherning T, et al. Correlation of global N-acetyl aspartate with cognitive impairment in multiple sclerosis. Arch Neurol 2006; 63:533–6.

104. Staffen W, Zauner H, Mair A, et al. Magnetic resonance spectroscopy of memory and frontal brain region in early multiple sclerosis. J Neuropsychiatry Clin Neurosci 2005;17:357–63.

105. Huber SJ, Paulson GW, Shuttleworth EC, et al. Magnetic resonance imaging correlates of dementia in multiple sclerosis. Arch Neurol 1987;44:732–6.

106. Huber SJ, Bornstein RA, Rammohan KW, et al. Magnetic resonance imaging correlates of neuropsychological impairment in multiple sclerosis. J Neuropsychiatry Clin Neurosci 1992;4:152–8.

107. Pozzilli C, Passafiume D, Anzini A, et al. Cognitive and brain imaging measures of multiple sclerosis. Ital J Neurol Sci 1992;13:133–6.

108. Tsolaki M, Drevelegas A, Karachristianou S, et al. Correlation of dementia, neuropsychological and MRI findings in multiple sclerosis. Dementia 1994;5:48–52.

109. Benedict RH, Bruce JM, Dwyer MG, et al. Neocortical atrophy, third ventricular width, and cognitive dysfunction in multiple sclerosis. Arch Neurol 2006;63: 1301–6.

110. Houtchens MK, Benedict RH, Killiany R, et al. Thalamic atrophy and cognition in multiple sclerosis. Neurology 2007;69:1213–23.

111. Benedict RH, Ramasamy D, Munschauer F, et al. Memory impairment in multiple sclerosis: correlation with deep grey matter and mesial temporal atrophy. J Neurol Neurosurg Psychiatry 2009;80:201–6.

112. Tekok-Kilic A, Benedict RH, Weinstock-Guttman B, et al. Independent contributions of cortical gray matter atrophy and ventricle enlargement for predicting neuropsychological impairment in multiple sclerosis. Neuroimage 2007;36: 1294–300.

113. da Pozzo S, Manara R, Tonello S, et al. Conventional and diffusion-weighted MRI in progressive multifocal leukoencephalopathy: new elements for identification and follow-up. Radiol Med 2006;111:971-7.

114. Vadacca M, Buzzulini F, Rigon A, et al. Neuropsychiatric lupus erythematosus. Reumatismo 2006;58:177-86.

115. Weiner SM, Otte A, Schumacher M, et al. Diagnosis and monitoring of central nervous system involvement in systemic lupus erythematosus: value of F-18 fluorodeoxyglucose PET. Ann Rheum Dis 2000;59:377-85.

116. Handa R, Sahota P, Kumar M, et al. In vivo proton magnetic resonance spectroscopy (MRS) and single photon emission computerized tomography (SPECT) in systemic lupus erythematosus (SLE). Magn Reson Imaging 2003;21:1033-7.

117. Castellino G, Padovan M, Bortoluzzi A, et al. Single photon emission computed tomography and magnetic resonance imaging evaluation in SLE patients with and without neuropsychiatric involvement. Rheumatology 2008;47:319-23.

118. Chen JJ, Yen RF, Kao A, et al. Abnormal regional cerebral blood flow found by technetium-99m ethyl cysteinate dimer brain single photon emission computed tomography in systemic lupus erythematosus patients with normal brain MRI findings. Clin Rheumatol 2002;21:516-9.

119. Peterson PL, Axford JS, Isenberg D. Imaging in CNS lupus. Best Pract Res Clin Rheumatol 2005;19:727-39.

120. Sibbitt WL Jr, Haseler LJ, Griffey RR, et al. Neurometabolism of active neuropsychiatric lupus determined with proton MR spectroscopy. AJNR Am J Neuroradiol 1997;18:1271-7.

121. Sundgren PC, Jennings J, Attwood JT, et al. MRI and 2D-CSI MR spectroscopy of the brain in the evaluation of patients with acute onset of neuropsychiatric systemic lupus erythematosus. Neuroradiology 2005;47:576-85.

122. Pohjasvaara T, Mäntylä R, Ylikoski R, et al. Comparison of different clinical criteria (DSM-III, ADDTC, ICD-10, NINDS-AIREN, DSM-IV) for the diagnosis of vascular dementia. National Institute of Neurological Disorders and Stroke-Association Internationale pour la Recherche et l'Enseignement en Neurosciences. Stroke 2000;31(12):2952-7.

123. Bowler J. Modern concept of vascular cognitive impairment. Br Med Bull 2007; 83:291-305.

124. Jellinger K. Morphologic diagnosis of "vascular dementia"–a critical update. J Neurol Sci 2008;270:1-12.

125. Guermazi A, Miaux Y, Rovira-Cañellas A, et al. Neuroradiological findings in vascular dementia. Neuroradiology 2007;49:1-22.

126. Román G. Senile dementia of the Binswanger type. JAMA 1987;258(13):1782-8.

127. Lanna M, Alves C, Sudo F, et al. Cognitive disconnective syndrome by single strategic strokes in vascular dementia. J Neurol Sci 2012;322(1-2):176-83.

128. Fazekas F, Chawluk J, Alavi A, et al. MR signal abnormalities at 1.5 T in Alzheimer's dementia and normal aging. AJNR Am J Neuroradiol 1987;149:351-6.

129. Wahlund L, Barkof F, Fazekas F, et al. A new rating scale for age-related white matter changes applicable to MRI and CT. Stroke 2001;32:1318-22.

Imaging of Chiari Type I Malformation and Syringohydromyelia

Jennifer W. McVige, MD[a],*, Jody Leonardo, MD[b,c]

KEYWORDS

- Chiari malformation • Syringohydromyelia • Syrinx • Headaches • Neuroimaging

KEY POINTS

- Chiari malformations are anatomic anomalies that comprise a broad spectrum of neurologic conditions.
- The most common malformation, a Chiari type I malformation (CMI), can present with a variety of signs and symptoms, most frequently an occipital Valsalva-induced headache.
- Cranial and spinal magnetic resonance (MR) imaging is used to identify the degree of tonsillar descent and document the presence of syringohydromyelia.
- Furthermore, this imaging serves as a baseline study that can be used for future comparison, particularly after a surgical procedure.
- The advent of cine-MR flow imaging (cine as in "cinema") has provided new insight as to the dynamic process involved in the evolution of this pathophysiology.
- It has also proved to be a useful tool to identify potential surgical candidates and evaluate postoperative progress.

Learning Objectives

1. Review the pathophysiology of Chiari malformations (CM) and syringohydromyelia (SH).

2. Recognize clinical signs and symptoms associated with CM and SH.

3. Radiographically define CM, SH, and associated pathologic condition.

4. Briefly discuss the medical and surgical treatments of CM and SH.

5. Understand the use of neuroimaging in preoperative and postoperative analysis of CM and SH.

Financial Relationships/Potential Conflicts of Interest: Nil.
[a] Pediatric Neurology, Adult and Pediatric headache, and Neuroimaging, Dent Concussion Center, Dent Neurologic Institute, 3980 Sheridan Drive, Amherst, NY 14226, USA; [b] School of Medicine and Biomedical Sciences, University at Buffalo, State University of New York, Buffalo, NY, USA; [c] University at Buffalo Neurosurgery, 3980A Sheridan Drive, Buffalo, NY, USA
* Corresponding author.
E-mail address: jmcvige@dentinstitute.com

INTRODUCTION

The general term "Chiari malformation" (CM) refers to caudal displacement of the cerebellar tonsils through the foramen magnum; however, this is a heterogeneous disorder with varying degrees of pathology associated with a broad spectrum of signs and symptoms. The most common presentation is CMI; therefore, this is the primary focus of this article. The anatomy and pathophysiology of CMI and syringo-hydromyelia (SH), as well as the clinical signs and symptoms associated with these disorders, are presented. Radiological classification and diagnostic criteria of CMs and SH are reviewed. Finally, medical treatment and indications for surgery are also discussed.

BRIEF HISTORY

The diagnosis and treatment of CMI has been a topic of great debate in the literature since Austrian pathologist Hans Chiari (1851–1916) first discussed the disease at the end of the nineteenth century. Recent advances in neuroimaging and neurosurgery have provided new knowledge regarding the underlying pathophysiology, but the topic remains controversial because of the poor correlation between traditional neuro-imaging modalities and clinical presentations.

The first case presented in Hans Chiari's initial work in 1891 described a 17-year-old girl who died of typhoid fever. She was found on autopsy to have "elon-gation of the [cerebellar] tonsils and medial divisions of the inferior lobules of the cerebellum into cone-shaped projections which accompany the medulla oblon-gata into the spinal canal." Chiari initially believed that herniation of the cerebellar tonsils was caused by chronic hydrocephalus.[1] This condition later became known as CMI.

Chiari subsequently described different but related conditions later termed Chiari types II (CMII) and III (CMIII). In further papers, he determined that the degree of hydro-cephalus did not always correlate with the amount of cerebellar and spinal pathology. He hypothesized that poor growth of the bone in the posterior occipital region contrib-uted to the likelihood of hindbrain herniation.[2] He cited both Cleland and Arnold in an 1896 publication discussing CMII.[2] Cleland[3] in 1883 had reported a case of an infant with hydrocephalus and spina bifida, and Arnold,[4] in 1894, a case of an infant with spina bifida and elongation of the cerebellar tonsils. Later, a series of cases of CMII malformations was reported by students of Arnold who referred to this as an "Arnold-Chiari malformation."[5] There was a great deal of confusion regarding the nomenclature, so, in 1971, Dreisen and Schmidt[6] proposed using only the term "Chiari malformation" to describe the type II presentation, which is currently the accepted terminology.

CLASSIFICATION

Diagnostic MR imaging criteria for CMI and CMI variants have been redefined by both age and associated pathology (**Box 1**, **Fig. 1**, **Table 1**). The presentation and severity of symptoms can change with age and time.[7] The measure of the cerebellar tonsils in normal individuals has been observed to decrease with age as measured on MR imaging by Mikulis and colleagues.[8] The measure can also increase with related intracranial pathologic changes such as hydrocephalus, mass lesion, and hypotension.

Imaging criteria for Chiari types II–IV are provided in **Box 1**, and representative images are shown in **Fig. 2**.

Box 1
Diagnostic MRI characteristics for Chiari type I/variants and Chiari types II-IV

Chiari 0: The cerebellar tonsils do not descend greater than 3 mm below the basion-opistion line on sagittal images. Syringohydromyelia is present. There can be crowding of the foramen magnum with caudal displacement of the obex and a slight tilt of the pons and medulla.

Chiari I: The fourth ventricle remains in normal position. Syringomyelia (or syringohydromyelia) is present in 30% to 70% of cases. The degree of cerebellar tonsillar extension below the basion-opistion line on sagittal MR images defines the type of pathology.

- Less than 3 mm below the line is considered normal and can be referred to as "ectopia."

- About 3–5 mm below the line is considered to be "borderline Chiari type I malformation" and can be abnormal if there are co-occurring pathologies (e.g., syringohydromyelia) or symptoms.

- Greater than 5 mm below the line is considered pathologic in individuals older than 15 years.

- Greater than 6 mm is considered pathologic in individuals younger than 15 years.

Chiari I.5: Caudal displacement of the cerebellar tonsils with herniation. Caudal displacement of the brain stem and fourth ventricle. Bulbocervical kinking without spina bifida.

Chiari II: Herniation of the cerebellar vermis into the upper cervical canal. Almost always associated with myelomeningocele, usually lumbar. Elongation of the pons, medulla, and fourth ventricle. Cervicomedullary kinking (in 70% of cases), syringohydromyelia (in 50%), and hydrocephalus in most. Agenesis or hypogenesis of the corpus callosum (in 70%–90%). Other possible associations include stenogyria, lacunar skull, tectal beaking, and colpocephaly.

Chiari III: Herniation of the posterior fossa contents through the foramen magnum into the upper cervical canal, often with a high cervical or suboccipital myelocystocele or encephalocele with features of Chiari II. Cervicomedullary kinking. Tectal beaking.

Chiari IV: Primary cerebellar agenesis or hypoplasia. Cerebellar remnants present, without cerebellar herniation. No myelomeningocele. Normal sized or small brain stem.

Data from Refs.[7,9–11]

SH is a longitudinally oriented cerebrospinal fluid (CSF)-filled cavity with associated gliosis in the spinal cord (**Fig. 3**).[9] The terminology used when reviewing the MR images defines the location of the syrinx (i.e., the fluid-filled cavity or cyst) within the cord (**Box 2**). Milhorat and colleagues[12] in 1995 described different types of SH based on the histopathology, which depicted the location and presence or absence of communication.

PATHOPHYSIOLOGY

The cause of CM is multifactorial. The essence of the pathology involves the cerebellum and how it relates to the compartment in which it is contained, the posterior fossa. There are primary genetic and physiologic causes, as well as secondary acquired developments due to physiologic change, such as SH. The pathologies seen in the CM spectrum have been attributed to many causes (**Box 3**). When reviewing the theories, it becomes apparent that one theory cannot adequately account for all the associated findings within the Chiari spectrum.

In some individuals, a genetic predisposition is associated with secondary developmental physiologic changes either in utero or postnatally. However, many presentations are thought to occur de novo. "A polygenic model of inheritance seems plausible in a majority of CMI cases."[13] In many syndromes associated with CM, it

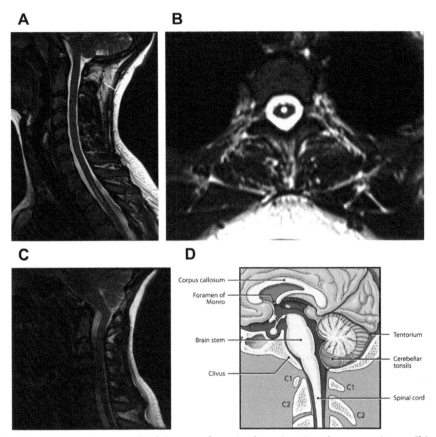

Fig. 1. Magnetic resonance (MR) image of cervicothoracic spine demonstrating a Chiari 0 malformation. (*A*) Sagittal T2 images revealing thoracic syringohydromyelia (SH) without evidence of cerebellar tonsillar descent. (*B*) Axial T2 image showing thoracic SH at T2-3. (*C*) Sagittal T2 MR image demonstrating a Chiari I.5 malformation with tonsillar herniation with cervicomedullary kinking. (*D*) Drawing of normal anatomy, for comparison. ([*C*] *From* Tubbs RS, Iskandar BJ, Bartolucci AA, et al. A critical analysis of the Chiari 1.5 malformation. J Neurosurg 2004;101:181; with permission.)

Table 1
Diagnostic quick reference for Chiari type I malformation and variants

Definition	Measurement of Tonsillar Descent Below the Basion-Opistion Line on MR Sagittal Images
Cerebellar tonsillar ectopia (considered normal)	<3 mm
Chiari 0	<3 mm with syringomyelia or syringohydromyelia
Borderline Chiari I	3–5 mm
Chiari I (>15 y)	>5 mm
Chiari I (<15 y)	>6 mm

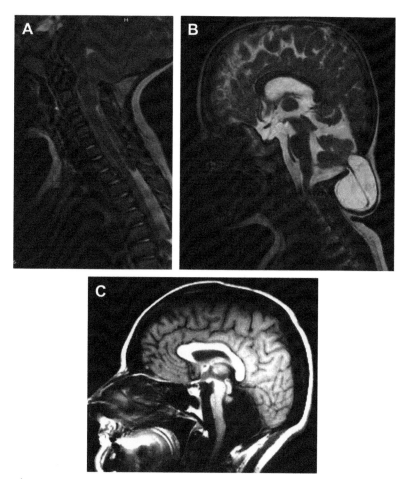

Fig. 2. Chiari types II–IV malformations. (*A*) Chiari II. Sagittal T2 MR image of cervical spine. Notice the cerebellar vermian and medullary descent along with cervicomedullary kinking. (*B*) Chiari III. Sagittal T2 MR image showing an occipital encephalocele. (*C*) Chiari IV. Sagittal T1 MR image showing cerebellar hypoplasia with cerebellar remnant and small brain stem. ([*B*] *Courtesy of* Dr Paresh K Desai. Available at: http://radiopaedia.org/cases/chiari-type-iii-malformation-1. Accessed March 23, 2013, with permission; and [*C*] *From* Hadley DM. The Chiari malformations. J Neurol Neurosurg Psychiatry 2002;72(Suppl 2):ii38–40, with permission.)

is difficult to tell whether the CM is a primary congenital presentation or secondary to acquired morphologic changes associated with the syndrome. Examples of associated syndromes are displayed in **Box 4** and **Figs. 4** and **5**. It is essential for a neuroimager to look for features seen with associated syndromes for proper diagnosis.

Hydrodynamic theories regarding abnormal CSF pressures in CM deserve special attention, given the relationship to SH formation. Gardner[14] in 1965 was the first to hypothesize that the fourth ventricle and central canal communicate because of failure of the fourth ventricle foramen to open in utero. Forces from CSF pulsations create a "water-hammer" effect, forming the syrinx. In the 1970s, Williams[15] elaborated on this theory, hypothesizing that intrathoracic pressure, such as a cough, creates a

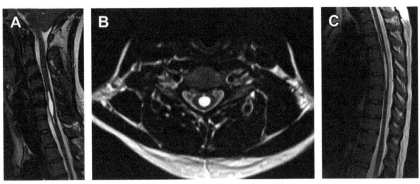

Fig. 3. MR images showing syringohydromyelia. (*A*) Cervical MR T2 sagittal image. (*B*) Cervical MR T2 axial image. (*C*) Thoracic MR T2 sagittal image.

cranial-spinal pressure gradient causing CSF to get "sucked" into the central canal of the cord. Still other theories at that time suggested that CSF enters the canal via perivascular spaces (Ball and Dayan[16]) or that cord production of CSF and stenosis contributed (Aboulker[17]). The most recent theory (1999) comes from Heiss and colleagues,[18] who demonstrated intraoperatively that the cerebellar tonsils act like a piston occluding the subarachnoid space, moving with the heart beat. The cerebellar tonsils descend in systole and ascend in diastole. This finding has been reproduced outside of the operating room with cine-MR imaging studies.[19]

CLINICAL PRESENTATION

The prevalence of CMI has been reported to range from 0.56% to 1.0%.[20–22] CMI usually presents in adults and older children. The clinical presentation is not always

---

Box 2
Syrinx definitions and types

Definitions

  Hydromyelia: A dilated central canal

  Syringomyelia: Cavitation of the cord extending laterally or independent of the central canal

  Syringohydromyelia: Involves both hydromyelia and syringomyelia

  Syringobulbia: Extends to medulla

Types

  Type 1: Dilated central canal communicates with fourth ventricle (associated with hydrocephalus)

  Type 2: Dilation of central canal below syrinx free segment (associated with Chiari and arachnoiditis)

  Type 3: Extracanalicular cysts arise in cord parenchyma, but the syrinx does not communicate with canal. Located in watershed areas (associated with trauma, infarct, and transverse myelitis)

Data from Barkovich AJ. Pediatric neuroimaging. 4th edition. Philadelphia: Lippincott; 2005. p. 932.

Box 3
Pathophysiology theories

- Hypoplasia of the occipital bones
- Premature fusion of the skull bones (craniosynostosis)
- Dysgenesis of the cerebellum, brainstem, and spinal cord
- Dysregulation of craniospinal pressures
- Intracranial hypertension
- Intracranial hypotension
- Genetic causes (chromosomes 9 and 15, paired box-containing genes [Pax genes], fibroblast growth factor receptor 2)

---

correlated with the degree of cerebellar tonsillar ectopia.[20,21] Frequently, cases of CMI are diagnosed incidentally on MR imaging, after a head injury, accident, and infection or during pregnancy.[7] In 2011, Massimi and colleagues[7] mentioned that there is a high frequency of a temporal association between minor head injury and CMI symptom onset.

CMI symptoms and signs are widely varied (**Boxes 5** and **6**). One of the most frequent symptoms in CMI is headache. This headache is of a specific type, presenting as a paroxysmal escalation of sharp or throbbing pain during cough, Valsalva maneuvers, or physical exertion.[23] The pain is localized to the posterior occipital or upper cervical area and is usually not associated with radicular signs in the upper extremities.

SH is associated with CMI in 30% to 70% of cases.[24] It is commonly seen in adolescents and early adulthood. It can be associated with specific clinical symptoms and signs that may wax and wane (**Box 7**). Scoliosis is a common sign observed in patients with CMI with SH.

Box 4
Syndromes associated with Chiari malformation

- Craniosynostosis syndromes (Apert, Crouzon, and Pfeiffer)
- Osteopathic syndromes (Paget disease, acromegaly, achondroplasia, osteopetrosis, and rickets)
- Connective tissues disorders (Ehlers-Danlos syndrome, Marfan syndrome, and Shprintzen-Goldberg syndrome)
- Vertebral anomalies (Klippel-Feil anomaly (see **Fig. 4**), PHACE (see **Fig. 5**), VACTERL)
- Craniofacial anomalies (Pierre-Robin syndrome, Goldenhar syndrome)
- Williams syndrome
- Noonan syndrome
- Neurofibromatosis

Abbreviations: PHACE, posterior fossa, hemangioma, arterial lesions, cardiac anomalies, eye abnormalities; VACTERL, vertebral, anal, cardiac tracheoesophageal fistula, renal limb.

Data from Massimi L, Novegno F, di Rocco C. Chiari type I malformation in children. Adv Tech Stand Neurosurg 2011;37:143–211.

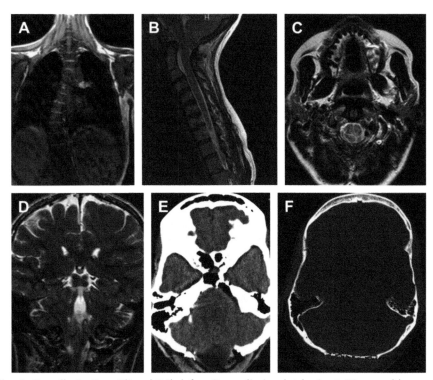

Fig. 4. Case illustration: Klippel-Feil deformity, scoliosis, platybasia. A 32-year-old woman developed cervicothoracic pain and progressive occipital headaches after a motor vehicle accident. On examination, she was found to have a hyperreflexive patellar response (+4) with multiple beats of clonus in both lower extremities with inability to tandem gait. She underwent a suboccipital craniectomy, C1 laminectomy, tonsillar exploration and fenestration of adhesions, bovine pericardial dural patch graft placement, and partial cranioplasty. (*A*) Thoracic coronal MR images showing right scoliotic curvature. Cervical preoperative MR images: (*B*) Sagittal T2 depicting CMI, platybasia, and Klippel-Feil deformity showing fusion of C2-C3, and (*C*) Axial T2 at the level of C1 showing crowding of tonsils. (*D*) Preoperative coronal T2 MR image of brain showing tonsillar descent caudal to foramen magnum. Postoperative CT scan: (*E*) Axial soft tissue windows demonstrating new retrocerebellar space with dural patch graft and (*F*) Axial bone windows depicting postoperative partial cranioplasty (Stryker cranial plate) at rostral level of decompression.

DIAGNOSTIC NEUROIMAGING

Diagnostic neuroimaging has been an essential tool in elucidating the pathophysiology and treatment of CMI. The advent of MR imaging transformed the way this controversial disorder is diagnosed and managed. The newer dynamic neuroimaging cine-MR imaging flow studies have furthered the understanding of CSF flow and pressure gradients, thus creating an in vivo way of measuring normal and abnormal physiologic processes and allowing more refined treatment protocols.

The first radiographic studies published regarding CM used computed tomographic (CT) myelography[25] in an attempt to differentiate and measure the severity of this anatomic anomaly.[26] It was initially hypothesized that evaluating these studies for severity could help dictate treatment strategies. This hypothesis was later proved to

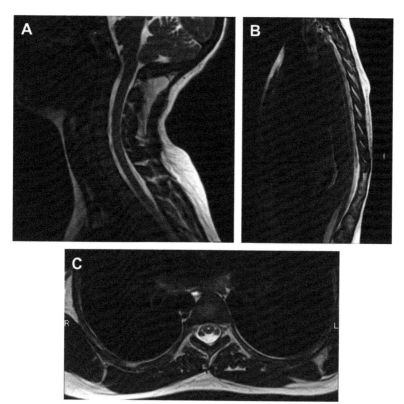

Fig. 5. Case illustration: PHACE (posterior fossa, hemangioma, arterial lesions, cardiac anomalies, eye abnormalities) syndrome. This patient is a 21-year-old woman with a past medical history of tetralogy of Fallot status-post repair, hemangioma involving the trigeminal division of the V3 dermatome, cerebral palsy with hypotonia, and mild mental retardation. The patient complained of headaches, back pain, and paresthesias. (*A*) Sagittal T2 MR image of cervical spine with crowded posterior fossa without caudal cerebellar tonsillar herniation. (*B*) Sagittal T2 MR image of thoracic spine demonstrating fusion of the T9-11 vertebral bodies. (*C*) Axial T2 MR image of thoracic spine showing syringohydromyelia.

be incorrect.[21] After much scientific debate in the 1980s and 1990s, a measurement protocol defining the type of CM was agreed upon (see **Box 1** and **Table 1**). The anatomic measurement landmarks were taken from the historic paper by Baker in 1963,[26] recommending that a line be drawn from the tip of the clivus to the base of the foramen magnum on sagittal MR imaging of the brain (**Fig. 6**). A second line is then drawn from the middle of the cerebellar tonsils where they meet line 1, inferiorly at the lowest point of the tonsil. The same method is used with coronal sequences to evaluate for tonsillar asymmetry (**Fig. 7**).

Frequently, a CMI disorder is discovered incidentally on CT or MR imaging of the head or spine. Routine CT scans done for headache symptoms or in children with craniosynostosis should always be reviewed for evidence of cerebellar tonsillar crowding (**Fig. 8**), as this is easily missed. If CM is suspected on CT scan of the head, MR imaging of the brain and spinal axis (cervical, thoracic, and lumbar) should be obtained.[7] When assessing the images, the neuroimager should comment on

---

Box 5
Symptoms associated with Chiari type I malformations

- Headache (typically a suboccipital headache exacerbated by Valsalva maneuvers)
- Neck, back, and/or face pain
- Cape pain (severe pain in neck, upper back, and shoulders)
- Nonradicular limb pain
- Weakness
- Limb dysesthesias or paresthesias
- Double vision
- Tinnitus
- Dizziness
- Vertigo
- Nausea
- Hearing loss
- Disequilibrium
- Slurred speech
- Syncopal episodes
- Facial numbness
- Difficulty swallowing
- Difficulty sleeping
- Urinary incontinence

---

cerebellar tonsillar crowding, anatomic variants, presence/absence of syrinx or hydrocephalus, breach on the integrity of the spinal canal or cord causing myelocele, and the possibility of secondary syndromes or causes. If surgical intervention is being considered, contrast material should be used to exclude the presence of neoplastic processes. If the patient has already undergone surgical intervention, contrast material, use of susceptibility-weighted imaging or gradient-refocused echo, diffusion-weighted imaging, and apparent diffusion coefficient sequences are advised to assess for hemorrhage, infection, or infarct. Standard diagnostic imaging protocols are summarized in **Table 2**.

A small infratentorial to supratentorial space ratio in CMI has been well documented.[27] Patients with a smaller posterior cranial fossa have been observed to present earlier with symptoms and respond better to decompressive surgical intervention.[27] Despite the finding of small posterior fossa, "brain tissue volume remains the same."[7] It is important to evaluate the orientation of the clivus, as this can determine the size of the posterior fossa. Abnormal skull-based flattening, defined as greater than 143° angle when measuring from the anterior cranial fossa to the clivus, is termed platybasia (see **Fig. 4**). Other skeletal abnormalities associated with CMI, such as basilar invagination (upward projection of the odontoid process through the foramen magnum), atlanto-occipital assimilation, Klippel-Feil syndrome (vertebral fusion usually in the upper cervical area C2-3) (see **Fig. 4**), and Sprengel deformity (elevated scapula with Klippel-Feil) should also be recognized.

Box 6
Signs associated with Chiari type I malformations

Cranial nerve dysfunction

- Nystagmus
- Hoarseness
- Dysphagia
- Dysarthria
- Dysphonia
- Palatal weakness
- Tongue atrophy
- Cough
- Stridor
- Sleep apnea (obstructive)
- Abnormal vocal cord movement

Brain stem compression

- Nystagmus (downbeat pattern due to cervicomedullary compression; worsens on lateral gaze)
- Sleep apnea (central)
- Hiccups
- Sensorineural hearing loss
- Sinus bradycardia
- Hypertension
- Sinus tachycardia
- Syncope

Cerebellar

- Truncal ataxia
- Head titubation
- Dysmetria
- Dysdiadokinesia

Spinal cord

- Hyperactive upper and/or lower extremity reflexes
- Babinski reflex
- Hoffman reflex
- Spastic gait
- Clonus
- Urinary incontinence, urgency, and/or frequency
- Hand atrophy
- Upper and/or lower extremity weakness
- Fasciculations

Box 7
Symptoms and signs of syringohydromyelia

- Neck and back pain
- Paresthesias
- Upper and/or lower extremity weakness
- Unsteady or spastic gait
- Scoliosis
- Loss of pain and temperature
- Urinary incontinence, urgency, and/or frequency
- Hyperactive upper and/or lower extremity reflexes
- Babinski reflex
- Hoffman reflex
- Clonus
- Hand atrophy

Secondary causes of CMI must also be excluded, such as neoplasm (especially in the posterior fossa) (**Figs. 9** and **10**), hemorrhage, hydrocephalus, intracranial hypotension (as evidenced by leptomeningeal enhancement on brain MR imaging with contrast), or benign intracranial hypertension (which can be correlated with empty sella turcica in some cases).

Cine-MR imaging flow studies are used as a dynamic measure of the severity of compression in the posterior fossa. Bhadelia and Wolpert[19] in 2000 compared 18 CMI patients with 18 normal control subjects. They found that "foramen magnum obstruction leads to increased systolic spinal cord motion and impaired diastolic spinal cord recoil and diastolic motion." They evaluated multiple levels in the brain and upper spine and found that the abnormal flow in the C2-3 area correlated with SH. They argue that it is essential to look at both axial and sagittal views when obtaining

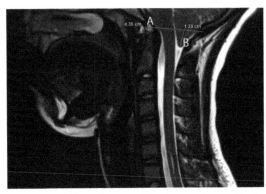

Fig. 6. Sagittal measurements delineating tonsillar descent in a patient with CMI. Foraminal line "A" is drawn from the tip of clivus to the undersurface of the suboccipital bone. Tonsillar line "B" is drawn from the foraminal line to the caudal projection of the tonsils on the midline sagittal view.

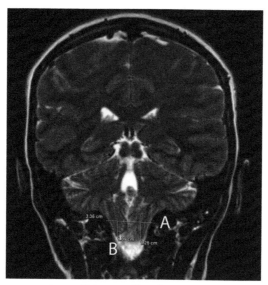

Fig. 7. Coronal measurements specifying tonsillar descent in a patient with CMI. Foraminal line "A" is made across the foramen magnum underneath the occipital bone. Tonsillar lines "B" are measured 90° from the foraminal line to the most caudal projection of tonsillar descent.

cine studies. They observed that, in CMI, CSF flow is increased in the anterolateral subarachnoid space and decreased in the posterolateral subarachnoid space. This finding has been replicated in several studies.[28-31] Researchers have also evaluated changes in cine images postoperatively to predict outcomes. They found improvement after Chiari decompression surgery, which was more obvious in patients with an associated syrinx.[30,32]

Future research recommendations involve a more pragmatic approach to cine-MR and other dynamic flow studies. Assessing flow sagittally and at multiple levels intracranially and intraspinally offers a more comprehensive picture of altered CSF flow patterns, but cine-MR protocols should be standardized. Lastly, single-photon emission computed tomography or proton chemical shift imaging has been used in many disorders, such as normal pressure hydrocephalus[33] to evaluate for chemical alterations in brain parenchyma. Elevated lactate level peaks have been found in brain parenchyma, which has been compromised. Future studies could use this technique to evaluate the cerebellum as other studies have found aberrant neuroectodermal development in the cerebellum in individuals with CMI and seizures.[34]

CLINICAL MANAGEMENT OF CHIARI I MALFORMATIONS

Medical and surgical management can be used to treat CMI. Initially, medical management is attempted via pharmacotherapy, physical therapy, and therapeutic injections. As headaches are the most common presenting symptom of CMI, they are typically treated according to presenting phenotype. The decision for surgical intervention is based on a combination of the clinical presentation, neuroimaging and/or physiologic studies such as somatosensory evoked potentials, swallow evaluations,

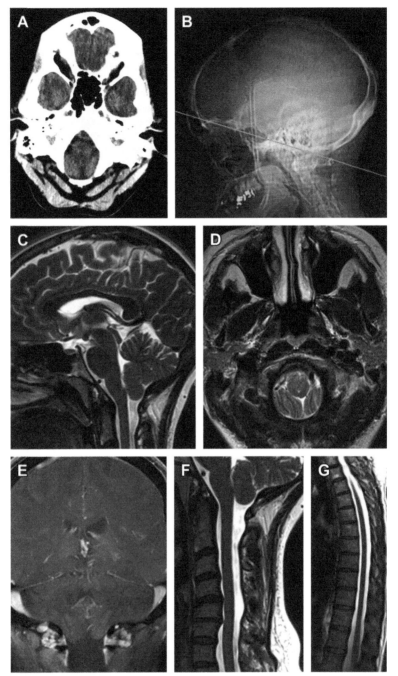

Fig. 8. Tonsillar crowding in CMI. The patient is a 48-year-old woman with a history of progressive occipital headaches worsening with Valsalva maneuvers, as well as subjective clumsiness in the upper and lower extremities. She was found to have a myelopathy on examination, with left-sided Hoffman reflex, hyperreflexic patellar reflexes at +3, and inability to tandem walk. Head CT scan without contrast: (*A*) Axial soft-tissue windows showing crowding between foramen magnum and C1. (*B*) Axial plane of scout images from which image A was taken. Brain MR images: (*C*) Sagittal T2 image showing CMI. (*D*) Axial T2 image showing crowding of tonsils at foramen magnum. (*E*) Coronal T1 image with contrast showing tonsillar descent past the foramen magnum. (*F*) Cervical MR sagittal T2 image without evidence of syrinx. (*G*) Thoracic MR sagittal T2 image without evidence of syrinx.

Table 2
Standard diagnostic imaging protocols

Study	Utility
CT scan of head without contrast enhancement (axial)	Visualize tonsillar crowding
MR imaging of brain with/without contrast (axial, sagittal, and coronal)	Measure tonsillar descent. Exclude intracranial/skull-based pathology or anomalies
MR imaging of spinal axis with/without contrast (axial and sagittal)	Measure tonsillar descent. Identify presence of syrinx. Exclude skull-based/spinal/skeletal pathology or anomalies
Cine-MR imaging study	Visualize CSF flow anterior and posterior to cerebellar tonsils and in cerebral aqueduct if hydrocephalus is present
X-ray of spinal axis	Evaluate for vertebral anomalies and scoliosis

and sleep studies. **Fig. 11** provides a flow chart for clinical management of CMI. If surgical intervention is necessary, most neurosurgeons prefer performing a suboccipital craniectomy with cervical laminectomy with or without duroplasty as the primary surgical treatment.

Following a Chiari decompression, a postoperative CT scan is usually performed within the first 24 hours to document adequate decompression and to identify any hemorrhage, hydrocephalus, or pneumocephalus. No further imaging is performed after the decompression as long as the preoperative symptoms resolve. However, in cases of SH, postoperative MR imaging of the brain and the spinal axis are obtained approximately 3 months later to determine whether the SH has resolved and to serve as a future baseline.

POSTOPERATIVE COMPLICATIONS AND ASSOCIATED IMAGING FINDINGS

After a Chiari decompression, postoperative imaging is instrumental in identifying early postoperative complications and assessing the adequacy of the decompression overall (**Table 3**).

Hemorrhage in the epidural, subdural, subarachnoid, intraparenchymal, or intraventricular space must be recognized early so that the patient can be carefully monitored with serial imaging and neurologic examinations. Eventual surgical decompression may be necessary if symptoms arise or if there is radiographic progression. Given the fixed volume within the posterior fossa compartment, hemorrhage in the posterior fossa can restrict the outflow of spinal fluid from the fourth ventricle, leading to acute obstructive hydrocephalus. Even the presence of minuscule retained blood products from surgery or persisting compression at the skull base can lead to postoperative hydrocephalus. Once discovered, any radiographic finding of hemorrhage or ventriculomegaly should be communicated immediately to the neurosurgeon as either malady can progress rapidly and be fatal. Hydrocephalus may also occur in the delayed postoperative period and is often the driving force leading to formation of pseudomeningoceles or CSF leaks (**Figs. 12 and 13**).

A subdural hygroma, an abnormal collection of CSF in the subdural space, can also occur in the immediate postoperative period. Subdural hygromas are likely due to an alteration of CSF flow caused by the introduction of CSF into the subdural

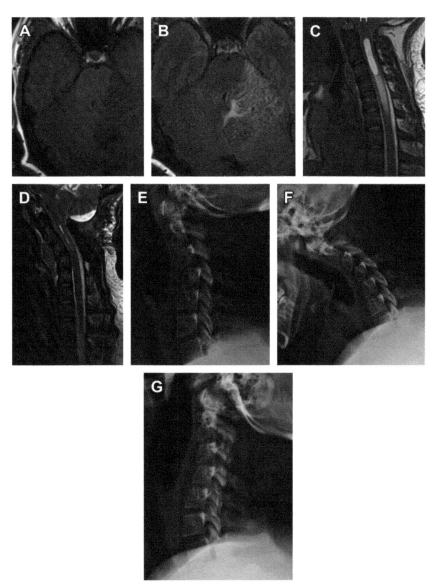

Fig. 9. Case illustration: secondary Chiari. The patient is a 25-year-old man with a history of Lhermitte-Duclos disease. The patient developed a secondary CMI with associated cervical syrinx due to mass effect caused by left-sided dysplastic cerebellar gangliocytoma. Preoperative MR images. (*A*) Axial T1 imaging showing left-sided cerebellar gangliocytoma. (*B*) Axial fluid attenuated inversion recovery image. (*C*) Sagittal T2 image depicting CMI and SH with surrounding edema. (*D*) Postoperative sagittal T2 image revealing creation of cisterna magna following decompression and dural patch graft placement and dramatic resolution of preoperative SH. Upright plain radiographs in (*E*) neutral, (*F*) flexion, and (*G*) extension positions documenting cervical kyphotic deformity at C2-C3 with increased angulation on flexion.

compartment as a result of arachnoid fenestration. A subdural hygroma appears hypodense on a CT scan (see **Fig. 12**; **Fig. 14**). Subdural hygromas are usually asymptomatic and should be monitored via serial imaging if there is any concern that they could be compressive. In rare cases, subdural hygromas actually require shunting and have been found to potentiate acute hydrocephalus following subocci-pital decompression.[35]

In patients found to have an acute neurologic deficit immediately after Chiari decompression, MR imaging of the brain and cervical spine should be performed. MR fluid attenuated inversion recovery imaging of the brain is useful in detecting parenchymal damage, whereas short T1 inversion recovery imaging of the spine may demonstrate myelomalacia. In addition, consideration should be given to obtain-ing a CT or MR perfusion imaging study to identify any ischemic changes arising from vascular injury (**Fig. 15**).

Pneumocephalus is often present on immediate postoperative imaging because of air retained underneath the dural patch graft that can dissipate through the subarach-noid space (**Fig. 16**). Appearing as intense hypodensities in the intraventricular, sub-arachnoid, and even subdural spaces, pneumocephalus is easily identifiable on soft tissue or bone windows. Although the amount of pneumocephalus is usually minimal, extensive pneumocephalus can occur and is usually treated by administering 100% oxygen via nasal cannula to help displace the retained air. If excessive pneumocepha-lus is present causing compression associated with neurologic change, the patient may be experiencing a tension pneumocephalus and urgent needle or surgical decompression may be required.

In the early postoperative period, a pseudomeningocele or CSF leak may occur. Imaging should be obtained to delineate the cause and exclude hydrocephalus, as hydrocephalus often serves as a driving force for the development of pseudomeningo-celes and CSF leaks. Pseudomeningoceles present clinically as a fluctuant subcu-taneous fluid collection beneath the incision (see **Fig. 12**). The pseudomeningocele is usually managed conservatively unless it is associated with a CSF leak or becomes aesthetically unpleasing.

Infections can occur in the form of bacterial meningitis, superficial or deep wound infections, or even frank abscesses within the first month to 3 months of surgery. Although the diagnosis of bacterial meningitis is made based on a lumbar puncture, MR imaging of the brain and cervical spine with and without contrast media must be obtained to identify an associated wound infection or postsurgical abscesses. In cases in which postoperative wound infection is suspected, MR imaging of the brain and cervical spine is necessary to determine not only the anatomic location of the infection but also the severity or extent to guide the neurosurgeon's decision making in terms of treatment. For example, small suprafascial infections may be treated with oral or intravenous antibiotics, whereas larger subfascial infections require surgical exploration. Inflammatory reactions involving dural grafts may also cause postopera-tive enhancement.[36]

Occipital-cervical and/or cervical instability may occur months to years after Chiari decompression, requiring neuroradiologists to pay close attention to the occipital-cervical junction and cervical alignment on postdecompression images. Instability may occur as a direct result of osseous and ligamentous disruption, particularly an overzealous craniectomy or laminectomy. This condition may pre-sent as occipital-cervical instability, atlantoaxial instability, cervical kyphosis (see **Fig. 9**), or cervical spondylolithesis. Only upright cervical spine plain films portray a patient's true alignment, as the images are acquired in an upright fashion compared with CT or MR imaging in which patients lie supine during the

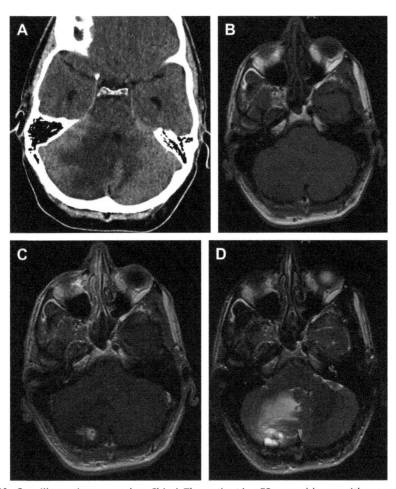

Fig. 10. Case illustration: secondary Chiari. The patient is a 53-year-old man with progressive occipital Valsalva maneuver–induced headaches with persistent occipital pressure sensation. A head CT scan revealed a ring-enhancing lesion with a mural nodule and associated edema causing right-sided tonsillar descent. He underwent a right cerebellar craniectomy and resection of the lesion, which was found to be a hemangioblastoma. His headaches completely resolved after surgery. (*A*) Preoperative noncontrast head CT scan showing right cerebellar edema and effacement of fourth ventricle with obstructive hydrocephalus. Preoperative MR images of the brain: (*B*) axial T1 without contrast, (*C*) axial T1 with contrast showing enhancing mural nodule, (*D*) axial T2 showing extensive surrounding edema and cystic portion of lesion, and (*E*) coronal T1 with contrast showing right-sided cerebellar tonsillar descent. Postoperative MR images of the brain with contrast performed 2 years after operation. (*F*) Axial T1 showing postoperative cavity without recurrence. (*G*) Coronal T1 with contrast showing almost complete resolution of right tonsillar descent.

image-acquisition process. Serial plain films can also be used in surveillance for progressive deformity.[37]

Cerebellar sag, also referred to as cerebellar ptosis, was described initially by Williams[38] in 1978. This condition may be a delayed postoperative complication after an overzealous craniectomy, leading to "sag" of the cerebellum through the generously

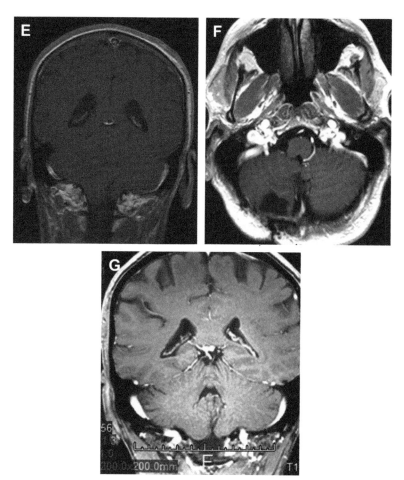

Fig. 10. (*continued*)

decompressed foramen magnum, which appears radiographically as filling of the decompression site by the cerebellum obliterating the cisterna magna. Patients experiencing cerebellar sag often present clinically with headaches caused by dural tension from the sagging cerebellum.[39] These headaches are usually distinct from the classic Valsalva-induced occipital headaches, as they occur most commonly in the frontal, orbital, or mandibular regions. Dural innervation by the nociceptive cranial nerve fibers, specifically of cranial nerves V, IX, and X, incites this pain as the dura encounters an excessive stretching force.[40,41] In addition to headaches incurred by dural strain, the patient may also develop a return of the original Chiari complaints due to blockage of posterior fossa spinal fluid egress pathways and resultant syringomyelic cavity reexpansion.[39] In the study conducted by Zhang and colleagues,[42] 7.2% of 69 patients undergoing a larger posterior decompression had symptomatic deterioration postoperatively because of cerebellar sag. As cautioned by Batzdorf and colleagues,[43] patients with a near-parallel orientation of the clivus in relation to the tentorium are at a high risk for developing cerebellar sag (see **Fig. 13**). Failure to recognize these imaging characteristics preoperatively led to reoperation in 3 patients for

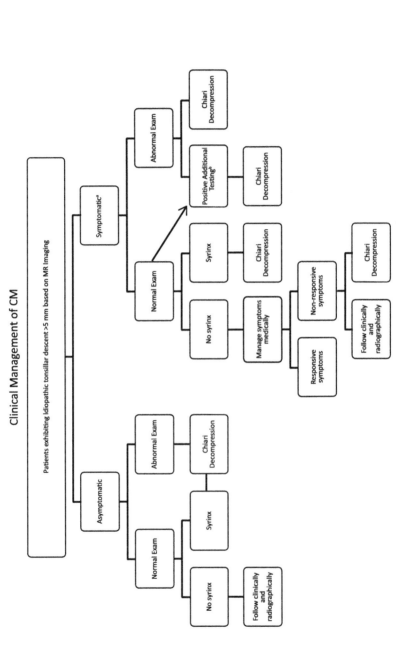

Fig. 11. Clinical management of Chiari malformation I (CMI). [a] Please refer to **Box 5** for symptoms. [b] Tests to include brain stem auditory-evoked potentials, polysomnography, motor-evoked potential/somatosensory-evoked potential monitoring, swallow evaluation, and nystagmography.

Table 3
Postoperative complications and associated imaging findings[a]

Complication	Assessment, Findings
Hydrocephalus	Ventricular enlargement compared with preoperative ventricular size
Hemorrhage	Density on CT scan of head or intensity on MR brain according to age of bleed, hypointense on GRE/SWI
Subdural hygroma	Hypodense on CT scan of head; isointense on MR brain relative to CSF on T1 and T2
Pneumocephalus	Hypodensities on CT soft-tissue and bone windows
Stroke	DWI/ADC series to detect ischemia CT or MR perfusion to assess for volume of brain affected CT or MR angiography of brain and cervical spine to evaluate for specific arterial injury
Parenchymal injury	FLAIR changes in brain parenchyma STIR changes in spinal parenchyma
Pseudomeningocele/seroma	Nonenhancing, isodense to CSF on CT/isointense to CSF on MR imaging
Infection	
Cerebellar abscess	Closed-ring enhancing lesion on CT or MR imaging; DWI positive on MR imaging
Wound abscess	Suprafascial or subfascial enhancing fluid collection
Bacterial meningitis	Leptomeningeal enhancement on CT or MR imaging (Leptomeningeal enhancement may also reflect intracranial hypotension caused by CSF leak or pseudomeningocele)
Instability	Spondylolithesis or abnormal curvature on neutral/flexion/extension plain films Boney misalignment on CT of head and neck Hyperintensities in cervical ligaments on MR of spine; STIR suggests instability

Abbreviations: ADC, apparent diffusion coefficient; DWI, diffusion-weighted imaging; FLAIR, fluid attenuated inversion recovery; GRE, gradient-focused echo; STIR, short T1 inversion recovery; SWI, susceptibility-weighted imaging.
[a] Postoperative MR imaging should always include contrast material, SWI or GRE, DWI, and ADC sequences.

cerebellar ptosis in their series, prompting the investigators to argue for judicious craniectomies and partial reconstruction of the posterior fossa by supportive plating. A cine-MR study to assess flow posteriorly around the cerebellar tonsils after a decompressive procedure can also facilitate diagnosis.

Retethering of the cerebellum via dense arachnoid adhesions within the postoperative cavity may manifest as a delayed complication after decompressive surgery occurring either primarily or as sequelae of cerebellar sag. Minimal cisterna magna reconstruction with cine-MR study evidence of poor flow posterior to the cerebellar tonsils may prompt clinician concerns that retethering occurs when a patient experiences recurrence of clinical symptoms of a CM postoperatively (see **Fig. 13**).

In patients with known SH, postoperative MR imaging should be obtained within 3 months of the decompression. In approximately 70% of patients, the syrinx cavity decreases following surgery.[40] However, some syrinxes may persist[41,44,45] and others may worsen.[46–48] If the SH does not improve, further evaluation via a cine MR study

116

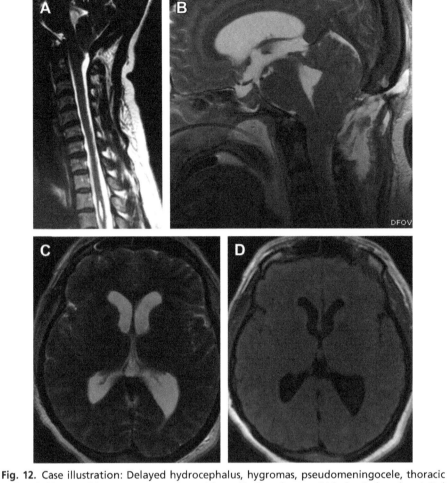

Fig. 12. Case illustration: Delayed hydrocephalus, hygromas, pseudomeningocele, thoracic syrinx. A 40-year-old woman presenting with medically refractory Valsalva-induced occipital headaches was found to have CMI with associated thoracic syrinx. The patient underwent a suboccipital craniectomy and C1 laminectomy. During the dural opening, a venous lake was encountered, and the patient suffered a venous air embolism. Due to developing cardiac instability, the dural opening was rapidly completed to provide tonsillar decompression, and a synthetic dural matrix was placed over the cerebellum without sewing of a dural patch graft. The patient was neurologically at her baseline on awakening. Approximately 1 month after surgery, she developed hydrocephalus due to posterior fossa outlet obstruction and was successfully treated with an endoscopic third ventriculostomy (ETV). (*A*) Sagittal T2 MR image showing CMI and associated thoracic syrinx. MR images acquired immediately after craniectomy and laminectomy: (*B*) Sagittal T2 with postoperative changes at the decompression site. (*C*) Axial T2 establishing baseline postoperative ventricular size. (*D*) Axial fluid attenuated inversion recovery (FLAIR) image without any significant transependymal FLAIR changes. One-month postoperative MR images: (*E*) Sagittal T2 showing interval progression of superior cerebellar hygroma and hydrocephalus. (*F*) Axial T2 documenting clear progression of ventriculomegaly compared with immediate postoperative imaging. (*G*) FLAIR T2 now showing obvious transependymal FLAIR changes. (*H*) Axial T2 documenting bilateral inferior cerebellar hygromas. (*I*) Axial T2 showing interval progression of pseudomeningocele. (*J*) Axial T1 without contrast (for comparison). (*K*) Axial T1 with contrast illustrating pseudomeningocele with normal postoperative enhancement without evidence of abscess. (*L*) Head CT scan obtained 2 years postdecompression procedure without contrast noting persistent resolution of hydrocephalus after ETV.

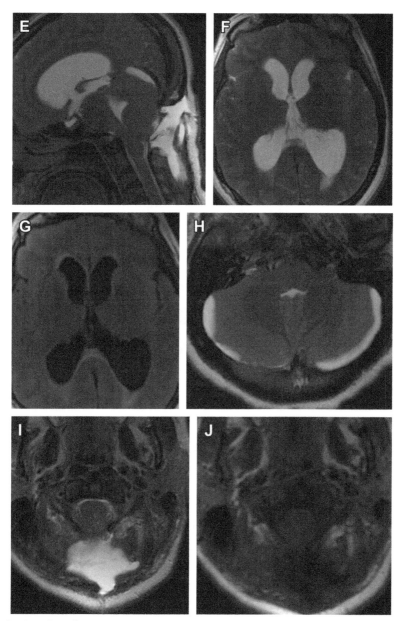

Fig. 12. (*continued*)

should be performed to look for evidence of persistent compression, retethering, or cerebellar sag.

What the referring physician needs to know
- Recognize the symptoms and signs of CMI and SH.
- Develop a pragmatic approach to medical and surgical management.

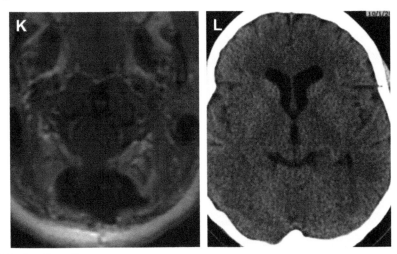

Fig. 12. (*continued*)

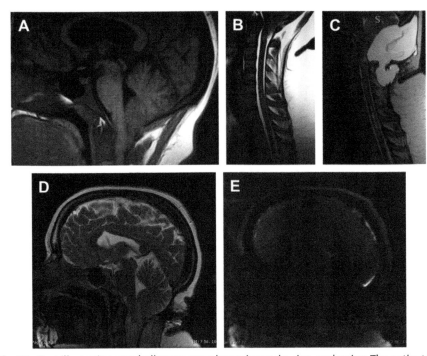

Fig. 13. Case illustration: cerebellar sag, pseudomeningocele, cine, and syrinx. The patient is a 26-year-old woman with a history of CMI and associated cervical syrinx status-post suboccipital craniectomy and decompression. She required repetitive procedures due to persisting pseudomeningocele despite cerebrospinal fluid shunting and eventually developed cerebellar sag and postoperative retethering. (*A*) Sagittal T1 MR image of brain illustrating CMI. Note the almost parallel orientation of the clivus to the tentorium, which is a risk factor for the development of cerebellar sag postoperatively. (*B*) Sagittal T2 image of cervical spine documenting baseline cervical syrinx. (*C*) Postoperative sagittal T2 MR image depicting pseudomeningocele compressing the cerebellum. (*D*) Sagittal T2 MR image in same patient now experiencing symptomatic recurrence with postdecompressive development of cerebellar "sag" and further expansion of syringobulbia with surrounding edema. (*E*) Cine MR imaging showing paucity of cerebrospinal fluid flow posterior to the tonsils further suggesting possible tethering.

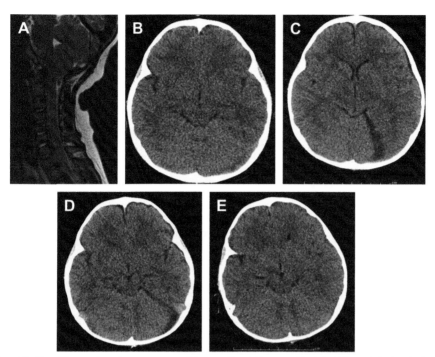

Fig. 14. Case illustration: hygroma, peglike tonsils. A 5-year-old girl with occipital Valsalva-induced headaches was found to have a Chiari I malformation without syringromyelia that was refractory to medical management. (A) Preoperative T2 sagittal MR image with tonsillar descent to C2 lamina. (B) Immediate postoperative CT scan of head. Brain CT without contrast obtained after patient returned to office complaining of progressive occipital headaches approximately 10 days after Chiari decompression: (C) Supracerebellar left subdural hygromas. (D) Lateral extension of left subdural hygroma along petrous surface of cerebellum. (E) Noncontrast head CT scan 1 month after original procedure showing almost complete spontaneous resolution of hygroma.

- MR imaging and cine-MR studies are the gold standard for diagnosis and monitoring of CMI and SH.
- Be aware of secondary causes of CMI and SH.

Imaging pearls
- Look for tonsillar crowding on an axial CT scan of the head in patients with headache.
- Coronal MR imaging is useful in anatomic assessment of tonsillar position.
- Image the craniospinal axis if CMI or SH is identified.
  - Obtain contrast-enhanced cranial imaging to exclude cause of secondary CMs such as neoplastic, inflammatory, or infectious processes.
  - All postoperative imaging should be obtained with contrast enhancement.
- Monitor patients with known SH carefully via serial postoperative imaging studies to assess for stabilization or resolution. Persistence or worsening of syrinx may be due to inadequate decompression, requiring further surgery.
- Obtain cine-MR study to determine flow posterior to tonsils preoperatively and postoperatively to guide decision making.

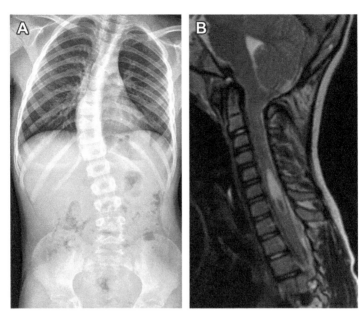

Fig. 15. Case illustration: scoliosis, syrinx, and cine. A 10-year-old boy with history of progressive scoliosis found to have a CMI with associated cervicothoracic syrinx. The patient was otherwise asymptomatic with a nonfocal neurologic examination. He underwent a suboccipital craniectomy, C1 laminectomy, and pericranial dural patch graft. During the next year, the patient's scoliotic curvature persisted without any decrease in the size of the syrinx. The patient developed occipital headaches and bilateral paresthesias of the hands and feet. MR imaging showed slight increase in the size of the syrinx with poor flow posterior to the tonsils on a cine study. He then underwent reexploration with lysis of adhesions and bovine pericardial graft placement. At the time of surgery, the cerebellum was densely adherent to the previously placed graft. (A) Preoperative coronal upright scoliosis plain film showing a 38° right thoracic curvature. (B) Preoperative T2 sagittal MR image with CM and associated cervicothoracic syrinx. (C) Postoperative T2 sagittal MR image performed approximately 1.5 years after initial surgery and before the detethering procedure (mentioned later), showing slight increase in size of the syrinx. (D) Cine study showing paucity of retrotonsillar flow. Postoperatively after the second decompression surgery, the patient exhibited mild right hemiparesis and dysmetria, as well as ataxia that resolved almost completely within 1 week. No hemorrhage was seen on CT scans of the head and cervical spine performed immediately on awakening of the patient from surgery. Immediate postoperative MR imaging excluded a stroke and showed postoperative changes associated with detethering. No clear cause of the patient's postoperative neurologic changes was found. Postoperative MR images: (E) Sagittal T1 without evidence of hemorrhage, (F) Sagittal T2 with hyperintensities along the inferior cerebellar hemisphere and posterior cervical cord, (G) Axial fluid attenuated inversion recovery MR imaging of brain showing hyperintensities along inferior cerebellum where detethering occurred, (H) diffusion-weighted imaging and apparent diffusion coefficient correlate showing no evidence of ischemia.

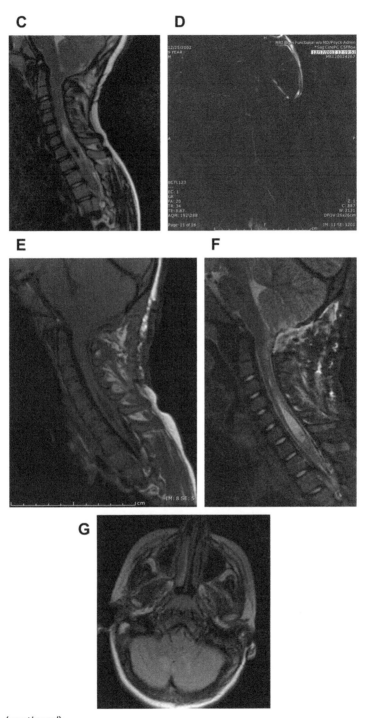

Fig. 15. (*continued*)

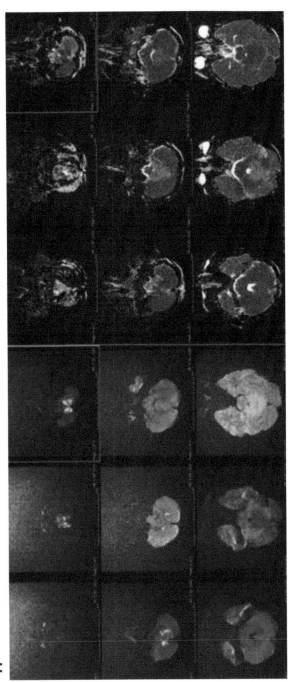

Fig. 15. (continued)

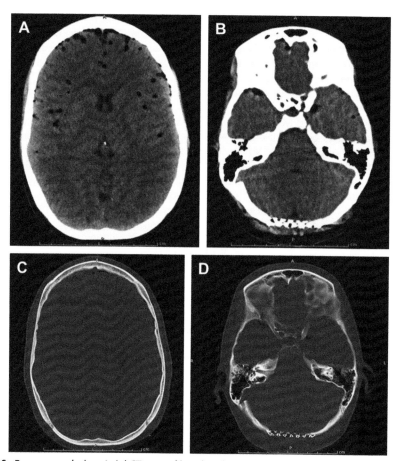

Fig. 16. Pneumocephalus. Axial CT scan of head without contrast performed within 24 hours of surgery showing evidence of pneumocephalus throughout the intracranial subarachnoid space. Soft-tissue windows at cerebral convexity (A) and skull base (B) showing pronounced pneumocephalus. Bone windows further demonstrating pneumocephalus at level of convexities (C) and skull base (D). Notice the titanium plate, which was placed after decompression to provide cerebellar support and decrease postoperative adhesions.

SUMMARY

CM and SH are a fascinating and diverse group of pathologic conditions. Neuroimaging has been instrumental in developing current diagnostic and treatment protocols, as well as elucidating the neurophysiological mechanisms behind these phenomena. The advent of MR imaging and the novel application of cine-MR studies have not only broadened clinician's understanding of these pathologies but have also enhanced patient care. As these imaging modalities become more advanced in the future, the diagnosis and treatment of CM and SH will become even more refined.

REFERENCES

1. Chiari H. Uber Veranderungen des Kleinhirns infolge von Hydrocephalies des Grosshrins. Dtsch Med Wochenschr 1891;17:1172–5.

2. Chiari H. Uber Veranderungen des Kleinhirns, der Pons und der Medulla oblongata in Folge von congenitaler Hydrocephalie des Grosshrins. Denkschr Akad Wissensch Math Naturw Cl 1896;3:71–116.
3. Cleland J. Contribution to the study of spina bifida, encephalocele, and anencephalus. J Anat Physiol 1883;17:257–92.
4. Myelocyste AJ. Tranposition von Gewebskeimen und Sympodie. Beitr Pathol Anat 1894;16:1–28.
5. Schwalbe E, Gredig M. Uber Entwicklungsstoungen des Kleinhrins, Hirnstamms und Halsmarks bei Spina bifida (Arnold'sche und Chiari'sche Missbildung). Beitr Pathol Anat 1907;40:132–94.
6. Dreisen W, Schmidt H. Malformations in structures of the posterior fossa. In: Krayenbuhl H, Maspes PE, Sweet WH, editors. Progress in neurological surgery. Basel (Switzerland): Karger; 1971. p. 102–32.
7. Massimi L, Novegno F, di Rocco C. Chiari type I malformation in children. Adv Tech Stand Neurosurg 2011;37:143–211.
8. Mikulis DJ, Diaz O, Egglin TK, et al. Variance of the position of the cerebellar tonsils with age: preliminary report. Radiology 1992;183:725–8.
9. Barkovich AJ. Pediatric neuroimaging. 4th edition. Philadelphia: Lippincott; 2005. p. 932.
10. Barkovich AJ, Wippold FJ, Sherman JL, et al. Significance of cerebellar tonsillar position on MR. AJNR Am J Neuroradiol 1986;7:795–9.
11. Hadley DM. The Chiari malformations. J Neurol Neurosurg Psychiatry 2002; 72(Suppl 2):ii38–40.
12. Milhorat TH, Capocelli AL Jr, Anzil AP, et al. Pathological basis of spinal cord cavitation in syringomyelia: analysis of 105 autopsy cases. J Neurosurg 1995;82: 802–12.
13. Urbizu A, Toma C, Poca MA, et al. Chiari malformation type I: a case-control association study of 58 developmental genes. PLoS One 2013;8: e57241.
14. Gardner WJ. Hydrodynamic mechanism of syringomyelia: its relationship to myelocele. J Neurol Neurosurg Psychiatry 1965;28:247–59.
15. Williams B. Cerebrospinal fluid pressure-gradients in spina bifida cystica, with special reference to the Arnold-Chiari malformation and aqueductal stenosis. Dev Med Child Neurol Suppl 1975;(35):138–50.
16. Ball MJ, Dayan AD. Pathogenesis of syringomyelia. Lancet 1972;2:799–801.
17. Aboulker J. Syringomyelia and intra-rachidian fluids. X. Rachidian fluid stasis. Neurochirurgie 1979;25(Suppl 1):98–107 [in French].
18. Heiss JD, Patronas N, DeVroom HL, et al. Elucidating the pathophysiology of syringomyelia. J Neurosurg 1999;91:553–62.
19. Bhadelia RA, Wolpert SM. CSF flow dynamics in Chiari I malformation. AJNR Am J Neuroradiol 2000;21:1564.
20. Aitken LA, Lindan CE, Sidney S, et al. Chiari type I malformation in a pediatric population. Pediatr Neurol 2009;40:449–54.
21. Meadows J, Kraut M, Guarnieri M, et al. Asymptomatic Chiari type I malformations identified on magnetic resonance imaging. J Neurosurg 2000;92:920–6.
22. Speer MC, Enterline DS, Mehltretter L, et al. Chiari I malformation with or without syringomyelia: prevelance and genetics. J Genet Couns 2003;12:297–311.
23. Silberstein SD, Lipton RB, Dodick DW. Wolff's headache and other head pain. New York: Oxford University Press; 2008. p. 760.
24. Guinto G, Zamorano C, Dominguez F, et al. Chiari I malformation: part I. Contemp Neurosurg 2004;26:1–7.

25. Adams RD, Schatzki R, Scoville WB. The Arnold-Chiari malformation. Diagnosis, demonstration by intraspinal lipoidal and successful surgical treatment. N Engl J Med 1941;225:125–31.
26. Baker HL Jr. Myelographic examination of the posterior fossa with positive contrast medium. Radiology 1963;81:791–801.
27. Badie B, Mendoza D, Batzdorf U. Posterior fossa volume and response to suboccipital decompression in patients with Chiari I malformation. Neurosurgery 1995; 37:214–8.
28. Alperin N, Sivaramakrishnan A, Lichtor T. Magnetic resonance imaging-based measurements of cerebrospinal fluid and blood flow as indicators of intracranial compliance in patients with Chiari malformation. J Neurosurg 2005;103:46–52.
29. Tominaga T, Koshu K, Ogawa A, et al. Transoral decompression evaluated by cine-mode magnetic resonance imaging: a case of basilar impression accompanied by Chiari malformation. Neurosurgery 1991;28:883–5.
30. Ventureyra EC, Aziz HA, Vassilyadi M. The role of cine flow MRI in children with Chiari I malformation. Childs Nerv Syst 2003;19:109–13.
31. Vurdem UE, Acer N, Ertekin T, et al. Analysis of the volumes of the posterior cranial fossa, cerebellum, and herniated tonsils using the stereological methods in patients with Chiari type I malformation. ScientificWorldJournal 2012;2012:616934.
32. Sivaramakrishnan A, Alperin N, Surapaneni S, et al. Evaluating the effect of decompression surgery on cerebrospinal fluid flow and intracranial compliance in patients with Chiari malformation with magnetic resonance imaging flow studies. Neurosurgery 2004;55:1344–51.
33. Kizu O, Yamada K, Nishimura T. Proton chemical shift imaging in normal pressure hydrocephalus. AJNR Am J Neuroradiol 2001;22:1659–64.
34. Elster AD, Chen MY. Chiari I malformations: clinical and radiologic reappraisal. Radiology 1992;183:347–53.
35. Elton S, Tubbs RS, Wellons JC 3rd, et al. Acute hydrocephalus following a Chiari I decompression. Pediatr Neurosurg 2002;36:101–4.
36. Rosen DS, Wollman R, Frim DM. Recurrence of symptoms after Chiari decompression and duraplasty with nonautologous graft material. Pediatr Neurosurg 2003;38:186–90.
37. Mazzola CA, Fried AH. Revision surgery for Chiari malformation decompression. Neurosurg Focus 2003;15:E3.
38. Williams B. A critical appraisal of posterior fossa surgery for communicating syringomyelia. Brain 1978;101:223–50.
39. Udani V, Holly LT, Chow D, et al. Posterior fossa reconstruction using titanium plate for the treatment of cerebellar ptosis following decompression for Chiari malformation. World Neurosurg 2013 Jan 19. http://dx.doi.org/10.1016/j.wneu.2013.01.081. pii: S1878-8750(13)00142-3.
40. Depreitere B, Van Calenbergh F, van Loon J, et al. Posterior fossa decompression in syringomyelia associated with a Chiari malformation: a retrospective analysis of 22 patients. Clin Neurol Neurosurg 2000;102:91–6.
41. Tubbs RS, Webb DB, Oakes WJ. Persistent syringomyelia following pediatric Chiari I decompression: radiological and surgical findings. J Neurosurg 2004;100:460–4.
42. Zhang Y, Zhang N, Qiu H, et al. An efficacy analysis of posterior fossa decompression techniques in the treatment of Chiari malformation with associated syringomyelia. J Clin Neurosci 2011;18:1346–9.
43. Batzdorf U, McArthur DL, Bentson JR. Surgical treatment of Chiari malformation with and without syringomyelia: experience with 177 adult patients. J Neurosurg 2013;118:232–42.

44. Kalb S, Perez-Orribo L, Mahan M, et al. Evaluation of operative procedures for symptomatic outcome after decompression surgery for Chiari type I malformation. J Clin Neurosci 2012;19:1268–72.

45. Pare LS, Batzdorf U. Syringomyelia persistence after Chiari decompression as a result of pseudomeningocele formation: implications for syrinx pathogenesis: report of three cases. Neurosurgery 1998;43:945–8.

46. Ma J, You C, Chen H, et al. Cerebellar tonsillectomy with suboccipital decompression and duraplasty by small incision for Chiari I malformation (with syringomyelia): long term follow-up of 76 surgically treated cases. Turk Neurosurg 2012; 22:274–9.

47. McGirt MJ, Attenello FJ, Datoo G, et al. Intraoperative ultrasonography as a guide to patient selection for duraplasty after suboccipital decompression in children with Chiari malformation type I. J Neurosurg Pediatr 2008;2:52–7.

48. Wetjen NM, Heiss JD, Oldfield EH. Time course of syringomyelia resolution following decompression of Chiari malformation type I. J Neurosurg Pediatr 2008;1:118–23.

Neuroimaging of Infectious Disease

Patrick M. Capone, MD, PhD[a,b,c],*, Joseph M. Scheller, MD[b,c]

KEYWORDS

- Central nervous system • Infection • Magnetic resonance imaging
- Computerized tomography • Abscesses • Meningitis

KEY POINTS

- Fifty percent of neuroimaging studies of acute meningitis show no specific abnormalities.
- Imaging is warranted to exclude space-occupying lesions, provide evidence of the source of infection, and better categorize the specific organism.
- Several sources of encephalopathy such as human immunodeficiency virus, JC virus, toxoplasmosis, and Creutzfeldt-Jakob disease have distinct imaging features that can be diagnostic.
- Properly tailored protocols are vital for imaging studies such as short tau inversion recovery or other fat-saturation sequences to properly visualize disorders.
- Metastatic disease, tumefactive demyelinating disease, resolving cerebral hemorrhages, subacute infarctions, and gliomas can appear similar to cerebral abscesses on standard T1-weighted and T2-weighted scan sequences but can generally be distinguished with advanced imaging modalities including diffusion, magnetic resonance (MR) perfusion, and MR spectroscopy.

The modalities of modern neuroimaging are invaluable tools for the diagnosis and treatment of patients with infectious diseases of the central nervous system (CNS). These modalities supplement the clinical assessment of patients as to the type and specific anatomic location along with providing objective measures of the response to antibiotic therapy or the need for other modalities such as surgical intervention. There are a myriad of infectious diseases that invade the CNS. A detailed review of the multitude of CNS infections is beyond the scope of this article. However, there are a limited number of cellular responses that can be produced.[1]

Disclosures: None.

[a] Virginia Commonwealth University, Richmond, VA, USA; [b] Department of Neurology and Medical Imaging, Winchester Medical Center, 1840 Amherst Street, Winchester, VA 22601, USA; [c] Winchester Neurological Consultants, Inc, 125-A Medical Circle, Winchester, VA 22601, USA
* Corresponding author. Winchester Neurological Consultants, Inc, 125-A Medical Circle, Winchester, VA 22601.
E-mail address: pcapone@winchesterneurological.com

Neurol Clin 32 (2014) 127–145
http://dx.doi.org/10.1016/j.ncl.2013.07.009   **neurologic.theclinics.com**
0733-8619/14/$ – see front matter © 2014 Elsevier Inc. All rights reserved.

Infections can be classified by the location within the CNS, the pattern of cellular response, type of infectious organism, and severity.[2,3] These features overlapping for several disease causes such as with pyogenic or fungal abscesses. At times imaging shows more specific disease features that may allow an exact diagnosis, as in cases of herpes simplex encephalitis or neurocysticercosis.[4–9]

In the approach to treatment of patients who present with symptoms suggesting a CNS infection, such as intractable headache, altered sensorium, fever, and/or seizures, the primary modalities of modern neuroimaging are computed tomography (CT) and magnetic resonance imaging (MRI). These modalities provide exquisite anatomic detail along with providing differing but complementary information. These modalities can provide information that may preclude a lumbar puncture as a result of a significant space-occupying lesion or provide an alternative cause for the patient's presentation. CT has the advantage of rapid availability, easier access than MRI, and little to no contraindications if studies are provided without contrast. MRI has significantly better anatomic detail along with imaging features that better show the pathophysiologic changes that may significantly decrease the differential diagnosis and that are at times pathognomonic.[10] Familiarity with the imaging findings for CNS infections on CT or MRI is vital for neurologists who treat these patients.

This article describes our approach to using these imaging modalities and illustrates their findings with several selected clinical examples. An imaging overview is provided of several of the common CNS infections as organized by broad disease location and classifications.

MENINGITIS

Meningitis is the most frequent infection of the CNS.[3,11,12] Patients with the cardinal features of meningitis (headache, fever, altered sensorium, and meningismus) are presumed to have meningitis until proved otherwise. Approximately half of the imaging studies of acute meningitis show no specific imaging abnormalities.[13] Nevertheless, imaging is indicated to exclude space-occupying lesions; to exclude an alternate cause such as a subarachnoid hemorrhage; to assess for hydrocephalus; and to evaluate the potential sources of infection that might necessitate intervention beyond medical therapy, such as sinusitis, mastoiditis, or an empyema.[13]

The normal leptomeninges have a pattern of light and discontiguous enhancement along with the enhancing cortical vasculature. Familiarity with the normal range of contrast enhancement is essential for recognition of what are often subtle abnormalities that may prove diagnostic. Viral causes are the most common, with most being enteroviruses, herpes viruses, arboviruses, and human immunodeficiency virus (HIV). The most common bacterial organisms are *Streptococcus pneumoniae*, *Neisseria meningitides*, *Listeria monocytogenes*, group B streptococci, and *Haemophilus influenzae*.[3,11]

Fig. 1 shows examples of 2 separate patients with pneumococcal meningitis.

Imaging studies of patients with meningitis as in **Fig. 1** frequently show a normal pattern of contrast enhancement in spite of markedly abnormal cerebrospinal fluid (CSF) findings and cultures or may show increase signal on the fluid-attenuated inversion recovery (FLAIR) view and contiguous meningeal enhancement with similar CSF findings.[13–15]

Fig. 2 shows a more markedly abnormal dural enhancement in a patient with multiple episodes of recurrent bacterial meningitis. **Fig. 2** gives an example of FLAIR views, showing the thickened meninges and inflammatory changes to a high degree of sensitivity. These changes are however nonspecific and can be seen in conjunction

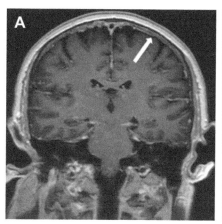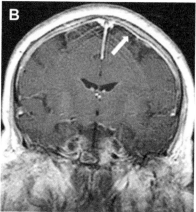

Fig. 1. T1 postcontrast coronal views of 2 patients with acute pneumococcal meningitis, showing the meninges (*arrows*). (*A*) A normal pattern of light and discontiguous contrast enhancement of the meninges and cortical vessels. (*B*) Abnormal prominent and contiguous meningeal contrast enhancement.

with multiple other causes of pachymeningitis, as seen with intracranial hypotension, sarcoidosis, other granulomatous diseases, or carcinomatous meningitis. Most acute meningitides that show imaging changes present with a predominately leptomeningitis pattern with enhancement along the pia mater throughout the sulci, fissures, and cisterns.

Studies and reviews of imaging features are available that provide additional guidelines to differentiate normal from abnormal meningeal enhancement and help to identify differing causes of meningitis.[15–18]

Other imaging features of meningitis beyond dural enhancement may include cerebral edema with a resultant blurring of the cortical sulci, fissures, and cisterns, along with hydrocephalus, pneumocephalus, ventriculitis, and ischemic lesions.[14,19]

Fig. 3 shows a patient with acute listeria meningitis with hydrocephalus most marked within the temporal horns along with ventriculitis, which is well seen with enhancement of the ependymal margin of the ventricles along with markedly increased signal of the FLAIR views within the lateral and third ventricles.[20,21]

A frequent imaging finding with bacterial meningitis is ischemic lesions as a result of vasculitis. These lesions can be small or large vessel infarctions.[14,22] **Fig. 4** shows small cortical infarctions along the left cerebellum in a patient with pneumococcal meningitis with no other imaging abnormalities to suggest a CNS infection.[23]

INFECTIONS OF THE ORBITS, SINUSES, AND SOFT TISSUES

Neuroimaging provides guidance for patient management and both a frequent assessment of response to treatment along with an assessment of adjacent structures that are potential sources of CNS infection, as in some of the following examples.

The most common cause of sinusitis similar to meningitis is viral. The most frequent bacterial causes are *S pneumoniae*, *H influenzae*, and *Moraxella catarrhalis*.[24–26]

Mastoiditis causes are predominately the same bacterial species as mentioned for sinusitis, along with *Staphylococcus aureus*, *Streptococcus pyogenes*, and various fungal species.[27]

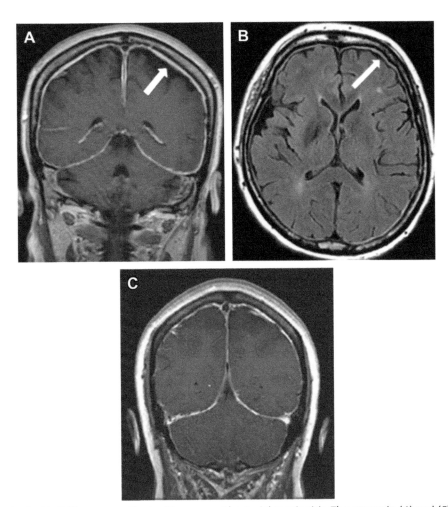

Fig. 2. (*A*, *B*) The same patient with recurrent bacterial meningitis. The *arrows* in (*A*) and (*B*) are pointing to the meninges. There is thickening of the pachymeninges shown on the coronal postcontrast T1-weighted view along with thickened and increased signal on the FLAIR-weighted view in *B*. (*C*) Postcontrast T1 view of a patient with intracranial hypotension with no infectious process.

Fig. 5 is a CT scan and MRI of a woman who presented with a meningitislike syndrome. The imaging shows acute mastoiditis and an empyema overlying the right hemisphere.

Diffusion-weighted imaging (DWI) is invaluable in showing acute ischemic lesions. It is also invaluable in showing many infectious processes. Both acute infarctions and pyogenic infections show restricted diffusion because of reduced brownian movement. In infections this is caused by the thick cellular debris. **Fig. 6** shows an acute thalamic infarction caused by vasculitis associated with the empyema and shows the increased diffusion-weighted signal within the empyema, which is a frequent hallmark of infections. The study shows the appearance of a right hemispheric empyema on the FLAIR-weighted views with bright signal along the pia and dura mater and the subdural collection of phlegmon. An empyema can be subdural, epidural, or both.

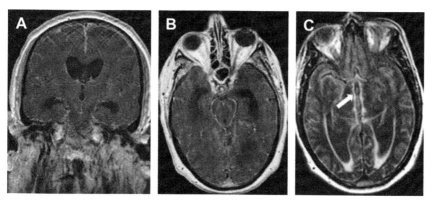

Fig. 3. Patient with listeria meningitis and ventriculitis. (*A, B*) Postcontrast T1-weighted views showing the moderate to severe hydrocephalus and meningeal enhancement. (*C*) FLAIR-weighted view showing marked inflammatory changes within the lateral and third ventricle, and the ependymal margin of the third ventricle with associated increased signal (*arrow*).

The restricted diffusion signal of purulent collections can also frequently aid in distinguishing a neoplastic from an infectious CNS lesion. Foci of intracranial free air in the setting of acute mastoiditis or sinusitis are also subtle findings that can suggest meningitis.

The paranasal sinuses are another frequent source of infection. **Fig. 7** shows an acute empyema arising in association with frontal sinusitis.[26,28]

Extracranial soft tissues may be a source of infection or additional infected regions to be noted on imaging studies. **Fig. 8** shows a patient with severe right frontotemporal cellulitis with associated orbital abscess and sinusitis within the maxillary and ethmoid sinuses.

Properly tailoring protocols to improve diagnostic yield is vital. Imaging sequences such as short T1 inversion recovery (STIR) and other fat-saturation techniques may be required to visualize disorders. The STIR sequence is designed to suppress signal

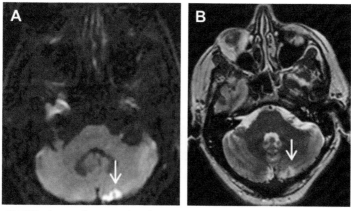

Fig. 4. (*A, B*) Diffusion and T2-weighted axial views of a patient with acute pneumococcal meningitis. The small acute infarctions (*arrows*) are the only imaging abnormalities on this study.

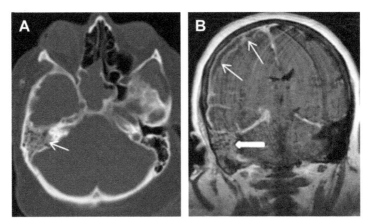

Fig. 5. (*A*) CT image showing bone windowing in a patient with acute mastoiditis. Note the infected right mastoid air cells (*arrow*) compared with the normally aerated left mastoid air cells. Sphenoid sinusitis is also evident. (*B*) Postcontrast coronal view of the same patient. Note the acute mastoiditis (*large arrow*) and an acute empyema overlying the right hemisphere with prominent enhancement of the leptomeninges (*smaller arrows*). Mass effect is also evident from the right lateral ventricle by some midline shift. Note also the infected the right mastoid air cells (*large arrow*) compared with the normally aerated left mastoid air cells.

from fat, and it also enhances the signal from tissue with long T1 and T2 relaxation times, such as neoplastic and inflammatory tissues. **Fig. 9** presents an example of a study that requires the addition of a fat-saturation sequence. The study shows contrasted enhancement in the right orbit in a patient with Lyme pseudotumor. Fat-saturated axial and coronal views of the orbits are required to negate normal bright T1 signal of intraorbital fat tissue.[29,30]

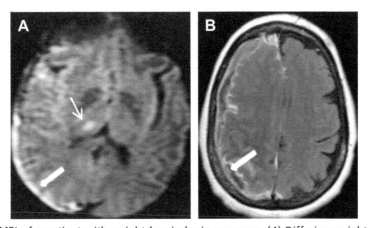

Fig. 6. MRI of a patient with a right hemispheric empyema. (*A*) Diffusion-weighted view showing the increased signal in the subdural states, caused by the purulent fluid (*large arrow*). There is also an acute infarction (*small arrow*) caused by vasculitis associated with the CNS infection. (*B*) FLAIR-weighted view showing increased signal along the pia and dura mater as a result of the purulent fluid (*large arrow*).

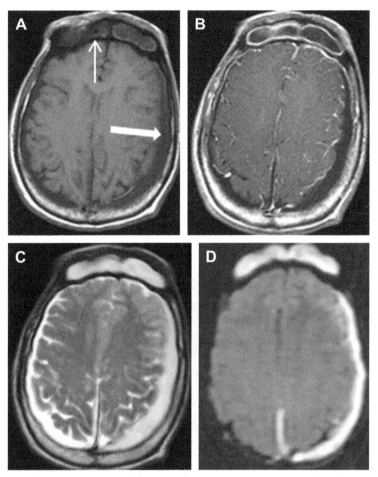

Fig. 7. MRI of a patient with a left hemispheric empyema associated with acute frontal sinusitis. (*A, B*) T1-weighted views without and with contrast, respectively. The *small arrow* points to the frontal sinusitis. The *larger arrow* points to the left hemispheric subdural empyema. (*C*) T2-weighted view showing the increased signal of the sinusitis and empyema. (*D*) Diffusion-weighted view showing the bright DWI signal associated with purulent infection.

It is incumbent on neurologists who manage these patients to be as observant of the adjacent extracranial structures as of the intracranial anatomy and be familiar with the optimal protocol for a given study.

MENINGOENCEPHALITIS AND ABSCESS

Abscesses may arise because of a myriad of bacterial, from fungal or parasitic causes, and they may be polymicrobial. Many infectious agents can present in several locations within the CNS, such as neurocysticercosis. Neurocysticercosis most commonly presents as parenchymal lesions in the gray-white junction. However, the cysticerci can accumulate throughout the meninges, the subarachnoid spaces, the intraventricular spaces, throughout the spinal canal, and within the orbit, which results in a wide range of complications depending on their size, stage of development, and location, such as seizure or hydrocephalus.[6,31]

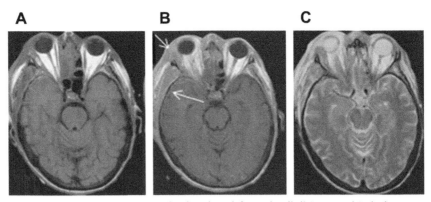

Fig. 8. MRI of a patient with a right facial and frontal cellulitis, an orbital abscess, and ethmoid sinusitis. (*A*) Noncontrast T1-weighted view and (*B*) postcontrast T1-weighted view showing the enhancing infection (*small arrow*) and the soft tissue cellulitis (*large arrow*). (*C*) T2-weighted view of the same region, again showing the swollen soft tissue and intraorbital inflammatory changes.

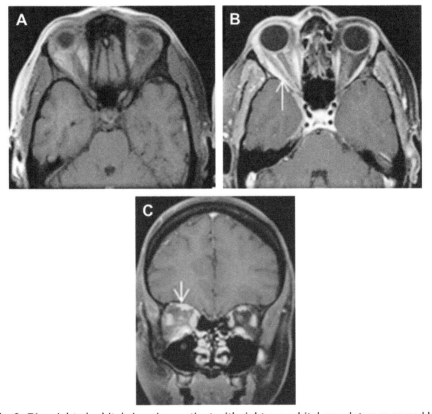

Fig. 9. T1-weighted orbital views in a patient with right eye orbital pseudotumor caused by Lyme disease. (*A*) Noncontrast T1-weighted view without the fat-saturation pulse. (*B, C*) Postcontrast fat-saturation T1-weighted views in the axial and coronal planes showing enhancement within the right orbital soft tissue, which is best shown by saturating the signal from the normal intracranial fat tissue. *Arrows* in (*B*) and (*C*) are pointing to the right orbital enhancement.

Fig. 10 shows neurocysticercosis presenting as cysts in various arachnoid spaces and meningeal infiltrations. The typical parenchymal involvement is shown in Fig. 11. Parenchymal cysts have a scolex that can often be visualized within the cyst walls. This appearance is nearly pathognomonic for this parasite. The only finding is often a calcified nodule representing a cysticercus, which is the degenerative end stage.[32,33]

Cerebral abscesses provide distinct clinical issues for the management and imaging concerns compared with meningitis. Cerebral abscesses are parenchymal collections of pus, immune cells, and other material that is typically surrounded by a vascular collagenous capsule of granulation tissue. These abscesses generally arise from a bacterial, fungal, or parasite source and evolve 1 or 2 weeks following the initial stage of cerebritis. On both CT and MRI scanning, an abscess typically appears as a capsular lesion with a rim of contrast.[14,34–36] Table 1 lists the temporal stages of abscess development in conjunction with the usual features on CT and MRI. Patient history and a clinical review of other organ systems often contribute to an accurate diagnostic interpretation.

Infections of the mastoid sinuses are associated with abscesses in the temporal lobes or the cerebellum, whereas those of the frontal, ethmoid, and sphenoid sinuses typically are associated with abscesses in the frontal lobes. Dental infections are a known cause in a small percentage of abscesses, and a more frequent suspected cause when the abscess is cryptogenic. Head trauma or neurosurgery procedures introduce infections into the brain parenchyma. These infections generally begin as cerebritis and evolve into abscesses.[26–28]

Blood-borne infections are responsible for a large percentage of brain abscesses. In this scenario the abscess is typically located in the distribution of the middle cerebral artery and most often it is found at the gray-white junction.

Immune deficiency states, such as in patients with HIV, organ transplantation, cancer, or immunosuppressive therapy, are more prone to fungal and protozoan causes of abscess. Third world travel can predispose to a host of less common infectious causes such as cysticercosis, which is endemic in Latin America, or tuberculosis, which is common in Africa and Asia.

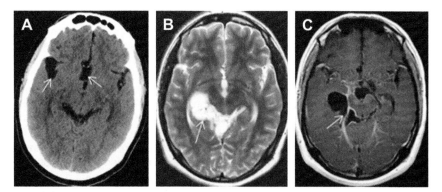

Fig. 10. (A) CT view with neurocysticercosis within the arachnoid spaces. There is cystic enlargement (small arrows) in the arachnoid spaces of the left sylvian and the interhemispheric fissures. (B, C) T2-weighted and postcontrast T1-weighted views, respectively, showing dural enhancement (small arrows in C) as a result of the meningeal infiltration by the parasites along with the prominent cystic enlargement of the perimesencephalic cisterns and right choroidal fissure (small arrows in B).

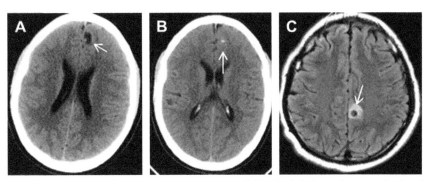

Fig. 11. (*A*) A typical small cyst on a noncontrast CT within the left frontal parasagittal region (*small arrow*). (*B*) A small calcified cyst (*small arrow*), likely an end-stage necrotic cysticerci. (*C*) A cyst (*small arrow*) similar to the cyst shown in (*A*) on an FLAIR-weighted view showing the associated inflammatory changes within the adjacent cortex and white matter.

On noncontrast CT scanning, an abscess in its early stages shows a lower density signal in its center, with surrounding vasogenic edema and mass effect. As time progresses, the edema and mass effect lessen. With contrast CT, the abscess rim is apparent, often appearing thicker closer to the cortex and thinner deeper in the brain parenchyma. As the capsule evolves, the abscess cavity grows smaller, and the rim thickens **Table 1**.

MRI is often helpful in further characterizing these lesions. T1-weighted views generally show a center of decreased signal relative to the surrounding white matter; the noncontrasted rim is isointense to hyperintense. T1 postcontrast views typical show a smooth enhancing rim. T2-weighted views show an isointense to hyperintense center with a hypointense rim. T2* or susceptibility-weighted imaging (SWI) generally does not suggest hemorrhage within the lesion (see **Table 1**).

Metastatic disease and glioblastoma multiforme can appear similar to brain abscesses on standard T1-weighted and T2-weighted sequences. However, neoplasms generally show thicker and more irregular walls compared with abscesses. Tumors are more likely to show hemorrhagic features, which are best seen as regions of markedly decreased signal on the T2* or susceptibility-weighted views. Abscesses generally produce high signal on diffusion-weighted sequences (DWI) and low apparent diffusion coefficient (ADC) values within the cystic cavity compared with what is generally low signal on diffusion views and high signal on ADC for necrotic or cystic tumors because of T2 shine through.[35,36]

However, there are several exceptions to this such as cysticercosis. These abscesses are generally isointense to mildly hyperintense on DWI, and high values on ADC and lymphoma caused by their high cellularity may show high DWI and decreased ADC values.

Some of the other lesions that may mimic abscesses on MRI scanning include tumefactive demyelinating disease, resolving intracerebral hemorrhage, and subacute infarctions. Tumefactive multiple sclerosis may show ring enhancement but this ring is often incomplete, opens toward the lateral ventricles, and does not have markedly bright signal on the diffusion-weighted views. An intracerebral hemorrhage shows blood products on the T2* or susceptibility-weighted views. Infarctions are typically localized to a vascular distribution.

When a brain abscess is suspected on imaging, the clinician should review the study for possible complications such as the formation of daughter abscesses, herniation,

Table 1
The temporal stages of abscess development in conjunction with the usual features on CT and MRI

Stage	NECT	CECT	T1WI	T2WI	DWI	T1C+
Early cerebritis 3–5 d	Ill defined Hypodense	Patchy enhancement	Poorly marginated Mixed hypointense/ isointense mass	Ill-defined hyperintense mass	Somewhat bright	Patchy enhancement
Late cerebritis 3 d to 2 wk	Central low density Peripheral edema Mass effect	Irregular rim enhancement	Hypointense center Isointense/ hyperintense rim	Hyperintense center Isointense rim Edema (hyperintense)	Somewhat bright	Intense but irregular rim enhancement
Early capsule >2 wk	Hypodense Moderate edema Mass effect	Low-density center Thin enhancing rim	Isointense/ hyperintense rim	Hypointense rim	Bright centrally	Well-defined, thin-walled enhancing rim
Late capsule Weeks to months	Less edema Less mass effect	Cavity smaller Capsule thicker	Cavity appears collapsed and capsule appears thick	Decrease edema and mass effect	Bright centrally	Cavity appears collapsed and capsule appears thick

Abbreviations: CECT, contrast-enhanced CT; DWI, diffusion-weighted imaging; NECT, nonenhanced CT; T1WI, T1-weighted imaging; T1C+, T1-weighted postcontrast; T2WI, T2-weighted imaging.

intraventricular rupture with ventriculitis, venous thrombosis, extra-axial fluid collections, and hydrocephalus.

Figs. 12 and **13** show the typical imaging feature of pyogenic cerebral abscesses. The lesions shown on CT and MRI were confirmed to be caused by *Fusobacterium*, which is a gram-negative anaerobic bacillus that likely resulted from periodontal disease in an otherwise healthy 36-year-old. These images show the typical noncontrast CT pattern of a cystic mass with a rim of increased density and adjacent prominent vasogenic edema, and MRI pattern of bright DWI signal, hypointense T2-weighted signal along the rim, and a rim with smooth margin of contrast enhancement.

Fig. 13 shows another pyogenic abscess as a result of *Nocaria*, which is gram-positive bacterium with fungal features. This infection is opportunistic and in this case developed in a 65-year-old with alcoholism and cirrhosis.

Fig. 14 shows a patient with 2 abscesses caused by toxoplasmosis in a patient with acquired immunodeficiency syndrome (AIDS).

The study shows a large abscess in the left basal ganglia and small abscess on the right with DWI signal within the abscess rim significantly less than adjacent unaffected

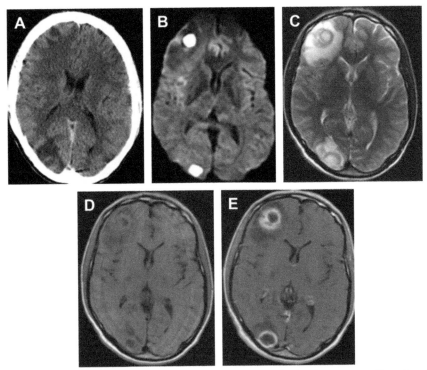

Fig. 12. (*A–E*) demonstrate a patient presenting with multiple abscesses confirmed to be Fusobacterium which is an anaerobic bacilli which likely resulted from periodontal disease in a young male. (*A*) CT noncontrast view showing the patient in the right frontal and the right occipital lobes with adjacent edema and a hyperdense rim. (*B*) Diffusion-weighted view showing the marked increased signal within the pyogenic infection. (*C*) T2-weighted view with the rim showing decreased T2-weighted signal with a perimeter of vasogenic edema and an essential area of increased signal. (*D, E*) T1-weighted views with and without contrast, respectively, showing a rim with increased T1-weighted signal on the noncontrast view and prominent contrast enhancement that is relatively smooth in (*E*), typical of an abscess.

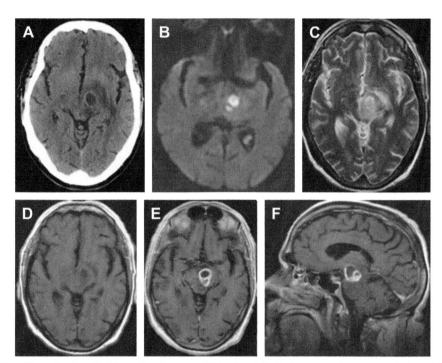

Fig. 13. patient with *Nocardia* abscess within the left thalamus and mesencephalon. (*A*) Noncontrast CT, again showing a rim with increased density compared to the core and adjacent vasogenic edema. (*B*) DWI view demonstrating the marked restricted diffusion within the pyogenic infection. (*C*) T2-weighted view. (*D–F*) T1-weighted views without and with contrast, respectively, depicting the smooth margin characteristic of a pyogenic infection. The lesion appears to be forming a satellite or daughter lesion, which is a common finding in *Nocardia* with its indolent development.

tissues. This pattern would not be expected in a pyogenic infection. Studies show that this is caused by the lack of purulent fluid within the necrotic center of this lesion.[36] The remainder of the imaging sequences appears near identical to a pyogenic infection. This pattern along with typically basal ganglia locations in an opportunistic host greatly help with the identification of this parasitic cause.

Encephalitis is a term that is generally used for viral infections of the brain. Herpes simplex encephalitis (herpes simplex virus [HSV]) is the most common lethal form in the United States, although it is treatable. Most cases are HSV-1, with a minority (predominately in neonates) HSV-2. Imaging findings typically involve the temporal lobes and ventral frontal lobes, at times bilaterally and occasional with insular and cingulate involvement.[37] Another treatable virus, Varicella zoster virus (VZV), presents as a meningoencephalitis, often with a vasculopathy, resulting in large and small vessel infarctions, vascular dissections, aneurysms, and intracranial hemorrhage.[37]

Fig. 15 shows a typical imaging presentation of a patient with HSV. The images show the increased DWI signal encompassing much of the left anterior and medial temporal lobe. The T2-weighted view shows the bright signal caused by the inflammation and edema from the acute infection. These lesions may or may now show contrast enhancement on initial presentation. If present, they tend to be gyriform, as in this case, and may show necrosis with hemorrhagic features best seen on the T2* or SWI views.

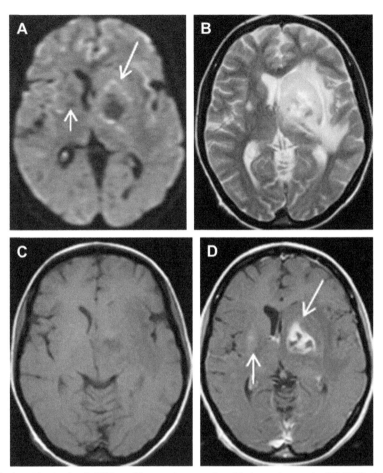

Fig. 14. A patient who is HIV positive and presents with toxoplasmosis. (*A*) DWI view that shows the decreased central diffusion signal with a perimeter of increased diffusion for these abscesses (*arrows*). Unlike pyogenic infections, some infections such as toxoplasmosis have necrotic centers that lack purulent fluid. They are nevertheless inflammatory, as shown in (*B*). The large left basal ganglion abscess shows marked increased signal and mass effect. (*C, D*) T1-weighted noncontrast and postcontrast views, respectively, showing the enhancing abscesses (*small arrows*).

INDOLENT INFECTIONS

HIV is another common neurotropic virus that produces indolent or latent encephalitis. Untreated, this can result in HIV encephalopathy or AIDS dementia complex, which on imaging shows cerebral atrophy with diffuse leukoencephalopathy and hydrocephalus ex vacuo. The leukoencephalopathy is thought to be caused by axonal degeneration. These changes result in symmetric periventricular and subcortical regions with increase T2-weighted signal best seen on T2-weighted and FLAIR-weighted views. **Fig. 16** shows a study of a 23-year-old woman with untreated AIDS and severe dementia. The images show severe cortical atrophy caused by neuronal loss and severe white matter disease.[38] JC virus is another latent neurotropic virus that develops as an opportunistic infection in immunocompromised individuals with AIDS, undergoing

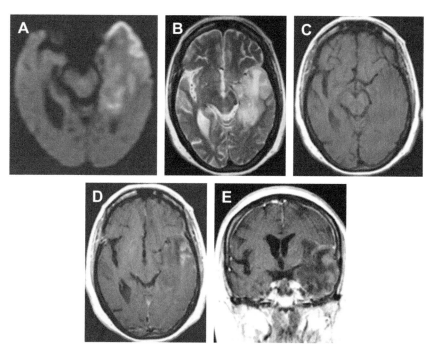

Fig. 15. A patient with acute herpes simplex encephalitis. (*A*) Diffusion-weighted view showing the marked increased signal along the cortical ribbon of the left medial anterior temporal lobe. (*B*) T2-weighted view showing increased signal in the region of the acute encephalitis with edema. (*C*) Noncontrast T1-weighted view showing a region of decreased signal that shows (*D, E*) enhancement along the cortical ribbon encircling the necrotizing encephalitis.

chemotherapy, or in treatment with natalizumab for multiple sclerosis or Crohn disease. This virus is associated with progressive multifocal leukoencephalopathy. These lesions can mimic demyelinating lesions and present as infiltrating focal white matter lesions with decreased density on CT and with increased signal on T2 and FLAIR

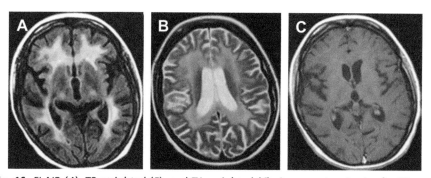

Fig. 16. FLAIR (*A*), T2-weighted (*B*), and T1-weighted (*C*) views, postcontrast, of a 23-year-old woman who presented with dementia. These views show severe cortical and subcortical volume loss along with severe diffuse white matter disease as a result of the untreated HIV virus, which is a neurotrophic virus.

studies, decreased T1 signal, and occasionally showing mild contrast enhancement and no mass effect.[34]

Creutzfeldt-Jakob disease is a spongiform encephalopathy and prion disease. It is a disorder that is best identified by MRI evaluation and in the proper clinical setting is pathognomonic. This disorder presents with evolving symmetric regions of high signal on DWI and FLAIR within the cortical ribbon, thalami, and basal ganglia. In the absence of a recent history of status epilepticus, anoxic encephalopathy, or acute viral encephalitis, which are disorders that can have similar MRI appearance, these imaging changes are considered pathognomonic.[39] **Fig. 17** shows a patient with sporadic Creutzfeldt-Jakob disease and shows the typical bright symmetric DWI signal within the thalami and throughout the cortical ribbon. In spite of imaging features that should be apparent to all neuroimaging specialists, the diagnosis is missed on two-thirds of radiology reports.[40]

Tuberculosis infections of the CNS are seen predominately in patients with immune compromise or in individuals after foreign travel, particularly to Asia and Africa. Its imaging characteristics range from basilar meningitis with thick nodular enhancing dural collections to, more rarely, tubercular abscesses in the brain parenchyma.[41] Hydrocephalus, cranial neuropathies, and vasculitis can result from the basilar meningitis. **Fig. 18** shows postcontrast T1-weighted views of a patient with CNS tuberculosis and HIV, and shows both nodular chronic basilar meningitis along the tentorium and sella region and small miliary abscesses.

Additional advanced imaging technologies, such as magnetic resonance (MR) perfusion and spectroscopy, can contribute to diagnosis accuracy. These techniques can aid in further distinguishing tumor from infection or infarctions. One important example of this is in patients with AIDS who present with subcortical mass lesions. Toxoplasmosis and lymphoma are the most common mass lesions in this patient population. These lesions can indistinguishable by standard CT and MRI imaging techniques in these patients. Studies show that lymphoma shows increased relative cerebral blood volume (rCBV) as a result of increased vascularity of the tumors, whereas toxoplasmosis abscesses have decreased rCBV and a lack of vascularization

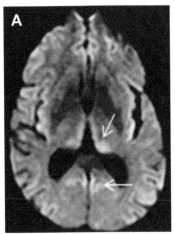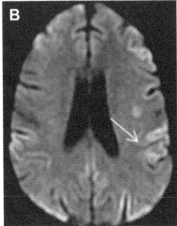

Fig. 17. (A, B) Diffusion-weighted views of a patient with sporadic Creutzfeldt-Jakob disease. The pulvinar sign (hockey-stick sign) showing the pulvinar (arrow). The increased DWI signal is present throughout the cortical ribbon (arrows).

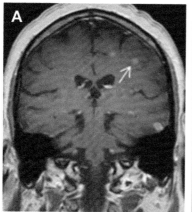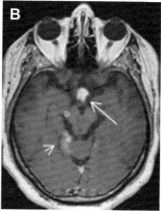

Fig. 18. Postcontrast T1-weighted coronal (*A*) and axial (*B*) views of a patient with AIDS, hepatitis, and tuberculosis. Small miliary abscesses of this indolent infection can be seen (*arrow in A*) along with basilar meningitis (*arrows in B*).

of the abscesses.[42,43] There is overlap on proton MR spectroscopic evaluation of lymphoma and toxoplasmosis for most metabolites; however, choline is generally significantly increased in lymphoma and decreased in toxoplasmosis.[44] Nuclear perfusion studies, including single-photon emission computed tomography or positron emission tomography can also be used to distinguish the decreased uptake in an abscess compared with a tumor typically showing increased uptake. CT perfusion is now widely available and should be similarly useful for these types of evaluations.[45]

SUMMARY

This article provides a brief overview of the imaging features for several commonly seen, and a few less commonly seen, CNS infections. More comprehensive reviews are available.[46–48]

It is incumbent on neurologists who provide acute care for patients to be completely familiar with the broad range of imaging findings with which patients with acute neurologic infections may present. They need to know what is the appropriate study in a given setting, the best protocol and views necessary to show the disorder, and they must be able to properly interpret them. This requirement applies particularly for CNS infections, as in stroke, in which a rapid appreciation of the exact cause of a patient's infection may play a major role in reducing mortality and morbidity.

REFERENCES

1. McKeever PE. Pathologic basis of central nervous system infections. Neuroimaging Clin N Am 2012;22:773–90.
2. Somand D, Meurer W. Central nervous system infections. Emerg Med Clin North Am 2009;27:89–100.
3. Riddell J, Shuman EK. Epidemiology of central nervous system infection. Neuroimaging Clin N Am 2012;22:543–56.
4. Akyldz BN, Gumus H, Kumandas S, et al. Diffusion-weighted magnetic resonance is better than polymerase chain reaction for early diagnosis of herpes simplex encephalitis: a case report. Pediatr Emerg Care 2008;24(6):377–9.

5. McCabe K, Tyler K, Tonobe J, et al. Diffusion-weighted MRI abnormalities as a clue to the diagnosis of herpes simplex encephalitis. Neurology 2003;61(7):1015–6.

6. Kimura-Hayama ET, Higuera JA, Corona-Cedillo R, et al. Neurocysticercosis; radiologic-pathologic correlation. Radiographics 2010;30:1705–19.

7. Noujaim SE, Rossi MD, Rao SK, et al. CT and MR imaging of neurocysticercosis. AJR Am J Roentgenol 1999;173:1485–90.

8. Zee CS, Go JL, Kim PE, et al. Imaging of neurocysticercosis. Neuroimaging Clin N Am 2000;10:391–407.

9. Ginier BL, Poirier VC. MR imaging of intraventricular cysticercosis. AJNR Am J Neuroradiol 1992;13:1247–8.

10. Kanamalla US, Ibarra RA, Jinkins JR. Imaging of cranial meningitis and ventriculitis. Neuroimaging Clin N Am 2000;10(2):309–31.

11. Leedom JM, Underman AE. Epidemiology of central nervous system infections. Neuroimaging Clin N Am 2008;10(2):297–308.

12. Rotbart HA. Viral meningitis. Semin Neurol 2000;20(3):277–92.

13. Mohan S, Jain KK, Arabi M, et al. Imaging of meningitis and ventriculitis. Neuroimaging Clin N Am 2012;22:557–83.

14. Quint DJ, Eldevik OP, Cohen JK. Magnetic resonance imaging of normal meningeal enhancement at 1.5 T. Acad Radiol 1996;6(3):463–8.

15. Smirniotopoulos JG, Murphy FM, Rushing EJ, et al. Patterns of contrast enhancement in the brain and meninges. Radiographics 2007;27(2):525–51.

16. Dietermann JL, Correia BR, Bogorin A, et al. Normal and abnormal meningeal enhancement: MRI features. J Radiol 2005;86(11):1659–83.

17. Kremer S, et al. Accuracy of delayed post-contrast FLAIR MR imaging for the diagnosis of leptomeningeal infectious or tumoral diseases. J Neuroradiol 2006;33(5):285–91.

18. Sage MR, Wilson AJ, Scroop R. Contrast media and the brain: the basis of CT and MR imaging enhancement. Neuroimaging Clin N Am 1998;8:695–707.

19. Mullins ME. Emergent neuroimaging of intracranial infection/inflammation. Radiol Clin North Am 2011;49:47–62.

20. Mylonakis E, Hohmann EL, Calderwood SB. Central nervous system infection with *Listeria monocytogenes*: 33 years' experience at a general hospital and review of 776 episodes from the literature. Medicine (Baltimore) 1998;77(5):313–36.

21. Faidas A, Shepard DL, Lim J, et al. Magnetic resonance imaging in listerial brain stem encephalitis. Clin Infect Dis 1993;16(1):186–7.

22. Bart R. Acute bacterial and viral meningitis. Continuum (Minneap Minn) 2012; 18(6):1255–70.

23. Kastenbauer S, Pfister HW. Pneumococcal meningitis in adults: spectrum of complications and prognostic factors in a series of 87 cases. Brain 2003;126(5): 1015–25.

24. Gwaltney JM. Acute community-acquired sinusitis. Clin Infect Dis 1996;23: 1209–25.

25. Durand M, Joseph M, Baker AN. Infections of the upper respiratory tract. In: Harrison's principles of internal medicine. 14th edition. 1998. p. 179–80.

26. Yousem DM. Imaging of sinonasal inflammatory disease. Radiology 1993;188: 303–14.

27. Vazquez E, Castellote A, Piqueras J, et al. Imaging of complications of acute mastoiditis in children. Radiographics 2003;23:359–72.

28. Hegde A, Mohan S, Pandya A, et al. Imaging in infections of the head and neck. Neuroimaging Clin N Am 2012;22:727–54.

29. Kapur R, Sepahdari AR, Mafee MF, et al. MR imaging of orbital inflammatory syndrome, orbital cellulitis, and orbital lymphoid lesions: the role of diffusion-weighted imaging. AJNR Am J Neuroradiol 2009;30:64–70.
30. Delfaut EM, Beltran J, Johnson G, et al. Fat suppression in MR imaging: techniques and pitfalls. Radiographics 1999;19:373–82.
31. Lerner A, Shiroishi MS, Zee C, et al. Imaging of neurocysticercosis. Neuroimaging Clin N Am 2012;22:659–76.
32. Del Brutto O. Neurocysticercosis. Continuum (Minneap Minn) 2012;18(6): 1392–416.
33. Razek AA, Watcharakorn A, Castillo M. Parasitic diseases of the central nervous system. Neuroimaging Clin N Am 2011;21:815–41.
34. Rath TJ, Hughes M, Arabi AM, et al. Imaging of cerebritis, encephalitis, and brain abscess. Neuroimaging Clin N Am 2012;22:585–607.
35. Ebisu T, Tanaka C, Umeda M, et al. Discrimination of brain abscess from necrotic or cystic tumors by diffusion-weighted imaging. Magn Reson Imaging 1996;14: 1113–6.
36. Falcon S, Post MJ. Encephalitis, cerebritis, and brain abscess: pathophysiology and imaging findings. Neuroimaging Clin N Am 2000;10(2):333–53.
37. Greenlee JE. Encephalitis in postinfectious encephalitis. Continuum (Minneap Minn) 2012;18(6):1271–89.
38. Kranick SM, Nath A. Neurologic complications of HIV-1 infection and its treatment in the era of antiretroviral therapy. Continuum (Minneap Minn) 2012;18(6): 1319–37.
39. Paterson RW, Torres-Chac CC, Kuo AL, et al. Differential diagnosis of Jakob-Creutzfeldt disease. Arch Neurol 2012;69(12):1578–82.
40. Geschwind MK, Kuryan C, Cattaruzza T, et al. Brain MRI and sporadic Jakob-Creutzfeldt disease is often misread [abstract]. Neurology 2010;74(9 Suppl 2).
41. Zunt JR, Balwin KJ. Chronic and subacute meningitis. Continuum (Minneap Minn) 2012;18(6):1290–318.
42. Ernst TM, Chang L, Witt MD, et al. Cerebral toxoplasmosis in lymphoma and AIDS: perfusion MRI imaging experience in 13 patients. Radiology 1998;208: 663–89.
43. Batra A, Tripathi RP, Gorthi SP. Magnetic resonance evaluation of cerebral toxoplasmosis in patients with acquired immunodeficiency syndrome. Acta Radiol 2004;45(2):212–21.
44. Chang L, Miller BL, McBride D, et al. Brain lesions in patients with AIDS, H-1 MRI spectroscopy. Radiology 1995;197:525–31.
45. Jain R. Perfusion CT imaging of brain tumors: an overview. AJNR Am J Neuroradiol 2011;32(9):1570–7.
46. Shah G. Central nervous system infections. Neuroimaging Clin N Am 2012; 22(4):xiii.
47. Scheld WM, Whitley RJ, Marra CM. Infections of the central nervous system. 3rd edition. Philadelphia: Lippincott Williams & Wilkins; 2004.
48. Gupta RK, Lufkin RB. MR imaging and spectroscopy of central nervous system infection. New York: Kluwer Academic/Plenum; 2001.

Imaging of Cancer Therapy-Induced Central Nervous System Toxicity

Jörg Dietrich, MD, PhD[a],*, Joshua P. Klein, MD, PhD[b],*

KEYWORDS

- Neurotoxicity • Cancer • Chemotherapy • Radiation therapy
- Central nervous system • Imaging

KEY POINTS

- Cancer treatment–related neurotoxicity can occur in patients with both central nervous system and non-central nervous system cancers, and clinical symptoms are nonspecific.
- On structural imaging techniques, such as computed tomography and magnetic resonance imaging, distinguishing volume gain versus volume loss can be helpful in differentiating edema, inflammation, and tumor growth from gliosis, necrosis, and atrophy.
- Comparison of a current imaging study with recent and more remote prior imaging is crucial for recognizing subtle changes that occur over time.
- Radiation necrosis, leukoencephalopathy, hydrocephalus, and ischemic and hemorrhagic vascular events can occur with highly variable delay following treatment.
- Perfusion imaging and positron emission tomography can potentially help differentiate tumor progression versus necrosis and leukoencephalopathy, and functional magnetic resonance imaging can be helpful in surgical planning.
- Recent advanced imaging research studies in patients with cancer have provided novel insights into the cause of cognitive impairment and other neurotoxic syndromes in patients with cancer.

INTRODUCTION

Cancer therapies can cause a wide range of acute and delayed treatment complications involving the central nervous system (CNS),[1,2] causing significant morbidity and mortality. Notably, these syndromes occur not only in patients with brain tumors but

[a] Division of Neuro-Oncology, Department of Neurology, Massachusetts General Hospital Cancer Center, Center for Regenerative Medicine, Harvard Medical School, 55 Fruit Street, Yawkey 9E, Boston, MA 02114, USA; [b] Department of Neurology, Brigham and Women's Hospital, Harvard Medical School, Room AB-124, 75 Francis Street, Boston, MA 02115, USA
* Corresponding author.
E-mail addresses: Dietrich.Jorg@mgh.harvard.edu; jpklein@partners.org

Neurol Clin 32 (2014) 147–157
http://dx.doi.org/10.1016/j.ncl.2013.07.004
0733-8619/14/$ – see front matter © 2014 Elsevier Inc. All rights reserved.
neurologic.theclinics.com

also in patients treated for cancer outside the CNS, such as systemic lymphoma, breast, and lung cancer.[3] With improved survival rates in patients with cancer and more aggressive and combined treatment modalities, neurologic treatment complications have been observed with increasing frequency. The clinical presentation of patients experiencing neurotoxicity is commonly nonspecific. Therefore, the diagnosis of neurotoxic syndromes often poses a major challenge to the treating physician. However, recognition of treatment-related neurologic complications is critically important to avoid unnecessary procedures, such as brain biopsy and lumbar puncture, and because symptoms may be confused with metastatic disease, tumor progression, paraneoplastic disorders, and infections of the CNS. Neuroimaging, including computed tomography (CT), magnetic resonance imaging (MRI), and positron emission tomography (PET), is an important diagnostic tool in patient evaluation and guidance of patient management. Moreover, advanced neuroimaging techniques with resting state and diffusion tensor MRI and functional MRI (fMRI) have most recently provided compelling evidence that both structural and functional brain changes occur in a substantial number of patients with cancer treated with chemotherapy and radiation.

In this review various imaging techniques and modalities that can be used in patients with cancer with suspected neurotoxic syndromes are highlighted and advantages and limitations of each imaging modality in the context of classical neurotoxic syndromes encountered in patients with cancer are discussed.

CT IN THE ASSESSMENT OF CANCER THERAPY–ASSOCIATED NEUROTOXIC SYNDROMES

CT is a technique that measures the attenuation of X-rays by different substances. Higher density materials absorb more x-rays than lower density materials and thus appear brighter (whiter). Two-dimensional images are reconstructed to display cross-sectional anatomy, and these individual images can be stacked so that one can view sequential images and appreciate the 3-dimensional contours of normal and abnormal structures. CT images can be acquired in any plane; for the brain, images are typically acquired in horizontal slices from the skull base to vertex. Slice thickness is variable, but most often approximately 5 mm per slice. Reformatted images in orthogonal planes (ie, coronal and sagittal) can be very useful in characterizing lesions. CT contrast is iodine-based; enhancement following contrast administration is seen in vascular structures and at sites of disruption of the blood-brain barrier.

The appearance of tumor on CT, as well as the effects of its treatment, depends on many variables. The contents of the tumor and the presence of surrounding edema, hemorrhage, necrosis, and postsurgical changes attenuate radiographs to a different extent. The degree of attenuation is measured on a scale of Hounsfield units (HU), which ranges from -1000 (air) to 0 (water) to $+1000$ (dense bone or metal). Intracranially, cerebrospinal fluid (CSF) measures about 15 HU; white matter measures 20 to 30 HU, and gray matter measures 35 to 45 (HU). Fat, as in myelin, does not strongly attenuate radiographs and has an HU range of -30 to -70; thus, white matter appears darker than gray matter. Vasogenic edema in tissue appears dark on CT because water has a lower Hounsfield unit value than normal brain tissue. Vasogenic edema will most often be associated with local or regional mass effect. Subtle evidence of mass effect includes effacement of cortical sulci and compression of ventricles. With more severe mass effect, loss of gray-white matter differentiation and herniation of brain tissue is seen.

Gliotic and necrotic tissue also appears hypodense compared with normal brain. Differentiation between vasogenic edema and gliosis or necrosis relies on assessment of whether there is associated volume gain (ie, mass effect from edema) versus volume loss (ie, tissue destruction). These 2 opposing effects are often seen on the same image and cannot easily be distinguished (**Fig. 1**). Comparison to prior scans, if available, can help assess for interval volume gain or loss. To further complicate matters, CT cannot differentiate edema clearly from infiltrating tumors such as low-grade glioma or lymphoma.

Hydrocephalus is an important imaging finding to recognize and occurs in 3 forms. With obstruction of ventricular outflow (noncommunicating hydrocephalus) or obstruction of CSF drainage into the venous circulation via arachnoid granulations (communicating hydrocephalus), there is elevated intracranial pressure. With cerebral atrophy and gliosis, ex vacuo ventricular dilatation occurs, and intracranial pressure may or may not be elevated. On CT, ventricular expansion with effacement of overlying cortical sulci is suggestive of noncommunicating hydrocephalus, and the most

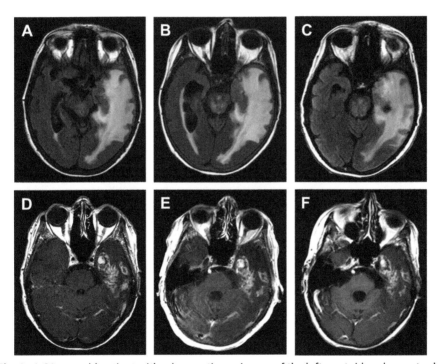

Fig. 1. A 64-year-old patient with adenocystic carcinoma of the left mastoid underwent subtotal tumor resection and subsequent proton beam radiation. Several years later, axial brain MRI showed extensive abnormal T2 hyperintensity extending throughout the white matter of the left hemisphere (*A*) with irregular enhancement within the left temporal lobe (*D*). Several months later, the patient suffered a seizure and repeat imaging showed interval development of hydrocephalus, seen here as expansion of the right lateral ventricle (*B*). There was no change in the pattern or extent of enhancement at this time (*E*). Placement of a ventricular shunt relieved the hydrocephalus as seen on MRI several weeks later (*C*). Again, there was no change in the pattern or extent of enhancement (*F*). The imaging findings are consistent with radiation necrosis and leukoencephalopathy, rather than tumor progression.

common sites of obstruction are where the conduits of intraventricular CSF flow are narrowest (ie, the cerebral aqueduct). Ventriculomegaly in proportion to widening of the overlying cortical sulci is more suggestive of an ex vacuo effect. In patients who have undergone combinations of surgical resection, chemotherapy, and radiation, the combined and opposing elements of volume loss and edema can produce various types of hydrocephalus (see **Fig. 1**). As always, careful comparison with prior scans and correlation with clinical symptoms are essential.

Despite these limitations, there are, in general, 3 settings in which imaging with CT may be a useful modality for patients with underlying cancer or known brain tumors: (1) with an abrupt change in neurologic examination, a CT can quickly and accurately assess for acute hemorrhage, herniation, or hydrocephalus; (2) if there is tumor extension into bone or if a tumor lies adjacent to bone, CT can be helpful to precisely delineate the margins of involvement and to assess for bony destruction (**Fig. 2**); (3) if a patient cannot undergo MRI because of metallic devices or some other reason, CT

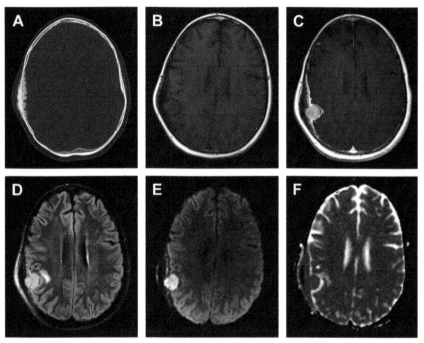

Fig. 2. A 27-year-old patient with a history of childhood acute lymphoblastic leukemia treated with methotrexate-based chemotherapy and later with prophylactic cranial radiation presented with a painless bump on his right parietal scalp more than 15 years after initial treatment. CT revealed a focus of hyperostotic irregular bone in the right parietal skull. (A) Axial T1 MRI before (B) and after (C) gadolinium contrast administration revealed a round and homogenously enhancing mass arising from the right parietal dura with a dural tail. Axial T2-FLAIR (fluid attenuation inversion recovery) MRI (D) showed displacement of underlying right parietal cortex, with abnormal T2 hyperintensity in the subcortical white matter. Hyperintensity on diffusion-weighted MRI (E) and corresponding hypointensity on apparent diffusion coefficient maps (F), consistent with reduced diffusivity, is a marker of the hypercellularity of the mass, which was found to be a World Health Organization II meningioma and was treated with resection and adjuvant radiation. Meningiomas can arise as a complication from remote radiation therapy.[4]

with contrast and supplementary techniques such as CT perfusion and PET can be used to characterize a tumor and its treatment response.

CT is highly sensitive for detecting hemorrhage, and acute hemorrhage and thrombus will appear hyperdense, typically at 60 to 80 HU. Blood becomes less hyperdense as it ages. Acute ischemia and infarction produce loss of gray-to-white matter differentiation and edema of involved tissue. Embolic or thrombotic occlusions of arteries and arterioles will most often produce wedge-shaped regions of hypodensity in corresponding arterial vascular distributions. Microvascular infarcts as seen with advanced atherosclerosis and lipohyalinosis following cranial radiation can occur in brain areas supplied by these tiny arteries, most often the basal ganglia and pons. Ischemic lesions disrupt the blood-brain barrier and will often enhance with contrast. Likewise, radiation necrosis is also commonly associated with abnormal contrast enhancement. This enhancement can be easily mistaken for tumor progression or recurrence and other imaging modalities can help differentiate these entities. Non-enhancing diffuse hypodensity within the cerebral white matter may indicate leuko-encephalopathy and is better evaluated on MRI. Venous hypertension resulting from obstruction of a cortical vein or venous sinus can produce a venous infarct, which does not respect arterial vascular distributions and often has a disproportionate amount of edema and sometimes hemorrhage.

MRI IN THE ASSESSMENT OF CANCER THERAPY–ASSOCIATED NEUROTOXIC SYNDROMES

MRI is obtained by aligning the natural atomic rotations of water molecules in the body within a strong magnetic field and superimposing brief radiofrequency pulses, to momentarily disalign their rotations. The manner in which molecules recover to their former alignment depends on the constituency of the tissue in which they are found and is what produces signal that can be reconstructed into images.

For assessing the neurotoxic effects of cancer therapy, MRI is usually preferred over CT, because MRI is more sensitive to detecting changes both in the microenvironment surrounding a resection cavity and in brain structures that may be remote from a tumor but that have been exposed to radiation or chemotherapy. With MRI, the effects of cancer therapy can be assessed both structurally and functionally. Routine structural MRI essentially includes T1-weighted, T2-weighted, diffusion-weighted, and susceptibility-weighted sequences.

With structural MRI, the principle of volume gain versus volume loss is the same as described for CT (**Fig. 3**). On T1-weighted sequences, white matter appears hyperintense (whiter) to gray matter because fat causes T1 shortening. Edema appears hypointense to normal white matter due to T1 prolongation of water within tissue. On T2-weighted sequences, white matter appears hypointense to gray matter because fat causes faster T2 signal decay. Edema appears hyperintense to normal white matter due to T2 prolongation of water within tissue (**Fig. 4**). Abnormal T2 prolongation is also seen in radiation-induced leukoencephalopathy and gliosis (see **Figs. 1** and **3**), which are commonly seen as delayed complication of CNS radiation therapy months to years after treatment.[5–7]

Diffusion-weighted imaging measures the ability of water molecules to diffuse freely within tissue. Restricted diffusion is seen in several scenarios including acute cytotoxic edema (ie, ischemic stroke), hypercellular tumors, and abscesses. Vasogenic edema, leukoencephalopathy,[2] and gliosis are more often associated with elevated diffusivity, the "T2 shine-through" phenomenon. The appearance of hemorrhage on MRI depends on the state of decomposition of hemoglobin[8] and can be

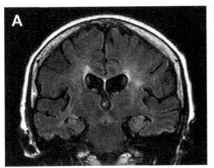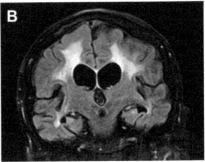

Fig. 3. A 66-year-old patient with a history of carcinoid lung cancer treated with lobectomy and adjuvant radiation and cisplatin-based chemotherapy, as well as prophylactic cranial radiation, presented several years later with progressive gait difficulties and cognitive decline. Coronal T2/FLAIR MRI at the time of cranial radiation (A) and at the time of re-presentation (B) show interval development of extensive abnormal T2 hyperintensity throughout the bi-hemispheric white matter, with loss of white matter volume and ex vacuo ventricular dilatation. There was no abnormal enhancement. The imaging findings are consistent with delayed leukoencephalopathy.

seen with tumor necrosis, radiation necrosis, primary hemorrhage, and hemorrhagic infarction (arterial and venous). Specialized sequences such as gradient echo and susceptibility-weighted imaging can detect microhemorrhages that are too small to be seen on T1-weighted and T2-weighted sequences. The added sensitivity of the gradient echo and susceptibility-weighted imaging sequences is due to "blooming artifact," which causes microhemorrhages to appear slightly larger than their true size.

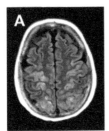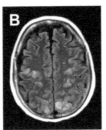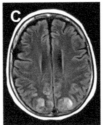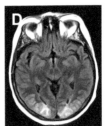

Fig. 4. A 58-year-old patient with multiple myeloma was treated with cyclophosphamide and dexamethasone, and after recurrence, underwent additional chemotherapy followed by autologous stem cell transplantation. The patient continued to have disease progression and was started on a proteasome inhibitor. Two days after infusion, the patient developed a headache, then blurred vision, and then had a generalized seizure. Axial T2-FLAIR MRI revealed multiple foci of abnormal T2 hyperintensity within the bilateral frontoparietal (A, B) and occipital (C, D) subcortical white matter and overlying gray matter, with cortical sulcal effacement. There was no abnormal enhancement or hemorrhage. These findings are consistent with posterior reversible leukoencephalopathy syndrome.[27,28] Of note, the patient was never found to be hypertensive and had no abrupt changes in blood pressure. The proteasome inhibitor was discontinued and symptoms improved over the next few weeks. Many cytotoxic immunosuppressant medications have been associated with posterior reversible leukoencephalopathy syndrome, including cyclosporin, tacrolimus, sirolimus, cisplatin, and bevacizumab.[3]

Like CT, contrast enhancement on MRI is seen in vascular structures and at sites of blood-brain barrier disruption. Increase or decrease in enhancement following specific therapies does not necessarily reflect tumor progression, which may complicate the interpretation of imaging findings in patients with cancer; instead, they may simply reflect changes in blood-brain barrier permeability, which is affected by both tumor and treatment. The phenomena of "pseudoprogression" and "pseudoresponse" have been described to bring attention to this potentially confounding aspect of image interpretation, which has been studied most extensively in glioblastoma.[9,10]

The principles of recognizing hydrocephalus are the same on MRI as on CT (see **Figs. 1** and **3**). With noncommunicating hydrocephalus, the additional finding of trans-ependymal flow of CSF appears as smooth "caps" of uniform and confluent abnormal T2 hyperintensity within the periventricular white matter. Also, like CT, radiation necrosis can induce variable edema as well as abnormal enhancement (**Figs. 5** and **6**).

FUNCTIONAL IMAGING IN THE ASSESSMENT OF CANCER THERAPY–ASSOCIATED NEUROTOXIC SYNDROMES

Advanced imaging modalities, such as perfusion imaging, PET, and fMRI, are being used with increasing frequency to assess tumors and their response to treatment. Perfusion imaging can be performed with both CT and MRI. The technique usually requires an infusion of contrast and measurement of changes in enhancement of tissue as contrast transits through it. A time-intensity curve is created, from which the interdependent measurements of blood volume, blood flow, and transit time can be calculated. Highly vascular tumors will demonstrate elevated blood volume, whereas necrotic or ischemic tissue will demonstrate reduced blood flow (ischemic) versus reduced blood volume (infarcted or necrotic).[11] This technique is particularly useful for assessing abnormal posttreatment enhancement that can occur as a result of both tumor recurrence or radiation necrosis.

The PET technique can be used to study cellular metabolism and pharmacology by generating a map of positron-emitting-radioisotope-labeled biomolecules in living tissues. In oncology, the radioisotope [18F]fluoro-deoxyglucose (FDG) is commonly used to measure glucose uptake as a surrogate marker of cellular metabolism. Highly metabolically active tissues such as the cerebral cortex have intrinsically high glucose

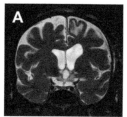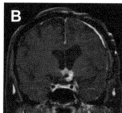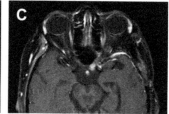

Fig. 5. A 65-year-old patient with melanoma metastatic to the left frontal lobe underwent resection and proton beam stereotactic radiosurgery and brachytherapy. The patient developed progressive loss of vision in the left and right eye several years after radiation therapy. Coronal T2 MRI revealed abnormal hyperintensity in the left greater than right optic chiasm as well as the pituitary infundibulum and inferior basal ganglia on the left (A). Coronal (B) and axial (C) T1 MRI following gadolinium contrast administration showed abnormal enhancement of the left optic chiasm and nerve. These findings are consistent with radiation-induced optic neuropathy.[29] The patient was initially treated with dexamethasone and later bevacizumab, with clinical and radiographic stabilization.

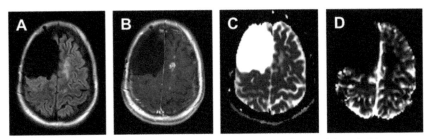

Fig. 6. A 23-year-old patient underwent resection of a right frontal lobe glioblastoma with adjuvant standard radiation and temozolomide. Subsequent brain imaging 3 to 4 years later revealed a large right frontal lobe resection cavity with interval development of multifocal areas of abnormal T2 hyperintensity (*A*) in the left frontal lobe with irregular enhancement on T1 postgadolinium MRI (*B*). There was no evidence of abnormal reduced diffusivity (hypointensity) on apparent diffusion coefficient maps (*C*), and no abnormal elevated blood volume (hyperintensity) on MR perfusion (*D*). These lesions have remained largely stable on subsequent imaging over 2 to 3 years, consistent with delayed radiation necrosis, rather than tumor recurrence.

utilization. Rapidly growing tumors can demonstrate elevated glucose utilization as well. PET can be coregistered with structural images acquired from CT and MRI, and in this setting, the metabolic state of a mass lesion can be assessed. Hypermetabolism suggests malignancy, whereas hypometabolism may represent necrosis or nonneoplastic inflammation.[12]

fMRI is used in surgical planning for tumors in or adjacent to eloquent areas of brain; fMRI signal generation is based on the concept of neurovascular coupling, whereby elevated local cerebral blood flow occurs in response to elevated activity of a population of neurons. Blood-oxygen–dependent changes are detected by comparing blood flow before and during a specific task. Motor, sensory, visual, and language areas of the brain can often be precisely localized, and the proximity of these areas to a tumor can be helpful in assessing the risk of tumor resection.

EMERGING IMAGING TECHNIQUES AND FUTURE DIRECTIONS IN CANCER THERAPY–ASSOCIATED NEUROTOXICITY

Several recent research studies using MRI, fMRI, and PET in the assessment of cancer therapy–associated neurotoxicity have provided evidence that structural and functional CNS changes occur in a significant number of patients with cancer treated with systemic chemotherapy.[13–16] For instance, structural MRI studies in patients with breast cancer treated with chemotherapy have revealed decreased regional volumes of gray and white matter, including the prefrontal and parahippocampal areas.[17] Consistent with these findings, recent MRI studies in a similar patient population identified reduction in overall brain volume,[18] and specifically in frontal, temporal, and cerebellar cortex in patients examined longitudinally before and after chemotherapy.[19]

Using diffusion tensor imaging, an MRI-based technique that makes vector-based, or directional, measurements of reduced diffusivity to reconstruct maps of white matter tracts, white matter damage related to systemic chemotherapy has been demonstrated.[13,20–22] In addition, a small number of recent fMRI studies supports the notion that systemic chemotherapy-induced cognitive impairment and decreased executive function correlates with regionally altered brain function.[23–25]

A functional imaging study using [15O] water and [18F]FDG-PET in a cohort of breast cancer survivors treated with tamoxifen-based chemotherapy 5 to 10 years before identified alterations in frontocortical, cerebellar, and basal ganglia metabolism.[26] Reduced resting glucose metabolism in inferior-frontal brain regions correlated with impaired short-term memory function. However, the lack of imaging data before chemotherapy was one of the major limitations of this study.

As this field of investigation is rapidly expanding, ongoing and future imaging research studies are likely to reveal novel biomarkers of neurotoxicity that will allow identification of patients with highest risk to develop neurotoxic syndromes as the consequence of their cancer treatment. Collectively, advanced imaging studies have identified both structural and functional brain changes as a consequence of cancer therapy, therefore challenging the previous dogma that the adult CNS is largely resistant to the toxic effects of systemic chemotherapy. With a growing understanding of the effects of chemotherapy and radiation in the brain, future clinical trials in patients with cancer are therefore expected to increasingly incorporate advanced imaging modalities along with other biomarker studies (eg, genetic, epigenetic, and metabolic) to assess and predict treatment-related neurotoxicity. In addition, steadily expanding knowledge about imaging biomarkers of neurotoxicity will facilitate identification and validation of neuroprotective strategies with the overall goal of improved management and quality of life of patients with cancer.

ACKNOWLEDGMENTS

The authors gratefully acknowledge the support of the American Academy of Neurology Foundation (J. Dietrich), the American Cancer Society (J. Dietrich), and the Stephen E. and Catherine Pappas Center Research Foundation (J. Dietrich). J. Dietrich is a Fellow of the Clinical Investigator Training Program (CITP) at Harvard Medical School.

REFERENCES

1. Dietrich J, Monje M, Wefel J, et al. Clinical patterns and biological correlates of cognitive dysfunction associated with cancer therapy. Oncologist 2008;13: 1285–95.
2. Arrillaga-Romany I, Dietrich J. Imaging findings in cancer therapy-associated neurotoxicity. Semin Neurol 2012;32:476–86.
3. Dietrich J, Wen P. Neurologic complications of chemotherapy. In: Schiff D, Kesari S, Wen P, editors. Cancer neurology in clinical practice. Totowa (NJ): Humana Press Inc; 2008. p. 287–326.
4. Galloway TJ, Indelicato DJ, Amdur RJ, et al. Second tumors in pediatric patients treated with radiotherapy to the central nervous system. Am J Clin Oncol 2012;35: 279–83.
5. Wang YX, King AD, Zhou H, et al. Evolution of radiation-induced brain injury: MR imaging-based study. Radiology 2010;254:210–8.
6. Rahmathulla G, Marko NF, Weil RJ. Cerebral radiation necrosis: a review of the pathobiology, diagnosis and management considerations. J Clin Neurosci 2013;20(4):485–502.
7. Yoshii Y. Pathological review of late cerebral radionecrosis. Brain Tumor Pathol 2008;25:51–8.
8. Bradley WG Jr. MR appearance of hemorrhage in the brain. Radiology 1993;189: 15–26.
9. Hygino da Cruz LC Jr, Rodriguez I, Domingues RC, et al. Pseudoprogression and pseudoresponse: imaging challenges in the assessment of posttreatment glioma. AJNR Am J Neuroradiol 2011;32:1978–85.

10. Tanaka S, Louis DN, Curry WT, et al. Diagnostic and therapeutic avenues for glioblastoma: no longer a dead end? Nat Rev Clin Oncol 2013;10:14–26.

11. Hu LS, Baxter LC, Smith KA, et al. Relative cerebral blood volume values to differentiate high-grade glioma recurrence from posttreatment radiation effect: direct correlation between image-guided tissue histopathology and localized dynamic susceptibility-weighted contrast-enhanced perfusion MR imaging measurements. AJNR Am J Neuroradiol 2009;30:552–8.

12. Chao ST, Suh JH, Raja S, et al. The sensitivity and specificity of FDG PET in distinguishing recurrent brain tumor from radionecrosis in patients treated with stereotactic radiosurgery. Int J Cancer 2001;96:191–7.

13. Deprez S, Amant F, Smeets A, et al. Longitudinal assessment of chemotherapy-induced structural changes in cerebral white matter and its correlation with impaired cognitive functioning. J Clin Oncol 2012;30:274–81.

14. Koppelmans V, Breteler MM, Boogerd W, et al. Neuropsychological performance in survivors of breast cancer more than 20 years after adjuvant chemotherapy. J Clin Oncol 2012;30:1080–6.

15. McDonald BC, Conroy SK, Ahles TA, et al. Alterations in brain activation during working memory processing associated with breast cancer and treatment: a prospective functional magnetic resonance imaging study. J Clin Oncol 2012; 30:2500–8.

16. McDonald BC, Conroy SK, Smith DJ, et al. Frontal gray matter reduction after breast cancer chemotherapy and association with executive symptoms: a replication and extension study. Brain Behav Immun 2013;30(Suppl): S117–25.

17. Inagaki M, Yoshikawa E, Matsuoka Y, et al. Smaller regional volumes of brain gray and white matter demonstrated in breast cancer survivors exposed to adjuvant chemotherapy. Cancer 2007;109:146–56.

18. Koppelmans V, de Ruiter MB, van der Lijn F, et al. Global and focal brain volume in long-term breast cancer survivors exposed to adjuvant chemotherapy. Breast Cancer Res Treat 2012;132:1099–106.

19. McDonald BC, Conroy SK, Ahles TA, et al. Gray matter reduction associated with systemic chemotherapy for breast cancer: a prospective MRI study. Breast Cancer Res Treat 2010;123:819–28.

20. Abraham J, Haut MW, Moran MT, et al. Adjuvant chemotherapy for breast cancer: effects on cerebral white matter seen in diffusion tensor imaging. Clin Breast Cancer 2008;8:88–91.

21. de Ruiter MB, Reneman L, Boogerd W, et al. Cerebral hyporesponsiveness and cognitive impairment 10 years after chemotherapy for breast cancer. Hum Brain Mapp 2011;32:1206–19.

22. Deprez S, Amant F, Yigit R, et al. Chemotherapy-induced structural changes in cerebral white matter and its correlation with impaired cognitive functioning in breast cancer patients. Hum Brain Mapp 2011;32:480–93.

23. Ferguson RJ, McDonald BC, Saykin AJ, et al. Brain structure and function differences in monozygotic twins: possible effects of breast cancer chemotherapy. J Clin Oncol 2007;25:3866–70.

24. Kesler SR, Bennett FC, Mahaffey ML, et al. Regional brain activation during verbal declarative memory in metastatic breast cancer. Clin Cancer Res 2009; 15:6665–73.

25. Kesler SR, Kent JS, O'Hara R. Prefrontal cortex and executive function impairments in primary breast cancer. Arch Neurol 2011;68:1447–53.

26. Silverman DH, Dy CJ, Castellon SA, et al. Altered frontocortical, cerebellar, and basal ganglia activity in adjuvant-treated breast cancer survivors 5-10 years after chemotherapy. Breast Cancer Res Treat 2007;103:303–11.

27. Bartynski WS, Boardman JF. Distinct imaging patterns and lesion distribution in posterior reversible encephalopathy syndrome. AJNR Am J Neuroradiol 2007; 28:1320–7.

28. Marinella MA, Markert RJ. Reversible posterior leucoencephalopathy syndrome associated with anticancer drugs. Intern Med J 2009;39:826–34.

29. Zhao Z, Lan Y, Bai S, et al. Late-onset radiation-induced optic neuropathy after radiotherapy for nasopharyngeal carcinoma. J Clin Neurosci 2013;20(5):702–6.

Neuroimaging of Neurocutaneous Diseases

Kaveer Nandigam, MD[a,b,*], Laszlo L. Mechtler, MD[b],
James G. Smirniotopoulos, MD[c]

KEYWORDS

- Neuroimaging • Neurocutaneous diseases • Neurofibromatosis • Schwannomatosis
- Tuberous sclerosis • von Hippel-Lindau • Sturge-Weber • Lhermitte-Duclos

KEY POINTS

- An in-depth knowledge of the imaging characteristics of the common neurocutaneous diseases (NCD) described in this article will help a neurologist understand the screening imaging modalities in patients with NCD.
- A neuroimager should be able to look for an associated neuroimaging stigmata in specific anatomic areas commonly involved, such as optic pathways in patients with neurofibromatosis type 1 to rule out optic pathway gliomas or high-resolution internal auditory canal images to rule out vestibular schwannomas.
- The detection of tumors and masses in NCD has greatly benefitted with improved availability of high-field strength 3T magnetic resonance imaging (MRI) machines in the past few years.
- Predicting cognitive impairment early on in children with NCS using imaging techniques, such as functional MRI, is not in the distant future.
- Neuroimaging will remain at the heart and soul of the multidisciplinary care of such complex diagnoses to guide early detection and monitor treatment.

INTRODUCTION

The neurocutaneous diseases (NCD) embrace an extensive group of developmental disorders with involvement of skin and central and/or peripheral nervous systems. The term *phakomatosis* was originally used by Jan Van der Hoeve[1] (an ophthalmologist) in 1933 to encompass the 3 known NCD at the time, known by their eponyms: Bourneville disease (tuberous sclerosis), Recklinghausen (neurofibromatosis type 1 [NF1]), and von Hippel-Lindau disease (VHL), referring to the lentiform retinal lesions (hamartomas) commonly seen in these 3 conditions. The subsequent inclusion of Sturge-Weber syndrome (SWS) in this group made this term less appropriate because

[a] Neurology and Stroke Associates, 640 E Oregon Rd, Lititz, Lancaster, PA, USA; [b] Dent Neurological Institute, Buffalo, NY, USA; [c] Uniformed Services University, Bethesda, MD, USA
* Corresponding author.
E-mail address: Kaveer@gmail.com

Neurol Clin 32 (2014) 159–192
http://dx.doi.org/10.1016/j.ncl.2013.07.003
0733-8619/14/$ – see front matter Published by Elsevier Inc.

neurologic.theclinics.com

it was not associated with similar retinal lesions, necessitating the introduction of the term *neurocutaneous syndromes*.[2] Over the years, not less than 60 such NCD have been described.[3] Apart from the 5 common conditions with pathognomonic neuroimaging findings, namely, NF1, neurofibromatosis type 2 (NF2), tuberous sclerosis complex (TSC), VHL, and SWS, the other described NCD are quite rare; the associated neuroimaging stigmata are often nonspecific. The pathologic features in NCD are either caused by problems related to neural crest cells migration and terminal differentiation or from tumor-suppressor gene dysfunction; both of these processes are genetically regulated. The diagnostic criteria and extensive clinicopathologic features of these conditions have been described in many reference texts.[3] The emphasis of this article is primarily on neuroimaging characteristics of the common NCD and appropriate use of advanced imaging for the diagnosis and monitoring of these conditions.

NF1 (VON RECKLINGHAUSEN DISEASE)

NF1 is the most frequent of the NCDs, although age-dependent presentation, clinical variability, and increased mortality in adulthood make it difficult to obtain precise population-based prevalence estimates. A 1956 population survey among Michigan residents showed an estimated incidence at birth of 30 to 40 cases per 100 000,[4] which was similar to that reported in a more recent German study among elementary school children, with an estimated incidence of 30 to 38 cases per 100 000 live births.[5] Moreover, it was demonstrated that NF1 can be diagnosed by 6 years of age in most cases by routine physical examination with special attention to the disease-associated skin stigmata. About 50% of cases are autosomal dominant, with virtually 100% penetrance by adulthood,[6] and the rest resulting from de novo germline mutations in the NF1 gene located at chromosome17qll.2, which encodes for a negative regulator of the RAS oncogene, neurofibromin.[7] About 90% of new mutations occur on the paternally derived chromosome.[8] Some of the clinical features seen in NF1 are attributed to neural crest dysfunction, such as café au lait macules secondary to abnormal melanocyte differentiation from the rhombencephalic neural crest, and an increased incidence of hypertelorism caused by incomplete formation of the intercanthal ligament caused by the involvement of prosencephalic neural crest derivatives. Subcutaneous connective tissue, including adipocytes, and Schwann cell tumors are also, in part, caused by prosencephalic neural crest dysfunction, although impaired tumor-suppressor gene function predisposes to neoplasia. The median age at death for patients with NF1 was 59 years on a review of US death certificates from 1983 to 1997.[9] Another analysis found about 50% of patients with NF1 can expect to live beyond 71 years of age,[10] with the main causes of early mortality directly attributed to the increased incidence of malignant neoplasms, especially the malignant peripheral nerve sheath tumor (MPNST) and glioma. Because there are no preventative treatments available, the primary strategy to prolong life expectancy in NF1 is ostensibly through early detection by screening neuroimaging and treatment of the malignancies.

Neuroimaging Abnormalities in NF1

Intracranial neoplasms

Patients with NF1 are 5.5 times more likely to have an intracranial neoplasm listed on their death certificate and about 8 to 11 times more likely among those younger than 40 years, compared with the general population.[9] The most common intracranial neoplasms in NF1 include glioma, cranial nerve schwannoma, and plexiform neurofibroma (PN). Secondary complications, such as obstructive hydrocephalus, are not infrequently encountered. NF1 deletion is associated with increased neuroglial progenitor stem cells in the brainstem but not in the cortex.[11] This association is consistent with an increased incidence of intracranial tumors affecting the optic pathway, hypothalamus, and brain stem in patients with NF1.

Optic pathway gliomas (OPG) are one of the dreaded and frequent neoplasms seen in about 20% of patients with NF1,[12] mostly children and young adults. These tumors are low-grade juvenile pilocytic astrocytoma (although they can be, rarely, high grade) and involve optic nerves or chiasm. OPG can occur in the non-NF1 population, although the presence of bilateral OPG is considered pathognomonic for NF1. Most OPG are diagnosed in children younger than 6 years,[13] especially in those undergoing screening neuroimaging because it can be difficult to reliably assess for vision symptoms in young children. Vision deficits tend to occur in less than 50% of patients,[14] leastwise in initial stages. The common symptoms include decreased visual acuity or loss of color vision and visual field defects. Although routine screening imaging of optic pathways is generally not recommended, it would be prudent to detect these tumors in the presymptomatic stage, especially in children with heedful imaging evaluation. Magnetic resonance imaging (MRI) is the best modality for the visualization of OPG. Special high-resolution fat-suppressed gadolinium-contrast thin-slice MRI sequences focused on optic nerves and chiasm in all 3 planes are most helpful in detecting small gliomas in an early stage. They appear as concentrically enlarged and sometimes irregular optic nerves or an enlarged chiasm, with hyperintense signal on T2-weighted (T2-W) sequence (**Fig. 1**). The degree of gadolinium contrast enhancement does not correlate with the tumor grade as is the case with spinal cord pilocytic astrocytoma. Thick-slice MRI sequences may miss the diagnosis for smaller OPG. The coronal plane tends to show the chiasm better, whereas optic nerve involvement is better appreciated on axial plane, with the ability to compare the thickness with the contralateral optic nerve. After the diagnosis, small or asymptomatic tumors are generally monitored with serial imaging every 3 to 6 months. Progressively enlarging and symptomatic OPGs are treated with chemotherapy, commonly with carboplatin and vincristine. No clear data regarding other chemotherapeutic medications, such as temozolomide, exist for these tumors. The outcomes of chemotherapy are not promising as reported in a recent study: only a third of the treated patients with NF1 showed improved visual acuity, a third remained unchanged, and a third declined.[15] Surgical excision is reserved for large OPG with a mass effect on adjacent structures, especially with chiasm tumors, which can cause endocrine abnormalities caused by a mass effect on the pituitary.

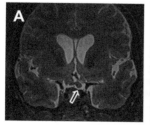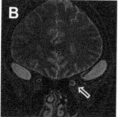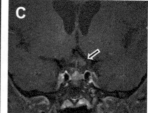

Fig. 1. Left optic pathway glioma (*arrow*) seen as enlarged left half of chiasm (*A*) and left optic nerve (*B*) on high-resolution T2-W coronal sequence with slice thickness of 0.9 mm. No contrast enhancement is seen (*C*).

Brainstem gliomas are the second most-frequent intracranial tumors in NF1.[16] Tectal glioma (**Fig. 2**) can cause a mass effect on the cerebral aqueduct and result in obstructive hydrocephalus. The hypothalamus is another commonly involved location. Corpus callosum neoplasms are seen in up to 5% of children with NF1[17,18] and must be suspected in callosal T2-hyperintense, nonenhancing lesions showing focal enlargement and/or a mild mass effect. Although these locations are more commonly involved, intracranial gliomas in general can occur in any parenchymal location, including in the cerebellum. Most of these tumors are low-grade astrocytomas and appear on MRI as focal areas of hyperintense signal change on T2-W or fluid-attenuated inversion recovery (FLAIR) sequence, with mild to moderate mass effect on adjacent sulci or cisterns (**Fig. 3**). Most of them are usually nonenhancing on post-contrast sequences. MR spectroscopy (MRS) can further assist in establishing a diagnosis, with an elevated choline (Cho)/ N-Acetyl aspartic acid (NAA) ratio seen in low-grade gliomas (**Fig. 4**). Serial imaging every 6 months is generally recommended after a glioma is discovered to monitor for progression and mass effect. A sudden, rapid increase in size or change in the enhancement pattern should raise suspicion for high-grade transformation. Tumor progression in a large case series was associated with either homogeneous or patchy contrast enhancement in 94% of the cases.[19] Chemotherapy and surgical resection remain the main therapeutic options. Gross-total resection is generally associated with improved progression-free survival.[19] Radiotherapy is avoided because of its known association with the development of secondary MPNST in the treatment field in patients with NF1.[20]

Meningiomas are far less common in NF1 compared with NF2.[21] Meningioma involving the optic nerve sheath can be seen, and one must be careful in differentiating it from an OPG. A rare case of both meningioma and OPG involving the same optic nerve in a 4-year-old patient with NF1 has been reported.[22] Childhood optic nerve sheath meningiomas tend to be associated with NF1 and are usually more aggressive than those found in adults. Cranial nerve sheath tumors are also less common compared with NF2. Orbitotemporal PN commonly presents with amblyopia in children.[23] Secondary intracranial PNs should be suspected in patients with NF1 who underwent prior radiation exposure. These tumors have a propensity to undergo malignant transformation. A case of intracerebral MPNST is reported in a patient with NF1 within the field of coil embolization of an middle cerebral artery (MCA) aneurysm, emphasizing the sensitivity to develop radiation-induced tumors.[24]

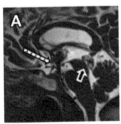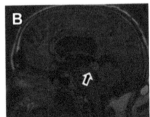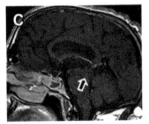

Fig. 2. Tectal glioma in a patient with NF1. Enlarged T2-hyperintense glioma in the midbrain tectum (*black arrow*) is seen on thin-slice T2-W (*A*) and T1-W (*B*) sagittal sequences. No gadolinium contrast enhancement is seen, as is typical with a low-grade glioma (*C*). Because of its location, it runs a risk of aqueductal obstruction leading to life-threatening obstructing hydrocephalus. A patent endoscopic third ventriculostomy (ETV) is noted (*A, white arrow*) for an alternate pathway for cerebrospinal fluid (CSF) flow. The prominent CSF flow artifacts through the ETV are seen with no flow artifacts through the aqueduct (*A*).

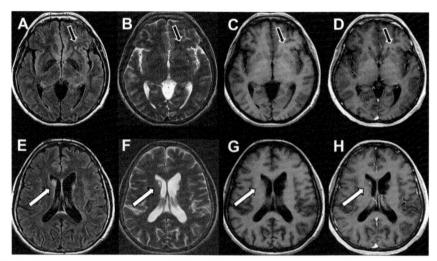

Fig. 3. Right caudate astrocytoma (*E–H, white arrow*) in a patient with NF1. This lesion is hyperintense on FLAIR (*E*) and T2-W (*F*) and hypointense on T1-W (*G*) axial images, with intense contrast enhancement of tumor nodule (*H*). Larger T2-hyperintense signal area on FLAIR (*E*) is contributed by peritumoral vasogenic edema causing mass effect on ventricular wall with asymmetric appearance of frontal horns of lateral ventricles. In comparison, the T2-hyperintense lesion in left frontal white matter (*A–D, black arrow*) shows no evidence of mass effect or contrast enhancement, which distinguishes it from a glioma.

Parenchymal T2-hyperintense lesions and volumetric anomalies

NF1 is well known to be associated with parenchymal T2-hyperintense signal changes, sometimes meretriciously referred to as *unidentified bright objects*. It is advisable to not use such ambiguous terms, which circumstantially gained some popularity in radiological literature. These T2-hyperintensities can be seen in up to 75% of pediatric patients with NF1, are even more common among children less than 7 years of age, and tend to decrease in prevalence with advancing age.[25] They can be seen in any parenchymal location, with basal ganglia, hypothalamus, brain stem, cerebellum, and subcortical white matter being commonly involved (**Fig. 5**). Cortical T2-hyperintensities are also not uncommon and are generally not associated with epilepsy[26] as opposed to seizures caused by cortical hamartomas or gliomas. These T2-hyperintensities are thought to result from vacuolar or spongiotic changes (intercellular edema) as seen on histology.[27] The absence of a mass effect may help differentiate it from a low-grade glioma, although early neoplastic changes can be very difficult to differentiate. Serial MRI follow-up, especially using MRS, in clinically asymptomatic patients is recommended.

More than 50% of children with NF1 have macrocephaly (ie, head circumference >95th percentile),[28] with increased overall white matter volume[29] and corresponding corpus callosum thickening,[30] which in turn is found to be associated with a lower IQ and poorer academic achievement.[31] The T2-hyperintensities involving the corpus callosum are frequently encountered in up to in 10% of patients with NF1 (see **Fig. 5**).[17] This may rarely lead to some concern to include other diseases commonly associated with callosal T2-hyperintensities, such as multiple sclerosis (MS), in the differential diagnosis, especially if neurofibromatosis is yet undiagnosed. Although rare, at least a dozen cases of patients with NF1 diagnosed with MS are reported.[32–34] Most of those reported cases were thought to be the primary progressive

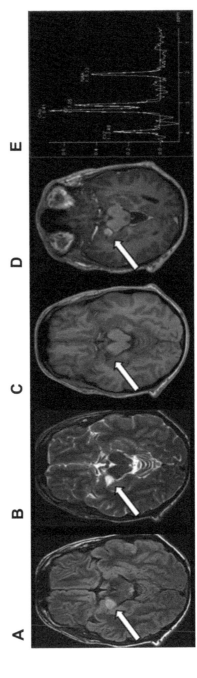

Fig. 4. Right mesial temporal astrocytoma in a patient with NF1 (*white arrow*). This lesion has the typical long T1 and T2 signal characteristics (*A–C*) with contrast enhancement (*D*). Mass effect is evident with effacement of adjacent right peri-mesencephalic cistern. The MR Spectroscopy (*E*) of the lesion shows elevated Cho with mildly reduced NAA, and reversal of Cho/NAA ratio, which is suggestive of a hypercellular lesion with mild neuronal loss, typical of a low-grade astrocytoma. These changes in NAA and Cho peaks will be amplified with increasing grade of the tumor and can be used in serial monitoring.

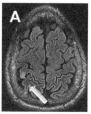
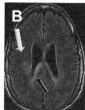
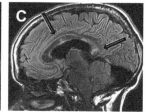
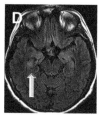

Fig. 5. Array of focal benign T2-hyperintense lesions in a patient with NF1. The FLAIR images show a right frontal cortical lesion without sulcal effacement. Such benign cortical lesions (*A, white arrow*) are generally are not associated with epilepsy as opposed to low-grade gliomas. A focal area of heterogeneous T2-hyperintense signal changes is seen in the right parietal periventricular white matter (*B, white arrow*). The focal corpus callosum lesions (*B, C, black arrows*) have a similar appearance as typically seen in multiple sclerosis. A right medial temporal lesion (*D, white arrow*) has a similar appearance as in mesial temporal sclerosis. These lesions must be monitored closely with serial MRIs (and MRS if attainable), for progressive increase in size or associated mass effect and for contrast enhancement, either of which may suggest a low-grade glioma.

type, with poor response to therapy. This diagnostic differential must be considered when clinically appropriate. Spinal cord parenchymal T2-hyperintensities in patients with NF1 are very rare (**Fig. 6**) and must be followed with serial MRI similar to brain lesions to evaluate for progressive enlargement or mass effect, which can suggest an astrocytoma. Ependymomas are not common in NF1 and are commonly associated with NF2.

Reliable association between parenchymal T2-hyperintensities and cognitive abilities in NF1 is arguable because of conflicting reports. Some studies suggest focal

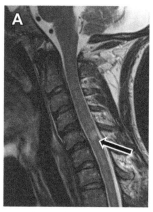
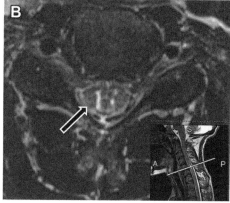

Fig. 6. Spinal cord focal T2-hyperintense lesions in a patient with NF1 (*black arrows*). The T2-hyperintense lesion at C5–6 level on sagittal T2-W image (*A, black arrow*) shows no expansion of cord or mass effect, which is typically seen with a glioma. The axial T2-W image (*B*) shows the same lesion as a right paracentral linear T2-hyperintesirty without mass effect (*black arrow*). A smaller left paracentral lesion is also seen. These spinal cord T2-hyperintense lesions should also be monitored closely with serial MRIs for progressive increase in size or associated mass effect and for contrast enhancement, either of which may suggest a low-grade glioma. Figure (*B*) right lower corner inset image shows the sagittal cervical spine MRI with the level of axial image marked with dotted horizontal line. A, anterior; P, posterior; S, Superior.

lesions in thalamo-striatal locations may be associated with more severe and generalized cognitive impairment,[35,36] with no clear association based on the total number of lesions.[36] As a result, attempts to identify new imaging surrogates to help quantify learning disabilities have been the main focus of the advanced structural neuroimaging techniques, such as diffusion tensor imaging (DTI) and functional imaging with bold functional MRI (fMRI). Using DTI measures, such as fractional anisotropy (FA), axial diffusivity parallel to axons as a marker for structural integrity, and radial diffusivity perpendicular to axon as a marker for myelination, it was found that alterations in white matter integrity were more pronounced in the frontal lobes.[29] The fMRI analysis of visual-spatial impairment, which is one of the hallmark cognitive deficits in NF-I, showed increased reliance on posterior cortex, further supporting evidence of frontal cortical impairment in NF-I.[37]

Cerebral and systemic vasculopathy

Cerebral vasculopathy in NFI is an underrecognized complication. It is reported to be present in about 5% of children diagnosed with NFI. It can be seen as moyamoya changes,[38] stenosis or occlusion of major intracranial arteries,[39] intracranial aneurysms, and arteriovenous malformations.[40] Most of these children with NF1 may be asymptomatic from a cerebrovascular standpoint. Recognizing this important risk will help incorporate vascular imaging, such as MR angiography (MRA) and susceptibility-weighted imaging (SWI), along with brain MRI for early detection of cerebrovascular disease.

Secondary hypertension is seen in up to 30% of young patients with NF1[41] and can lead to significant morbidity if not recognized early. The common causes include pheochromocytoma, renal artery stenosis, coarctation of aorta, and rarely renal artery aneurysms. A study reported the following common locations of arterial abnormalities: aorta (22%), renal arteries (16%), mesenteric (16%), extracranial carotid-vertebral arteries (13.5%), intracranial (5%), subclavian-axillary (4%), iliofemoral arteries (4%), and secondary vascular compression caused by PNST.[40] Most of them were aneurysms, whereas arterial stenosis was also commonly seen.[40] Vascular evaluation with MRA or ultrasonography (USG) is preferred as the screening modality for vascular anomalies. Because of the increased radiosensitivity of patients with NF1 as discussed previously, computerized tomographic angiography (CTA) should be considered only if MRA or USG is equivocal. A conventional angiography can be useful as both a diagnostic and therapeutic modality after an initial screening with noninvasive imaging. Sudden cardiac death in young children with NF1 caused by fatal coronary artery occlusion is reported.[42]

Sphenoid wing dysplasia

Sphenoid wing dysplasia (SWD) is one of the National Institutes of Health's (NIH) clinical criteria[43] for NF1 diagnosis. It is seen in up to 7% of patients with NF1.[44] It is considered a distinctive manifestation of NF1, although it can be seen in certain types of craniosynostosis. Primary SWD is secondary to mesencephalic neural crest dysfunction and manifests very early in life, such as macrocephaly. Secondary SWD is caused by tumors, such as PN, which result in progressive enlargement of temporal fossa, orbital fissure, and other cranial foramina. Most of SWD are thought to be secondary, because three-fourths of SWD tend to be associated with tumors such as PN.[45] Computed tomography (CT) with 3-dimensional (3D) reconstruction is the best modality for diagnosis. Newer 320-slice CT scanners not only offer high-resolution images, 0.1-mm slice thickness, and simultaneous images in multiple planes, which greatly improve 3D rendering capabilities, but are also better suited for patients with NF1 because of the lower radiation dose. MRI can show the enhancing nerve sheath tumors coursing through the enlarged skull base cranial foramina and orbital fissure, as commonly seen in secondary SWD. A similar mechanism of secondary calvarial defects can be seen because of the progressively enlarging PN and are often associated with dural ectasia.

Peripheral nerve sheath tumors (PNST)

The characteristic PNSTs seen in NF1 are neurofibromas. These PNSTs are benign. They can be found in subcutaneous or internal locations, including intradurally in the lumbosacral spinal canal. Most localized PNST are solitary. They show nonspecific signal intensities and variable contrast enhancement on MRI, better seen with fat-suppressed short inversion time inversion recovery (STIR) sequence. The described target-sign appearance of localized neurofibromas is referred to the hyperintense signal on a T2-weighted MRI sequence (T2-W) caused by peripheral myxoid material and a relatively low-signal intensity of the central fibrous component. It is seen in up to 70% of neurofibromas (compared with about 50% of schwannomas) and absent in MPNST.[46] A reverse target sign can be seen on a T1-W postcontrast sequence because of the enhancement of a central fibrous component and a relative lack of enhancement of the surrounding myxoid component. PNST involving cervical nerve roots can rarely extend into the canal causing compressive myelopathy. They cause enlargement of neural foramen, which can further help in detecting the spinal root PNST, especially if they are nonenhancing. A full-body STIR MRI can be useful as a screening tool to help in detecting PNST in deeper locations (**Fig. 7**). Monitoring the progression of the PNST by counting the number or volumetric analysis is cumbersome and generally not performed. Improved availability of commercial 3D-rendered software optimized for PNST evaluation may greatly assist in this aspect (**Fig. 8**). Because neurofibromas arise from the nerve fascicle without a capsule and are centrally located, they cannot be separated from the involved nerve, hence requiring resection of the nerve during surgical excision of asymptomatic neurofibromas.

The risk of mortality in patients with NF1 is highest from malignant transformation of the PNST. Certain imaging features on MRI, such as intratumoral lobulation, ill-defined margins, and irregular contrast enhancement, are associated with MPNST. Fluorine-18 fluorodeoxyglucose positron emission tomography (^{18}F-FDG PET) offers higher sensitivity in detecting MPNST, based on maximum standardized uptake value (SUVmax), mean standardized uptake value (SUVmean), and tracer uptake heterogeneity.[47,48] The presence of internal PNST increases the risk of MPNST (odds ratio [OR] 7.5).[49] A sex predilection is seen with females developing internal PNST earlier, with their prevalence increased during adolescence.[50] The factors that are independently associated with internal PNST include age (OR 1.16), xanthogranulomas (OR 5.85), and the presence of both subcutaneous and plexiform neurofibromas (OR 6.8).[50]

NEUROFIBROMATOSIS TYPE 2 (NF2)

NF2 is an autosomal dominant NCS characterized by schwannomas, meningiomas, ependymomas, and ocular abnormalities, such as presenile posterior subcapsular lenticular opacities (cataracts) and retinal hamartomas. The acronym MISME (**M**ultiple **I**nherited **S**chwannomas **M**eningiomas **E**pendymomas) can be used to remember these tumors in NF2.[51] Briefly on the history of NF2, J.H. Wishart[52] (a surgeon), in 1822, described a 21-year-old man with macrocephaly, deafness onset at 19 years of age, and seizures, who had multiple skull base tumors at autopsy. This description is regarded as the earliest description of NF2. Henneberg and Koch,[53] in 1903, described a patient with bilateral 8 cranial nerve tumors without skin lesions and

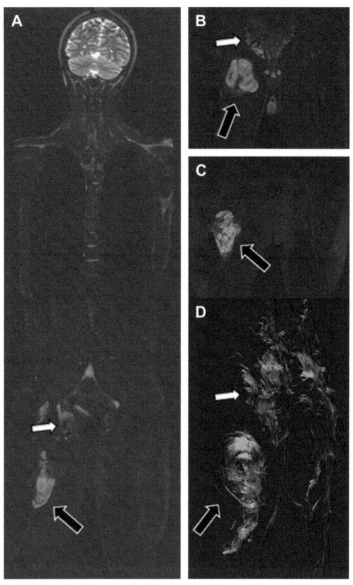

Fig. 7. Right thigh and groin area plexiform neurofibromas in a patient with NF1. A full-body STIR sequence (*A*) is very helpful as a screening imaging sequence, which facilitates detecting deep-tissue plexiform neurofibromas (*A–C*, STIR sequence, *black arrows*) as well as in confirming the diagnosis of those palpable superficially such as in groin (*A–C, white arrows*). Diffusion tensor tractography of these plexiform neurofibromas (*D, white and black arrows*) show clustered parallel fiber tracts within these lesions. The right femoral nerve is seen adjacent to the groin neurofibroma (*D, white arrow*). Refinement of the MRI tractography techniques in the future will further assist in diagnosis and surgical planning.

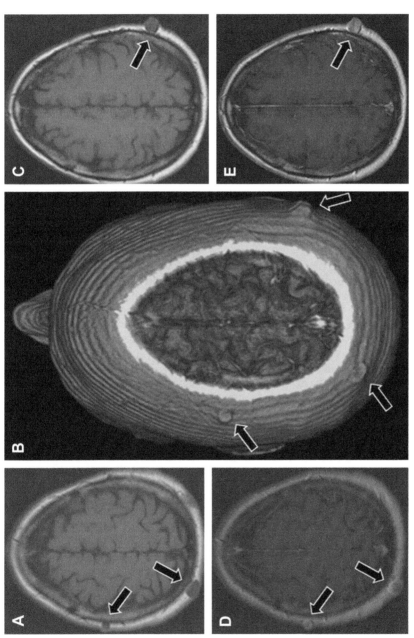

Fig. 8. Scalp subcutaneous neurofibromas in a patient with NF1 (*A, C, D, E, arrows*), with contrast enhancement (*D, E, arrows*). Three-dimensional (3D) reconstruction (*B, arrows*) techniques help in better visualization of such multiple small subcutaneous neurofibromas and can be used to monitor for increase in their size or new lesions. Similar 3D reconstructions can be performed for neurofibromas anywhere in the body, in theory using a full-body STIR MRI, for instance, although unfortunately current commercially available software packages do not have such automated capabilities.

introduced the term *central* NF to distinguish from the more common *peripheral* NF (ie, NF1). This distinction continued to remain ambiguous until the localization of distinct genes for the 2 diseases in early 1980s and was further facilitated by the introduction of gadolinium contrast in MRI in the late 1980s. The formal clinical delineation was completed at an NIH consensus meeting in 1987.[54] The estimated birth incidence of NF2 is 1 in 25 000.[55] The male-to-female ratio is nearly equal, with about 15% of patients with NF2 being mosaic.[56] More than 200 mutations in the NF2 gene (also known as neurofibromin-2), located in chromosome 22q12.2, have been identified. It encodes the protein merlin or schwannomin, which is a cytoskeletal protein that provides a functional link between the cell membrane and the actin cytoskeleton.[57] An important distinction from NF1 is that fewer than 5% of the patients with NF2 have more than 4 café au lait macules.[58]

Neuroimaging Abnormalities in NF2

Schwannomas

The presence of bilateral vestibular schwannomas (VS) is characteristic of NF2 (**Fig. 9**). About 7% of the patients with unilateral VS have NF2, and an estimated 1 per 1000 individuals will be diagnosed with VS in their lifetime.[55] Sporadic schwannomas and schwannomas in patients with NF2 are histopathologically indistinguishable. Spinal schwannomas are 2.5 times more common than VS in NF2, with most of these tumors (>90%) arising from dorsal root ganglia of sensory nerves.[59] VS arise from cells within the Scarpa ganglion, which is the sensory ganglion of the vestibular nerve located in the lateral aspect of the internal auditory canal (IAC). Cochlear nerve schwannomas arise from the spiral ganglion in the cochlea, and facial nerve schwannomas involve the geniculate ganglion. These two are relatively less frequent, composing about 10% to 20% of IAC schwannomas. As based on the location of the sensory ganglions described, the IAC schwannomas, thus, arise predominantly in the lateral aspect and tend to grow medially into the CP angle cistern. Trigeminal schwannomas almost always involve gasserian ganglion in the Meckel cave and are the next most common schwannomas after spinal and VS in NF2 (**Fig. 10**). The lower cranial nerve schwannomas are less common. The glossopharyngeal nerve has 2 ganglia that lie in the jugular foramen. The vagal nerve has 2 ganglia: the superior, which lies in the jugular foramen, and the inferior, which lies high in the neck. Hence, almost all of the vagal and glossopharyngeal schwannomas tend to occur in the jugular foramen or high in the neck associated with the ganglia.[59] The growth pattern of jugular foramen schwannomas may give rise to dumbbell-shaped tumors. In the spine, the dorsal root ganglia are commonly involved,[59] which are typically located within or just distal to the neural foramen. This location, again, often creates dumbbell-shaped schwannomas because of the bidirectional intraspinal canal and extraforaminal growth.

The MRI characteristics of schwannomas are similar to meningiomas in that they are mildly hypointense on T2-W, isointense on T1-weighted MRI sequence (T1-W), and enhance avidly with gadolinium contrast. Calcifications are uncommon compared with meningioma. A schwannoma is characteristically eccentric with respect to the affected nerve, with the nerve displaced to the periphery of the mass. This finding is helpful when present to differentiate from a neurofibroma, which is central and intimately related to the nerve; this distinction is found to be accurate in about 65% of cases.[60] This concentric versus eccentric relationship to nerve may not be easy to identify in small nerves. The target sign is less common compared with neurofibroma, although intratumoral cysts are more common.[46]

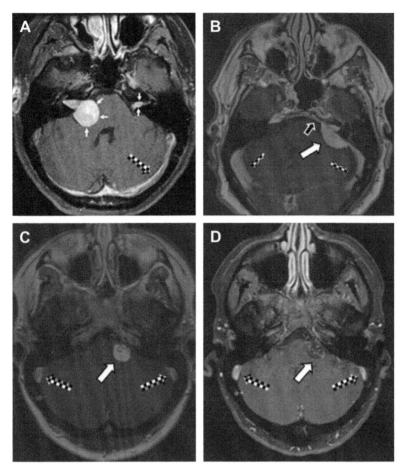

Fig. 9. Bilateral vestibular schwannomas in a patient with NF2 (*A, white arrows*), with homogenous contrast enhancing lesions (*white arrows*), which typically arise for Scarpa ganglion in lateral internal auditory canals. The checkered arrows indicate the vascular contrast enhancement in transverse and sigmoid venous sinuses (*A–D*). The major differential diagnosis for such extra-axial cerebellopontine (CP) angle lesions includes a meningioma (*B, white arrow*). Presence of a dural tail (*B, black arrow*) may occasionally help in differentiating a meningioma. CP-angle lipoma is another differential diagnosis, although it is easier to diagnose using a fat-suppressed sequence and typical hyperintense signal on T1-W sequence (*C, white arrow*) and absent contrast enhancement, as seen with fat-suppressed, postcontrast, T1-W image (*D, white arrow*). Note the subtle vascular enhancement of tiny vessels inside the lipoma.

Similar to meningiomas, surgical resection is the primary treatment option for symptomatic tumors, and serial imaging is performed to monitor asymptomatic lesions (**Fig. 11**). Schwannomas have a true capsule comprised of epineurium, which allows successful resection. Chemotherapy with bevacizumab for VS in a small 31-patient study showed hearing improvement and tumor shrinkage in more than 50% of progressive VS in patients with NF2.[61] Although this has been encouraging, larger clinical trials are hoped for before this treatment can be recommended.

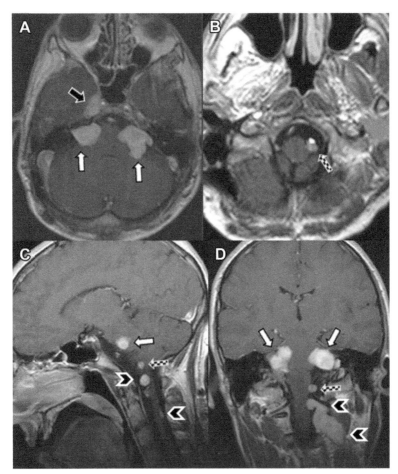

Fig. 10. A patient with NF2 with bilateral vestibular schwannomas (*A, C, D, white arrows*), a right trigeminal schwannoma (*A, black arrow*), left glossopharyngeal schwannoma (*B–D, checkered arrows*), and left C1-C3 spinal nerve root schwannomas (*C, D, black arrow heads*). Trigeminal schwannomas are next most common schwannomas after spinal and vestibular schwannomas in NF2 and almost always involve gasserian ganglion in the Meckel cave. Patients with schwannomatosis typically do not have bilateral vestibular schwannomas.

Meningioma

Intracranial meningiomas occur in about 50% of patients with NF2[56] and spinal meningiomas in up to one-third.[21] About 60% of patients develop at least one intracranial meningioma by 50 years of age; it increases to more than 70% by 60 years of age, with a greater proportion of males developing a cranial meningioma at less than 20 years of age compared with females.[56] These tumors can arise from any surface lined by dura, including the skull base, falx, and convexity, including from arachnoid cells in choroids plexus of the lateral ventricle. Most of the meningiomas associated with NF2 are histologically benign (World Health Organization [WHO] grade 1), with WHO grade II tumors found in about 29% and grade III tumors in less than 6%.[62] Patients with NF2 can have an average of 3 meningiomas, with a range of 1 to 10. These meningiomas are generally slow growing, at a rate of 1.0 to 1.5 mm per year, two-

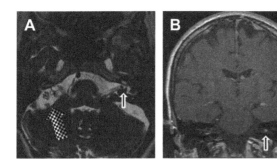
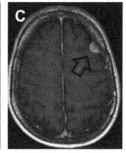

Fig. 11. Postoperative changes in right CP-angle cistern from resection of a right vestibular schwannoma (*A, checkered arrow*) in a patient with NF2. Small left VS (*A, B, white arrow*) was discovered several years after the original right VS surgery. This patient also has a left frontal convexity meningioma (*C, arrow*). Postoperative serial MRI monitoring to evaluate for ipsilateral recurrence or development of contralateral VS should be performed in patients with NF2. Moreover, about 7% of patients with unilateral VS have NF2.

thirds of which may not show significant growth over a year. Less than 10% of meningiomas grow faster than 20% a year, and about 10% develop de novo meningiomas during the annual follow-up.[62]

On MRI, they appear as extra axial mass lesions with mild hypointense signal on T2-W sequence because of the compact cellular structure, isointense on T1-W sequence, and mildly hyperintense on FLAIR. Variable degrees of calcifications are frequently seen. The contrast enhancement is usually inversely proportional to the degree of calcification. Calcified meningiomas will show a susceptibility blooming effect on SWI sequence. The mass effect depends on the size and location. Most benign meningiomas will not cause adjacent parenchymal signal changes. Scalloping of parenchyma caused by chronic slow growth can be seen.

Spinal meningiomas can be located in the neural foramen giving rise to a typical dumbbell-shaped tumor with widening of the foramen. Intraspinal canal tumors can cause compressive myelopathy. It can be difficult to distinguish a schwannoma from a meningioma, especially in the spine and in posterior fossa adjacent to lower cranial nerve foramen.

Surgical resection remains the primary treatment option for symptomatic meningiomas. In asymptomatic cases, at least annual imaging is recommended to monitor progression and de novo tumors. Chemotherapy with vascular endothelial growth factor (VEGF) inhibitor bevacizumab has not been encouraging, likely because of a different non-VEGF driven angiogenesis pathway in meningiomas.

Ependymomas
The association between NF2 and spinal ependymoma is well known.[63,64] Just more than 50% of patients with NF2 have intramedullary spinal cord tumors, with a relatively higher incidence among patients with nonsense and frame shift mutations.[65] Intramedullary ependymomas, in general, have a predilection for the cervical spinal cord such that 67% of tumors arise from or extend into this region.[66,67] Ependymomas of the cord are typically solitary tumors that arise from the ependymal lining of the central canal causing a diffuse enlargement of the cord over several levels and the associated syrinx in 50% of the cases. Spinal cord ependymomas have only a slight tendency to infiltrate the adjacent neural tissue and have a delicate capsule forming a plane of cleavage to separate the tumor from the spinal cord. The WHO recognizes 5 histologic variants of ependymoma, including the cellular, papillary,

epithelial, tanycytic,[68] and myxopapillary subtypes. Ependymomas are also commonly divided into typical, WHO grade II, or anaplastic WHO grade III varieties. In addition, 2 low-grade (WHO grade I) forms, myxopapillary ependymoma and subependymoma, have also been recognized. Anaplastic ependymoma (WHO grade III) are less common in the spinal cord and have additional pathologic features, such as increased cellularity, mitotic activity, pleomorphic nuclei, vascular hyperplasia, nuclear atypia, and necrosis.[69] Cellular ependymomas most often occur in the spinal cord.[70] The incidence of polar and tumoral cysts that are seen rostrocaudal to the tumor occurred in 50% to 90% of cases.[11] On T1-W images, cellular ependymomas tend to be isointense or slightly hyperintense to the spinal cord, and on T2-W images they seem to be hyperintense. Hemosiderin is seen as an area of hypointensity or a so-called cap sign, this may occur in 20% to 64% of cord ependymomas. STIR sequence shows hyperintensity, whereas 80% of these cases on T1-W enhance homogeneously with contrast. Minimal or no enhancement is actually relatively rare. Intratumoral hemorrhage is a common complication of ependymomas. Diffusion tensor imaging (DTI) may show that the tumor displaces the fiber tracts rather than disrupt them.[70]

SCHWANNOMATOSIS

Schwannomatosis is now considered the third major form of neurofibromatosis after NF1 and NF2.[70] It is characterized by multiple schwannomas, in the absence of bilateral VS typically seen with NF2. Constitutional mutations in the SMARCB1 (*SWI/SNF-related, matrix-associated, actin-dependent regulator of chromatin, subfamily b, member 1*) tumor suppressor gene are implicated in pathogenesis, which are found in 45% of familial and 7% of sporadic patients.[71] The SMARCB1 gene is located on chromosome 22q11.23, which is not too far from the NF2 gene. No clear pattern of inheritance has been found so far. This condition is rarer than NF2, with an incidence of around 1 per 40 000 individuals. Although the presence of VS has been excluded from diagnostic criteria for schwannomatosis, at least 2 cases with an identified SMARCB1 mutation were found to have unilateral VS.[72] This exclusion of VS needs to be redefined based on larger population studies. The revised diagnostic criteria are listed in the **Table 1**.[73]

Neuroimaging Abnormalities in Schwannomatosis

Similar to NF2, spinal schwannomas are more commonly found (in about 75%) compared with nonvestibular intracranial schwannomas seen in 10%. About 5% of patients have intracranial meningiomas. Peripheral schwannomas are the most common and seen in up to 90%. They are implicated in deep-seated chronic pain, which is a common presenting symptom in about 70% of patients with schwannomatosis.[74] The pain reported in patients with sporadic schwannomatosis is more severe compared with familial cases.[73] A rarer form called *segmental schwannomatosis* is seen in about one-third of patients with schwannomatosis, with an incidence of about 1 per 120 000. These individuals have tumors in an anatomically limited distribution, such as a single limb, or less than 5 contiguous segments of the spine.[75]

TUBEROUS SCLEROSIS COMPLEX (TSC) OR BOURNEVILLE DISEASE

TSC is an autosomal dominant NCS characterized by multisystem hamartomas, which are well-circumscribed groups of disorganized and dysplastic cells with a propensity to multiply excessively. They are benign tumors and may or may not cause symptoms. Neurologically, TSC is notorious for its association with seizures and cognitive

Table 1
Diagnostic criteria

Disease	NF1[43]	NF2[54]	Schwannomatosis[73]
	≥2 Features • ≥6 Café au lait macules (>5 mm in prepubertal, >15 mm in postpubertal) • ≥2 Neurofibromas of any type or one plexiform neurofibroma • Axillary or inguinal freckling • Optic pathway glioma • ≥2 Lisch nodules • A distinctive osseous lesion, such as sphenoid dysplasia or tibial pseudarthrosis • First-degree relative with NF1	One of the following • Bilateral VS • First-degree relative & unilateral VS or any 2 of the following: meningioma, schwannoma, glioma, neurofibroma, PSLO • Unilateral VS & any 2 of the following: meningioma, schwannoma, glioma, neurofibroma, PSLO • Multiple meningiomas & unilateral VS or any 2 of the following: schwannoma, glioma, neurofibroma	• ≥2 Nonintradermal schwannomas (one with pathologic confirmation), including no bilateral vestibular schwannoma by high-quality MRI of IAC with ≤3-mm slice thickness • One pathologically confirmed schwannoma or intracranial meningioma & affected first-degree relative • Possible diagnosis if ≥2 nonintradermal tumors but none has been pathologically proven to be a schwannoma; the occurrence of chronic pain in association with the tumors increase the likelihood of schwannomatosis • Exclusion: germline pathogenic NF2 mutation, fulfill diagnostic criteria for NF2, first-degree relative with NF2, or schwannomas in previous field of radiation therapy only • Molecular diagnosis: pathologically proved schwannomas or meningiomas & genetic studies of ≥2 tumors with chromosome 22 LOH and 2 different NF2 mutations or one pathologically proved schwannoma or meningioma & germline SMARCB1 pathogenic mutation
ICD-9	237.71	237.72	237.70
ICD-10	Q85.01	Q85.02	Q85.03

Abbreviations: ICD-9, International Classification of Diseases, Ninth Revision; ICD-10, International Classification of Diseases, Tenth Revision; LOH, loss of heterozygosity; PSLO, posterior, subcapsular lenticular opacities.

impairment. More than two-thirds of the cases are sporadic and the rest are familial. It is caused by more than 400 known DNA mutations involving either the TSC1 gene located on chromosome 9q34 encoding for protein *hamartin* or the TSC2 gene located on chromosome 16p13.3, which encodes the protein tuberin. Both *hamartin* and *tuberin* interact with each other to perform tumor suppressor function. The estimated prevalence is about 1 in 27 000 and twice that for children less than 10 years of age.[76] The clinical diagnostic criteria for tuberous sclerosis complex are well established and divide into definite, probable, or possible TSC based on the combination of major or minor clinical features as described in the **Table 2**.[77] These criteria are widely available for reference.

Neuroimaging Abnormalities in TSC

Cortical tubers (intracranial hamartomas)
These abnormalities are cortical hamartomas most commonly found in frontal lobes (53%), followed by parietal lobe (23%), temporal lobe (16%), and occipital lobe (8%).[78] Cerebellar tubers are relatively rare, although more than half of them change over time and may show de novo contrast enhancement with transformation to sub-ependymal giant cell astrocytomas (SEGA). As a result, a higher percentage of patients with TSC with cerebellar lesions tend to develop SEGA than those without cerebellar lesions.[79] Unlike cortical tubers, cerebellar tubers are usually wedge-shaped and not epileptogenic. Tubers in the brainstem or spinal cord are very rare. About 5% to 10% of the cortical tubers are epileptogenic. Increased interictal uptake in the tryptophan analogue, α-[^{11}C]methyl-L-tryptophan (AMT)–PET can help as an imaging marker to detect epileptogenic tubers. Lower FA values on DTI were also shown to correspond to epileptogenic tubers found on the AMT-PET.[80] Other neurologic symptoms may be caused depending on the location of tubers, including abnormalities in cognition, cranial nerve deficits, focal motor or sensory abnormalities, and cerebellar and gait abnormalities. Infantile spasms are highly prevalent among children with TSC. Multiple tubers of up to an average of 10 per patient are common. Large tubers are more likely to be symptomatic compared with smaller tubers, although smaller ones can be quite numerous.[81]

On MRI, the tubers appear hyperintense on T2-W and FLAIR images. The fast spin echo (FSE) T2-W sequence has a false-negative rate of 21% compared with less than 0.5% for FLAIR sequence in detecting cortical tubers.[78] Calcifications in tubers are very common, especially in adults. As a result, they show a susceptibility blooming effect on gradient echo T2* or SWI sequences (**Fig. 12**). The single-shot FSE T2-W sequence, which is not commonly used now, is reported to have high false-negative (56%) and false-positive (7%) rates for tuber detection.[78] Contrast enhancement is uncommon. High-field-strength 7-T MRI is reported to detect microtubers not visualized using a conventional 1.5-T MR scanner.[82]

Subependymal nodules or subependymal hamartomas
These nodules are hamartomas usually located throughout the lateral ventricular wall, more common along the caudate-thalamic groove (CTG). They are very common and seen in more than three-fourths of patients with TSC. Their location is thought to follow the course of the caudate nucleus. Moreover, the subependymal nodule (SEN) lesions along the CTG showed the potential to grow and transform into SEGA, compared with the stable size of non-CTG lesions over a 4-year follow-up.[83] The MRI appearance is described as *candle dripping appearance*, with T2-hypointese nodules, along the lateral ventricular wall. Contrast enhancement is typically absent, although enhancement may not necessarily correlate with gliomatous transformation. Calcifications

Table 2
Diagnostic criteria

Disease	TSC[77]	VHL	SWS
Criteria	Definite: 2 major or (1 major + 2 minor) Probable: 1 major and 1 minor Possible: 1 major or (≥2 minor) *Major Features* • Facial angiofibromas or forehead plaque • Nontraumatic periungual fibroma • Hypomelanotic macules (≥3) • Shagreen patch (connective tissue nevus) • Multiple retinal nodular hamartomas • Cortical tubers • Subependymal nodule • Subependymal giant cell astrocytoma • Cardiac rhabdomyoma • Lymphangiomyomatosis • Renal angiomyolipoma *Minor Features* • Multiple dental pits • Hamartomatous rectal polyps • Bone cysts • Cerebral white matter migration lines • Gingival fibromas • Nonrenal hamartoma • Retinal achromic patch • Confetti skin lesions • Multiple renal cysts	• ≥1 CNS hemangioblastomas Or • One CNS hemangioblastoma and visceral manifestations of VHL, which include pancreatic or renal cysts, retinal hemangioblastoma, renal cell carcinoma, pheochromocytoma, neuroendocrine tumor or serous cystadenoma of pancreas, papillary cystadenoma of epididymis Or • Any manifestation and a known family history of VHL • Molecular diagnosis with germline mutation in VHL gene	Clinical features • *Neurologic:* cortical/subcortical calcifications, leptomeningeal vascular malformations, cerebral atrophy • *Dermatologic:* nevus flammeus (port-wine facial stain) • *Ophthalmologic:* heterochromia of the iris, buphthalmos, glaucoma associated with choroidal capillary malformation
ICD-9	759.5	759.6	759.6
ICD-10	Q85.1	Q85.8	Q85.8

Abbreviations: CNS, central nervous system; ICD-9, *International Classification of Diseases, Ninth Revision;* ICD-10, *International Classification of Diseases, Tenth Revision.*

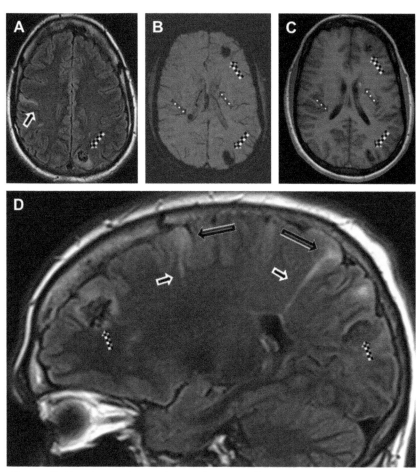

Fig. 12. MRI findings in a patient with TSC. The cortical hamartomas appear as focal areas of cortical thickening with FLAIR hyperintense signal, better seen in those without calcifications (*D, black arrows*). The calcified cortical hamartomas (*A–D, checkered arrows*) show a blooming artifact on SWI sequence (*B, checkered arrow*). The subependymal nodules are attached to ependymal surface in the lateral ventricular wall (*B, C, black dotted arrows*) and are usually calcified, better seen on SWI sequence because of their blooming artifact (*B, black dotted arrows*). The signal characteristic of a calcified nodule on T1-W sequence depends on the concentration of the particulate calcium.[123] The lesions with less than 30% by weight calcium will appear hyperintense on T1-W (*C, black dotted arrow*, left frontal subependymal nodule), compared with T1-hypointense signal in those with higher calcium content (*C, black dotted arrow*, right lateral ventricle subependymal nodule). The radial migration lines extending from cortical hamartomas to subcortical white matter are also characteristic of TSC (*A, D, white arrows*).

are common, especially in older children and adults, causing a blooming effect on SWI (see **Fig. 12**).

Sub ependymal giant cell astrocytomas (SEGA)

These tumors are well-demarcated intraventricular tumors seen in about 15% of patients with TSC.[84] They are comprised of variably sized astrocytic-appearing cells with less prominent mitosis and a low proliferation index. They can be indistinguishable from SEN histopathologically.[85] They can be differentiated from the SEN on MRI by the larger size and progressive increase in size during serial imaging (**Fig. 13**). They are slow-growing tumors and typically have no symptoms until obstructive hydrocephalus develops. Because they typically arise from SEN in the area adjacent to the foramen of Monroe and owing to their larger size, obstructive hydrocephalus is a dreaded complication. They are mostly confined to an intraventricular location and seldom invade brain parenchyma. They are slightly more common among patients with TSC with TSC2 gene mutations.[86] Rarely, degeneration into higher-grade or infiltrating neoplasms can occur, although most are WHO grade I. Rare intratumoral bleeding with intraventricular extension has been reported in 6 cases.[87] Earlier surgical resection of the tumors that show rapid growth is recommended to avoid the risk of obstructive hydrocephalus.[88] Everolimus (Afinitor) is a kinase inhibitor approved for use in pediatric and adult patients with TSC for the treatment of SEGA that requires therapeutic intervention but cannot be curatively resected. Class III evidence for everolimus to reduce tumor size in patients with TSC with SEGA for a median of 34 months was reported.[89]

Cerebral white matter radial migration lines
These lines are T2-hyperintense linear areas oriented in a radial fashion (see **Fig. 12**). They are thought to represent heterotopic glia and neurons along the expected path of cortical migration.[90] Although they are commonly seen in patients with TSC, their clinical importance is unknown.

VON HIPPEL-LINDAU DISEASE (VHL)

VHL is an autosomal dominant NCS characterized by retinal, cerebellar, brainstem, and spinal hemangioblastomas and endolymphatic sac tumors. Visceral lesions include renal cell carcinomas, renal cysts, pheochromocytomas, pancreatic cysts, and neuroendocrine tumors. It is caused by more than 370 known inherited germline mutations involving the VHL gene, or *von Hippel-Lindau tumor suppressorE3 ubiquitin protein ligase*, located on chromosome 3p25.3 encoding for proteins in the VCB-CUL2 protein complex. The VHL gene is a tumor suppressor gene. The estimated birth incidence of VHL is about 1 in 36 000 live births.[91]

Briefly on the history of VHL, Eugen von Hippel[92] (ophthalmologist) first described fundoscopic findings in a young man with vision loss in 1896, which were described subsequently in a series of other patients and were found to be congenital cystic capillaryangiomatosis or *angiomatosis retinae*. Arvid Lindau (who was a fellow under von Hippel at the time)[93] combined different features seen in VHL and called the syndrome *Angiomatosis des Zentral nervens systems* in 1926. Subsequent detailed descriptions by Cushing[94] in 1928 and Davison[95] in 1936 established the name of this syndrome as VHL.

Neuroimaging Abnormalities in VHL
Central nervous system hemangioblastomas
Central nervous system hemangioblastomas (CNS-HB) are one of the most common manifestations in VHL. These tumors are benign WHO grade 1 tumors. Cerebellum is the most common location seen in about 65% of all CNS-HB. The probability of a patient with VHL developing cerebellar HB by 60 years of age is 0.84.[96] They are also seen commonly in the brainstem (10%), spinal cord (25%), and pituitary fossa (1%). Patients with VHL with either brainstem or spinal cord HB have another HB more frequently than those with cerebellar HB.[97] Supratentorial location of HB is very rare

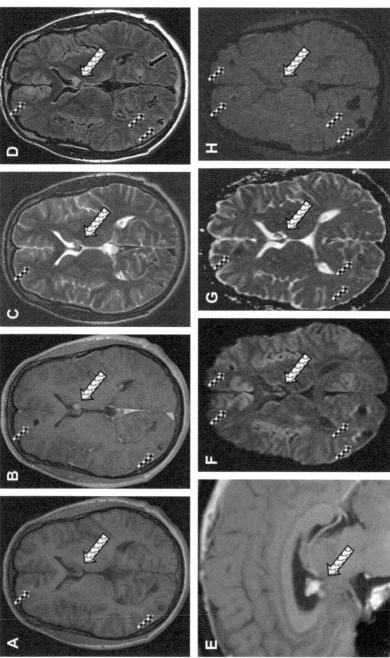

Fig. 13. Subependymal giant cell astrocytoma (*A–H, white arrow*) in a patient with TSC. Note the typical location just above the level of foramen of Monroe. These tumors are low-grade astrocytomas with hyperintense signal on T2-W (*C*) and FLAIR (*D*), isointense to gray matter on T1-W (*A*), and show avid contrast enhancement (*B, E*). Peripheral restricted-diffusion is seen on diffusion-weighted imaging (*F*) and Apparent diffusion coefficient (ADC) (*G*) images suggestive of hypercellularity, which is typical for gliomas. Calcification is less common, with no blooming artifact on SWI (*H*). Calcified cortical hamartomas are also seen (*A–D, F–H, checkered arrows*). A non-calcified cortical hamartomas is noted as a T2-hyperintense lesion (*D, black arrow*) in the left medial occipital cortex.

and more commonly associated with VHL disease compared with other locations.[98] These tumors are frequently seen in young patients with VHL in their 20s and 30s. Pregnancy has no effect on the development of new hemangioblastomas and peritumoral cysts or growth rate of existing tumors in young women with VHL.[99] The spinal intramedullary HB composes 2% to 8% of all intramedullary spinal cord tumors[100] and is frequently associated with VHL. Cervical and thoracic segments are commonly involved, with a predilection for dorsolateral cord surface. The tumors can be single or multiple and tend to be smaller than 10 mm in diameter in patients with VHL.[101] Grossly, they are well demarcated with a capsule and have characteristic abnormally dilated tortuous vessels on the surface.[102] The tumor mitotic activity measured as KI-67 activity, less than 1% for intramedullary tumors, compared with up to 25% for tumors that extend both into intramedullary and extramedullary space.[103]

On MRI (**Fig. 14**), these tumors are isointense on T1-W images and hyperintense on T2-W images.[101] They may have mixed heterogeneity if intralesional hemorrhage is present. The contrast enhancement on the tumor nodule is usually homogenous and well demarcated, with superficial heterogeneous enhancement within the flow voids. The surrounding vasogenic edema is usually mild. The flow voids are more common in tumors greater than 15 mm in size.[101] Because of the presence of dilated vessels, these tumors are often mistaken for a vascular malformation. A spinal cyst with enhancing mural nodule and nonenhancing cyst rim is another characteristic feature (**Fig. 15**). In terms of natural history, the cysts associated with the tumors

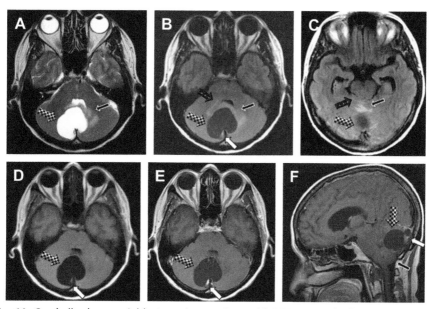

Fig. 14. Cerebellar hemangioblastoma in a patient with VHL. Note the large cystic lesion with cerebrospinal fluid characteristics (*A–F, checkered arrows*) and signal suppression on FLAIR (*B, C, checkered arrows*), which is often mistaken for an arachnoid cyst. Associated vasogenic edema (*A–C, black arrow*) and significant mass effect on the brain stem (*B, C, black dotted arrows*) highly indicates a neoplasm as opposed to benign arachnoid cyst. Contrast-enhancing mural nodule is seen in the posterior right paramedian cyst wall (*E, F, white arrow*; compare it with noncontrast T1-W, *D*). The mural nodule typically abuts pial surface, and can be seen as T2-hyperintese lesion on FLAIR images (*B, white arrow*). Note the cerebellar tonsillar ectopia (*F, black arrow*) secondary to mass effect from the tumoral cyst.

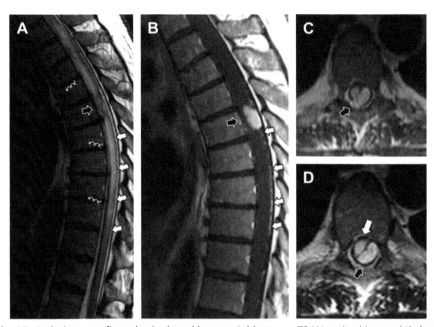

Fig. 15. Pathology-confirmed spinal cord hemangioblastoma. T2-W sagittal image (*A*) show a heterogeneous mass (*A, black arrow*) associated with extensive cord edema (*A, checkered arrows*). Note the hypointense linear structure consistent with a vessel posterior to the cord (*white arrows*). On the contrast sagittal T1-W image (*B*), an enhancing intramedullary bilobulated mass is seen (*B, black arrow*). An enhancing engorged vessel is seen posterior and caudal to tumor (*B, white arrows*). Axial T1-W contrast image shows an interesting bilobulated intramedullary and extramedullary snowman appearance (*C, black arrow*). The spinal cord hyperintensity on T2-W axial image (*D, white arrow*) is consistent with extensive holocord edema anterior to the tumor (*D, black arrow*). The cord edema resolved after surgery.

tend to grow faster than the tumor itself. The symptomatic mass effect is predominantly caused by the cysts (see **Fig. 14**). The tumor alternates between a growth phase separated by a quiescent phase with no growth. Hence, the tumor may remain the same size for several years in a quiescent phase.[104] Follow-up monitoring with serial imaging should be continued at regular intervals for this reason. The first-line treatment is microsurgical resection using the feeder vessels coagulation[105] or temporary arterial occlusion[106] techniques. Angiography can demonstrate enlarged feeding arteries, intense nodular stains, and early draining veins.[107] Cerebrospinal fluid (CSF) fistula is a common complication of the spinal surgery in less than 5% patients.[105] The presence of multiple tumors may necessitate a more aggressive approach with stereotactic radiosurgery.[108] There has been growing interest in the use of the VEGF inhibitor bevacizumab, which has shown to cause tumor regression in a single case study.[109] The prognosis in general is usually excellent,[110] although the intratumoral hemorrhage and tumor recurrence are common in patients with VHL.

Retinal HB
This tumor is one of the earliest manifestations because of the early symptoms of vision loss and has higher morbidity because of the visual deficits.[111] Retinal HB (R-HB) is the first manifestation in 45% of patients with VHL. The probability of a patient with VHL developing R-HB by 60 years of age is 0.7.[96] They appear as a small

discoloration on the retina in the early phase before progressing to a nodular appearance. Retinal hemorrhages leading to retinal detachment and visual loss are a dreaded complication. Early ophthalmologic screening and fundoscopic imaging are recommended.

Endolymphatic sac tumors

These tumors are locally invasive, slow-growing tumors of the *pars rugosa* of the endolymphatic duct or sac seen in up to 15% of patients with VHL.[112] The clinical findings are predominantly auditory, including high-frequency sensorineural hearing loss and tinnitus, and vestibular, such as vertigo or disequilibrium. MRI with high resolution 3D-Fast Spin Echo (FSE) technique with T2-weighted driven equilibrium pulse sequence (T2-DRIVE) can be used to produce up to 0.4-mm slice thickness images within a short imaging time in both axial and coronal planes for adequate visualization of the endolymphatic duct and sac. This sequence is performed by using a driven equilibrium pulse consisting of a 90° radiofrequency (RF) pulse in combination with a gradient refocusing pulse and a spoiling gradient. It rebuilds the vertical magnetization of fluids much faster. The repetition time (TR) is shortened by a factor of three to four times, while the fluids are still hyperintense in the images. Thus it allows achieving high resolution images with hyperintense fluids keeping rest of the tissues relatively isointense in a shorter scan time. The endolymphatic sac tumors can be seen as a hyperintense signal in an expanded and enlarged endolymphatic duct or sac.

STURGE-WEBER SYNDROME (SWS) OR ENCEPHALOTRIGEMINAL ANGIOMATOSIS

SWS is a sporadic congenital NCS characterized by capillary-venous vascular malformations of the brain and meninges and with involvement of the skin typically in the cranial nerve V1-V3 territory. It is one of the common NCS, after NF1 and TSC. The estimated incidence is 1 in 50 000.[113] Briefly on the history of SWS, William A. Sturge (trained under Jean Martin Charcot, considered the father of neurology discipline) presented a young girl to the Medical Society of London in 1879 who had right facial discoloration and left limb twitching seizures lasting 10 to 12 minutes. Frederick

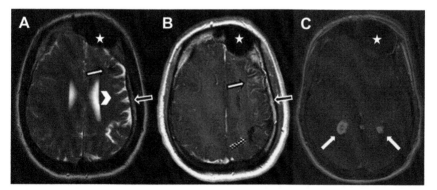

Fig. 16. Typical MRI findings in a patient with SWS, which includes left hemispheric hemiatrophy (*A, white arrow head*), enlarged ipsilateral left frontal paranasal sinus (*A–C, asterisk*), thickening of the ipsilateral frontal-parietal calvarium inner table (*A, B, black arrow with white margin*), ipsilateral left frontal leptomeningeal angiomatosis with contrast enhancement (*A, B, white arrow with black margin*), asymmetric enlarged choroid plexus (*C, white arrows*) and the ipsilateral gyral calcifications (*B, dotted arrow*). This patient has a nevus flammeus on the ipsilateral (left) forehead.

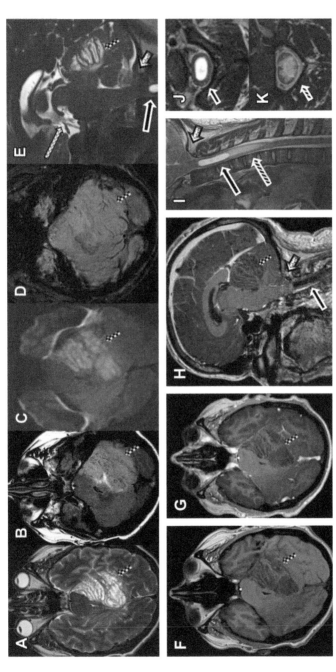

Fig. 17. Dysplastic gangliocytoma of the cerebellum (*A–H, checkered arrows*) in a patient with Lhermitte–Duclos disease. Note the enlarged cerebellum with a well-demarcated mass lesion in the superior cerebellum and vermis, with the characteristic striated folial pattern. The tumor is hyperintense on T2-W (*A, E, checkered arrow*) and FLAIR (*B*) sequences. It is hypointense on T1-W (*F*) with absent contrast enhancement (*G, H*). Mild restricted-diffusion is noted on diffusion-weighted imaging (*C*) ascribable to its hypercellularity. No evidence of tumoral calcifications or necrosis is noted on SWI (*E*), although increased vascularity is seen with abundance of tiny vessels in the tumor compared with the rest of cerebellum. Significant mass effect on the adjacent structures including the fourth ventricle and aqueduct are common and can lead to obstructive hydrocephalus. A third ventriculostomy is seen with CSF flow artifacts through it (*E, white arrow*). The mass effect also causes a secondary Chiari (*E, H, I, white dotted arrow*) with an associated large cervical spinal cord syrinx (*E, H–J, black arrow with white border*). Cord edema caudal to the syrinx can be seen (*I, K, white arrow*). The tumor itself is low grade, but the complications caused by its mass effect can be life threatening.

Parkes Weber,[114] a prolific writer with more than 1200 medical publications in his life-time, reported radiological features of brain atrophy on skull radiograph in 1922 in a patient with SWS.[114] He later described intracranial calcifications in 1929.[115]

Seizures are common and early clinical manifestation in most patients with SWS. They are typically focal motor seizures. Status epilepticus is not uncommon. Focal motor deficient on the side of the affected hemisphere can be seen. Vasculopathy in older patients with strokes are common. Mild cognitive impairment and migraine are associated neurologic clinical features.

Neuroimaging abnormalities in SWS

Patients with a typical facial port-wine stain and new-onset partial seizures should have high index of suspicion for SWS and undergo brain MRI. The tram-track calcifications described on skull radiographs is of historical significance, being associated with this condition for nearly half a century before the advent of MRI. The typical MRI features (**Fig. 16**) seen in SWS include hemiatrophy of cerebral hemispheres and ipsilateral leptomeningeal angiomatosis seen as vascular contrast enhancement and on SWI. Ipsilateral prominent choroid plexus in the lateral ventricle is also commonly seen. Ipsilateral calcifications are more severe and are better visualized on SWI because of their blooming artifact. Because of the capillary-venous vascular malformations, the cortical and white matter perfusion is altered in SWS, the degree of which is related to epilepsy.[116] Severe cortical calcification in the affected hemisphere is related to decreased parenchymal perfusion and is associated with more severe epilepsy in patients with SWS.[117]

Accelerated myelination is described in infants with SWS whereby the affected hemisphere shows areas of abnormal T2-W and FLAIR hypointensities in the white matter.[118] In older patients, white matter damage and loss in the affected hemisphere are seen, causing T2-hyperintense changes. DTI studies were reported to show reduced FA measures in both affected as well as the contralateral hemisphere, even in children, suggesting early onset of microstructural diffuse white matter damage.[119]

COWDEN DISEASE

Cowden disease (CD) is an autosomal dominant NCS characterized by multiple hamartomas. It is also associated with an increased risk of developing several types of systemic cancers at a young age. It has an estimated prevalence of 1 in 200 000 people. It is caused by more than 300 known mutations in the PTEN gene or *phosphatase and tensin homolog,* which is a tumor suppressor gene located on chromosome 10q23.3. Lhermitte-Duclos disease is a very rare condition, now recognized as part of CD, and characterized by dysplastic gangliocytoma of the cerebellum (**Fig. 17**), which results in headaches, cerebellar ataxia and cranial neuropathies, and may cause increased intracranial pressure.[120]

SUMMARY

In summary, an in-depth knowledge of the imaging characteristics of the common NCS described in this article will help a neurologist understand the screening imaging modalities in patients with NCS. A neuroimager should be able to look for an associated imaging stigmata in specific anatomic areas commonly involved, such as optic pathways in patients with NF1 to rule out OPG or high-resolution IAC images to rule out VS. The future of neuroimaging is geared toward developing and refining MRI sequences, which have incremental advantages, such as quantitative susceptibility mapping[121] and susceptibility tensor imaging,[122] which are highly sensitive to brain demyelination, a common finding in most of the NCS. The detection of tumors and masses in NCS has greatly benefitted with the improved availability of high-field-strength MRI machines in the past few years. Predicting cognitive impairment early on in children with NCS using imaging techniques, such as fMRI, is not in the distant future. Neuroimaging will remain at the heart and soul of the multidisciplinary care of such complex diagnoses to guide early detection and monitor treatment.

REFERENCES

1. Van der Hoeve J. Les phakomatoses de Bourneville, de Recklinghausen et de von Hippel-Lindau. J Belge Neurol Psychiatr 1933;33:752–62.
2. Yakovlev PI, Guthrie RH. Congenital ectodennoses (neurocutaneous syndromes) in epileptic patients. Arch Neurol Psychiatr 1931;26:1145–94.
3. Ruggieri M, Pascual Castroviejo I, Di Rocco C, et al. Neurocutaneous disorders phakomatoses and hamartoneoplastic syndromes. Wien (Germany); New York: Springer; 2008.
4. Crowe FW, Schull WJ, Neel JV. A clinical, pathological, and genetic study of multiple neurofibromatosis. Springfield (IL): Thomas; 1956.
5. Lammert M, Friedman JM, Kluwe L, et al. Prevalence of neurofibromatosis 1 in German children at elementary school enrollment. Arch Dermatol 2005;141(1): 71–4.
6. Huson SM, Compston DA, Clark P, et al. A genetic study of von Recklinghausen neurofibromatosis in south east Wales. I. Prevalence, fitness, mutation rate, and effect of parental transmission on severity. J Med Genet 1989;26(11): 704–11.
7. Cawthon RM, Weiss R, Xu GF, et al. A major segment of the neurofibromatosis type 1 gene: cDNA sequence, genomic structure, and point mutations. Cell 1990;62(1):193–201.
8. Jadayel D, Fain P, Upadhyaya M, et al. Paternal origin of new mutations in von Recklinghausen neurofibromatosis. Nature 1990;343(6258):558–9.
9. Rasmussen SA, Yang Q, Friedman JM. Mortality in neurofibromatosis 1: an analysis using U.S. death certificates. Am J Hum Genet 2001;68(5):1110–8.
10. Evans DG, O'Hara C, Wilding A, et al. Mortality in neurofibromatosis 1: in North West England: an assessment of actuarial survival in a region of the UK since 1989. Eur J Hum Genet 2011;19(11):1187–91.
11. Lee JS, Padmanabhan A, Shin J, et al. Oligodendrocyte progenitor cell numbers and migration are regulated by the zebrafish orthologs of the NF1 tumor suppressor gene. Hum Mol Genet 2010;19(23):4643–53.
12. Blazo MA, Lewis RA, Chintagumpala MM, et al. Outcomes of systematic screening for optic pathway tumors in children with neurofibromatosis type 1. Am J Med Genet A 2004;127A(3):224–9.
13. Listernick R, Charrow J, Greenwald M, et al. Natural history of optic pathway tumors in children with neurofibromatosis type 1: a longitudinal study. J Pediatr 1994;125(1):63–6.
14. Avery RA, Fisher MJ, Liu GT. Optic pathway gliomas. J Neuroophthalmol 2011; 31(3):269–78.
15. Fisher MJ, Loguidice M, Gutmann DH, et al. Visual outcomes in children with neurofibromatosis type 1-associated optic pathway glioma following chemotherapy: a multicenter retrospective analysis. Neuro Oncol 2012;14(6):790–7.
16. Pollack IF, Shultz B, Mulvihill JJ. The management of brainstem gliomas in patients with neurofibromatosis 1. Neurology 1996;46(6):1652–60.

17. Mimouni-Bloch A, Kornreich L, Kaadan W, et al. Lesions of the corpus callosum in children with neurofibromatosis 1. Pediatr Neurol 2008;38(6):406–10.
18. Pascual-Castroviejo I, Pascual-Pascual SI. Neurofibromatosis type 1 (NF1) associated with tumor of the corpus callosum. Childs Nerv Syst 2012;28(12):2177–80.
19. Udaka YT, Yeh-Nayre LA, Amene CS, et al. Recurrent pediatric central nervous system low-grade gliomas: the role of surveillance neuroimaging in asymptomatic children. J Neurosurg Pediatr 2013;11(2):119–26.
20. Kleinerman RA. Radiation-sensitive genetically susceptible pediatric sub-populations. Pediatr Radiol 2009;39(Suppl 1):S27–31.
21. Goutagny S, Kalamarides M. Meningiomas and neurofibromatosis. J Neurooncol 2010;99(3):341–7.
22. Buyukkapu-Bay S, Akca A, Karadogan M, et al. Concomitant meningioma and glioma within the same optic nerve in neurofibromatosis type 1. J Child Neurol 2013. [Epub ahead of print].
23. Avery RA, Dombi E, Hutcheson KA, et al. Visual outcomes in children with neurofibromatosis type 1 and orbitotemporal plexiform neurofibromas. Am J Ophthalmol 2013;155(6):1089–94.e1.
24. Ellis MJ, Cheshier S, Sharma S, et al. Intracerebral malignant peripheral nerve sheath tumor in a child with neurofibromatosis type 1 and middle cerebral artery aneurysm treated with endovascular coil embolization. J Neurosurg Pediatr 2011;8(4):346–52.
25. Sabol Z, Resic B, Gjergja Juraski R, et al. Clinical sensitivity and specificity of multiple T2-hyperintensities on brain magnetic resonance imaging in diagnosis of neurofibromatosis type 1 in children: diagnostic accuracy study. Croat Med J 2011;52(4):488–96.
26. Hsieh HY, Fung HC, Wang CJ, et al. Epileptic seizures in neurofibromatosis type 1 are related to intracranial tumors but not to neurofibromatosis bright objects. Seizure 2011;20(8):606–11.
27. DiPaolo DP, Zimmerman RA, Rorke LB, et al. Neurofibromatosis type 1: pathologic substrate of high-signal-intensity foci in the brain. Radiology 1995;195(3):721–4.
28. Payne JM, Moharir MD, Webster R, et al. Brain structure and function in neurofibromatosis type 1: current concepts and future directions. J Neurol Neurosurg Psychiatry 2010;81(3):304–9.
29. Karlsgodt KH, Rosser T, Lutkenhoff ES, et al. Alterations in white matter microstructure in neurofibromatosis-1. PLoS One 2012;7(10):e47854.
30. Margariti PN, Blekas K, Katzioti FG, et al. Magnetization transfer ratio and volumetric analysis of the brain in macrocephalic patients with neurofibromatosis type 1. Eur Radiol 2007;17(2):433–8.
31. Pride N, Payne JM, Webster R, et al. Corpus callosum morphology and its relationship to cognitive function in neurofibromatosis type 1. J Child Neurol 2010;25(7):834–41.
32. Pipatpajong H, Phanthumchinda K. Neurofibromatosis type I associated multiple sclerosis. J Med Assoc Thai 2011;94(4):505–10.
33. Feuillet L, Boudinet H, Casseron W, et al. Multiple sclerosis associated with neurofibromatosis type I. Rev Neurol (Paris) 2004;160(4 Pt 1):447–51 [in French].
34. Perini P, Gallo P. The range of multiple sclerosis associated with neurofibromatosis type 1. J Neurol Neurosurg Psychiatry 2001;71(5):679–81.
35. Chabernaud C, Sirinelli D, Barbier C, et al. Thalamo-striatal T2-weighted hyperintensities (unidentified bright objects) correlate with cognitive impairments in neurofibromatosis type 1 during childhood. Dev Neuropsychol 2009;34(6):736–48.

36. Hyman SL, Gill DS, Shores EA, et al. T2 hyperintensities in children with neurofibromatosis type 1 and their relationship to cognitive functioning. J Neurol Neurosurg Psychiatry 2007;78(10):1088–91.

37. Billingsley RL, Jackson EF, Slopis JM, et al. Functional MRI of visual-spatial processing in neurofibromatosis, type I. Neuropsychologia 2004;42(3):395–404.

38. Koss M, Scott RM, Irons MB, et al. Moyamoya syndrome associated with neurofibromatosis type 1: perioperative and long-term outcome after surgical revascularization. J Neurosurg Pediatr 2013;11(4):417–25.

39. Ghosh PS, Rothner AD, Emch TM, et al. Cerebral vasculopathy in children with neurofibromatosis type 1. J Child Neurol 2013;28(1):95–101.

40. Oderich GS, Sullivan TM, Bower TC, et al. Vascular abnormalities in patients with neurofibromatosis syndrome type I: clinical spectrum, management, and results. J Vasc Surg 2007;46(3):475–84.

41. Zinnamosca L, Petramala L, Cotesta D, et al. Neurofibromatosis type 1 (NF1) and pheochromocytoma: prevalence, clinical and cardiovascular aspects. Arch Dermatol Res 2011;303(5):317–25.

42. Kanter RJ, Graham M, Fairbrother D, et al. Sudden cardiac death in young children with neurofibromatosis type 1. J Pediatr 2006;149(5):718–20.

43. National Institutes of Health Consensus Development Conference statement: neurofibromatosis. Bethesda, Md., USA, July 13-15, 1987. Neurofibromatosis 1988;1(3):172–8.

44. Bognanno JR, Edwards MK, Lee TA, et al. Cranial MR imaging in neurofibromatosis. AJR Am J Roentgenol 1988;151(2):381–8.

45. Arrington DK, Danehy AR, Peleggi A, et al. Calvarial defects and skeletal dysplasia in patients with neurofibromatosis type 1. J Neurosurg Pediatr 2013; 11(4):410–6.

46. Beaman FD, Kransdorf MJ, Menke DM. Schwannoma: radiologic-pathologic correlation. Radiographics 2004;24(5):1477–81.

47. Derlin T, Tornquist K, Munster S, et al. Comparative effectiveness of 18F-FDG PET/CT versus whole-body MRI for detection of malignant peripheral nerve sheath tumors in neurofibromatosis type 1. Clin Nucl Med 2013;38(1):e19–25.

48. Tsai LL, Drubach L, Fahey F, et al. [18F]-Fluorodeoxyglucose positron emission tomography in children with neurofibromatosis type 1 and plexiform neurofibromas: correlation with malignant transformation. J Neurooncol 2012;108(3): 469–75.

49. Zehou O, Bularca S, Bastuji-Garin S, et al. Neurofibromatosis 1 phenotype associated to malignant peripheral nerve sheath tumours: a case-control study. J Eur Acad Dermatol Venereol 2012;27(8):1044–7.

50. Sbidian E, Hadj-Rabia S, Riccardi VM, et al. Clinical characteristics predicting internal neurofibromas in 357 children with neurofibromatosis-1: results from a cross-selectional study. Orphanet J Rare Dis 2012;7:62.

51. Smirniotopoulos JG, Murphy FM. The phakomatoses. AJNR Am J Neuroradiol 1992;13(2):725–46.

52. Wishart J. Case of tumours in the skull, dura mater, and brain. Edinburgh Med Surg J 1822;18:393–7.

53. Henneberg H, Koch M. Über "zentrale" Neurofibromatose und die Geschwülste des Kleinhirnbrückenwinkels (Akustikusneurinome). Arch Psychiat 1903;36:251.

54. Neurofibromatosis. Conference statement. National Institutes of Health Consensus Development Conference. Arch Neurol 1988;45(5):575–8.

55. Evans DG, Moran A, King A, et al. Incidence of vestibular schwannoma and neurofibromatosis 2 in the North West of England over a 10-year

period: higher incidence than previously thought. Otol Neurotol 2005;26(1): 93–7.

56. Smith MJ, Higgs JE, Bowers NL, et al. Cranial meningiomas in 411 neurofibromatosis type 2 (NF2) patients with proven gene mutations: clear positional effect of mutations, but absence of female severity effect on age at onset. J Med Genet 2011;48(4):261–5.

57. Xu HM, Gutmann DH. Merlin differentially associates with the microtubule and actin cytoskeleton. J Neurosci Res 1998;51(3):403–15.

58. Mautner VF, Lindenau M, Baser ME, et al. Skin abnormalities in neurofibromatosis 2. Arch Dermatol 1997;133(12):1539–43.

59. Tryggvason G, Barnett A, Kim J, et al. Radiographic association of schwannomas with sensory ganglia. Otol Neurotol 2012;33(7):1276–82.

60. Stull MA, Moser RP Jr, Kransdorf MJ, et al. Magnetic resonance appearance of peripheral nerve sheath tumors. Skeletal Radiol 1991;20(1):9–14.

61. Plotkin SR, Merker VL, Halpin C, et al. Bevacizumab for progressive vestibular schwannoma in neurofibromatosis type 2: a retrospective review of 31 patients. Otol Neurotol 2012;33(6):1046–52.

62. Goutagny S, Bah AB, Henin D, et al. Long-term follow-up of 287 meningiomas in neurofibromatosis type 2 patients: clinical, radiological, and molecular features. Neuro Oncol 2012;14(8):1090–6.

63. Plotkin SR, O'Donnell CC, Curry WT, et al. Spinal ependymomas in neurofibromatosis type 2: a retrospective analysis of 55 patients. J Neurosurg Spine 2011;14(4):543–7.

64. Aguilera DG, Mazewski C, Schniederjan MJ, et al. Neurofibromatosis-2 and spinal cord ependymomas: report of two cases and review of the literature. Childs Nerv Syst 2011;27(5):757–64.

65. Patronas NJ, Courcoutsakis N, Bromley CM, et al. Intramedullary and spinal canal tumors in patients with neurofibromatosis 2: MR imaging findings and correlation with genotype. Radiology 2001;218(2):434–42.

66. Koeller KK, Rosenblum RS, Morrison AL. Neoplasms of the spinal cord and filum terminale: radiologic-pathologic correlation. Radiographics 2000;20(6): 1721–49.

67. Smith AB, Soderlund KA, Rushing EJ, et al. Radiologic-pathologic correlation of pediatric and adolescent spinal neoplasms: part 1, intramedullary spinal neoplasms. AJR Am J Roentgenol 2012;198(1):34–43.

68. Lim BS, Park SQ, Chang UK, et al. Spinal cord tanycytic ependymoma associated with neurofibromatosis type 2. J Clin Neurosci 2010;17(7):922–4.

69. Kahan H, Sklar EM, Post MJ, et al. MR characteristics of histopathologic subtypes of spinal ependymoma. AJNR Am J Neuroradiol 1996;17(1):143–50.

70. Mechtler LL, Nandigam K. Spinal cord tumors: new views and future directions. Neurol Clin 2013;31(1):241–68.

71. Smith MJ, Wallace AJ, Bowers NL, et al. Frequency of SMARCB1 mutations in familial and sporadic schwannomatosis. Neurogenetics 2012;13(2):141–5.

72. Smith MJ, Kulkarni A, Rustad C, et al. Vestibular schwannomas occur in schwannomatosis and should not be considered an exclusion criterion for clinical diagnosis. Am J Med Genet A 2012;158A(1):215–9.

73. Plotkin SR, Blakeley JO, Evans DG, et al. Update from the 2011 International Schwannomatosis Workshop: from genetics to diagnostic criteria. Am J Med Genet A 2013;161(3):405–16.

74. Merker VL, Esparza S, Smith MJ, et al. Clinical features of schwannomatosis: a retrospective analysis of 87 patients. Oncologist 2012;17(10):1317–22.

75. MacCollin M, Chiocca EA, Evans DG, et al. Diagnostic criteria for schwannomatosis. Neurology 2005;64(11):1838–45.

76. Sampson JR, Scahill SJ, Stephenson JB, et al. Genetic aspects of tuberous sclerosis in the west of Scotland. J Med Genet 1989;26(1):28–31.

77. Roach ES, Gomez MR, Northrup H. Tuberous sclerosis complex consensus conference: revised clinical diagnostic criteria. J Child Neurol 1998;13(12):624–8.

78. Griffiths PD, Hoggard N. Distribution and conspicuity of intracranial abnormalities on MR imaging in adults with tuberous sclerosis complex: a comparison of sequences including ultrafast T2-weighted images. Epilepsia 2009;50(12): 2605–10.

79. Vaughn J, Hagiwara M, Katz J, et al. MRI characterization and longitudinal study of focal cerebellar lesions in a young tuberous sclerosis cohort. AJNR Am J Neuroradiol 2013;34(3):655–9.

80. Tiwari VN, Kumar A, Chakraborty PK, et al. Can diffusion tensor imaging (DTI) identify epileptogenic tubers in tuberous sclerosis complex? Correlation with alpha-[11C]methyl-L-tryptophan ([11C] AMT) positron emission tomography (PET). J Child Neurol 2012;27(5):598–603.

81. Pascual-Castroviejo I, Hernandez-Moneo JL, Pascual-Pascual SI, et al. Significance of tuber size for complications of tuberous sclerosis complex. Neurologia 2012. [Epub ahead of print].

82. Chalifoux JR, Perry N, Katz JS, et al. The ability of high field strength 7-T magnetic resonance imaging to reveal previously uncharacterized brain lesions in patients with tuberous sclerosis complex. J Neurosurg Pediatr 2013;11(3): 268–73.

83. Katz JS, Milla SS, Wiggins GC, et al. Intraventricular lesions in tuberous sclerosis complex: a possible association with the caudate nucleus. J Neurosurg Pediatr 2012;9(4):406–13.

84. Ekici MA, Kumandas S, Per H, et al. Surgical timing of the subependymal giant cell astrocytoma (SEGA) with the patients of tuberous sclerosis complex. Turk Neurosurg 2011;21(3):315–24.

85. Takei H, Florez L, Bhattacharjee MB. Cytologic features of subependymal giant cell astrocytom: a review of 7 cases. Acta Cytol 2008;52(4):445–50.

86. Michelozzi C, Di Leo G, Galli F, et al. Subependymal nodules and giant cell tumours in tuberous sclerosis complex patients: prevalence on MRI in relation to gene mutation. Childs Nerv Syst 2013;29(2):249–54.

87. Sterman H, Furlan AB, Matushita H, et al. Subependymal giant cell astrocytoma associated with tuberous sclerosis presenting with intratumoral bleeding. Childs Nerv Syst 2013;29(2):335–9.

88. de Ribaupierre S, Dorfmuller G, Bulteau C, et al. Subependymal giant-cell astrocytomas in pediatric tuberous sclerosis disease: when should we operate? Neurosurgery 2007;60(1):83–9 [discussion: 89–90].

89. Krueger DA, Care MM, Agricola K, et al. Everolimus long-term safety and efficacy in subependymal giant cell astrocytoma. Neurology 2013;80(6): 574–80.

90. Griffiths PD, Bolton P, Verity C. White matter abnormalities in tuberous sclerosis complex. Acta Radiol 1998;39(5):482–6.

91. Maher ER, Iselius L, Yates JR, et al. Von Hippel-Lindau disease: a genetic study. J Med Genet 1991;28(7):443–7.

92. Von Hippel E. Vorstellung eines Patienten mit einer sehr ungenwohnlichen Netzhaut. XXIV Verstellung der ophthalmologischen Gesellschaft. Wiesbaden (Germany): JF Bergman Verlag; 1896. p. 269.

93. Lindau, A. Studien uiber Kleinhirncysten Bau, Pathogenese und Beziehungen zur Angiomatosis retinae. Acta patk. et microbiol. Scandinav, Suppl. I: 1926.
94. Cushing H, Bailey P. Tumors Arising from the Blood Vessels of the Brain. Baltimore (MD): Charles C. Thomas; 1928.
95. Davison C. Retinal and central nervous system hemangioblastomas with visceral changes (von HippelLindau's disease). Bull Neurol Instit 1936;NY 5:72–93.
96. Maher ER, Yates JR, Harries R, et al. Clinical features and natural history of von Hippel-Lindau disease. Q J Med 1990;77(283):1151–63.
97. Kanno H, Kuratsu J, Nishikawa R, et al. Clinical features of patients bearing central nervous system hemangioblastoma in von Hippel-Lindau disease. Acta Neurochir (Wien) 2013;155(1):1–7.
98. Mills SA, Oh MC, Rutkowski MJ, et al. Supratentorial hemangioblastoma: clinical features, prognosis, and predictive value of location for von Hippel-Lindau disease. Neuro Oncol 2012;14(8):1097–104.
99. Ye DY, Bakhtian KD, Asthagiri AR, et al. Effect of pregnancy on hemangioblastoma development and progression in von Hippel-Lindau disease. J Neurosurg 2012;117(5):818–24.
100. Lonser RR, Weil RJ, Wanebo JE, et al. Surgical management of spinal cord hemangioblastomas in patients with von Hippel-Lindau disease. J Neurosurg 2003;98(1):106–16.
101. Chu BC, Terae S, Hida K, et al. MR findings in spinal hemangioblastoma: correlation with symptoms and with angiographic and surgical findings. AJNR Am J Neuroradiol 2001;22(1):206–17.
102. Na JH, Kim HS, Eoh W, et al. Spinal cord hemangioblastoma: diagnosis and clinical outcome after surgical treatment. J Korean Neurosurg Soc 2007;42(6):436–40.
103. Imagama S, Ito Z, Wakao N, et al. Differentiation of localization of spinal hemangioblastomas based on imaging and pathological findings. Eur Spine J 2011; 20(8):1377–84.
104. Wanebo JE, Lonser RR, Glenn GM, et al. The natural history of hemangioblastomas of the central nervous system in patients with von Hippel-Lindau disease. J Neurosurg 2003;98(1):82–94.
105. Bostrom A, Hans FJ, Reinacher PC, et al. Intramedullary hemangioblastomas: timing of surgery, microsurgical technique and follow-up in 23 patients. Eur Spine J 2008;17(6):882–6.
106. Clark AJ, Lu DC, Richardson RM, et al. Surgical technique of temporary arterial occlusion in the operative management of spinal hemangioblastomas. World Neurosurg 2010;74(1):200–5.
107. Abul-Kasim K, Thurnher MM, McKeever P, et al. Intradural spinal tumors: current classification and MRI features. Neuroradiology 2008;50(4):301–14.
108. Daly ME, Choi CY, Gibbs IC, et al. Tolerance of the spinal cord to stereotactic radiosurgery: insights from hemangioblastomas. Int J Radiat Oncol Biol Phys 2011;80(1):213–20.
109. Omar AI. Bevacizumab for the treatment of surgically unresectable cervical cord hemangioblastoma: a case report. J Med Case Rep 2012;6(1):238.
110. Garces-Ambrossi GL, McGirt MJ, Mehta VA, et al. Factors associated with progression-free survival and long-term neurological outcome after resection of intramedullary spinal cord tumors: analysis of 101 consecutive cases. J Neurosurg Spine 2009;11(5):591–9.
111. Wong WT, Liang KJ, Hammel K, et al. Intravitreal ranibizumab therapy for retinal capillary hemangioblastoma related to von Hippel-Lindau disease. Ophthalmology 2008;115(11):1957–64.

112. Choo D, Shotland L, Mastroianni M, et al. Endolymphatic sac tumors in von Hippel-Lindau disease. J Neurosurg 2004;100(3):480–7.

113. Thomas-Sohl KA, Vaslow DF, Maria BL. Sturge-Weber syndrome: a review. Pediatr Neurol 2004;30(5):303–10.

114. Weber FP. Right-sided hemi-hypotrophy resulting from right-sided congenital spastic hemiplegia, with a morbid condition of the left side of the brain, revealed by radiograms. J Neurol Psychopathol 1922;3(10):134–9.

115. Weber FP. A note on the association of extensive haemangiomatous naevus of the skin with cerebral (meningeal) haemangioma, especially cases of facial vascular naevus with contralateral hemiplegia. Proc R Soc Med 1929;22(4): 431–42, 435.

116. Alkonyi B, Miao Y, Wu J, et al. A perfusion-metabolic mismatch in Sturge-Weber syndrome: a multimodality imaging study. Brain Dev 2012;34(7):553–62.

117. Wu J, Tarabishy B, Hu J, et al. Cortical calcification in Sturge-Weber syndrome on MRI-SWI: relation to brain perfusion status and seizure severity. J Magn Reson Imaging 2011;34(4):791–8.

118. George U, Rathore S, Nittala P. MR demonstration of accelerated myelination in early Sturge Weber syndrome. Neurol India 2010;58(2):336–7.

119. Alkonyi B, Govindan RM, Chugani HT, et al. Focal white matter abnormalities related to neurocognitive dysfunction: an objective diffusion tensor imaging study of children with Sturge-Weber syndrome. Pediatr Res 2011; 69(1):74–9.

120. Tan TC, Ho LC. Lhermitte-Duclos disease associated with Cowden syndrome. J Clin Neurosci 2007;14(8):801–5.

121. Liu C, Li W, Johnson GA, et al. High-field (9.4 T) MRI of brain dysmyelination by quantitative mapping of magnetic susceptibility. Neuroimage 2011;56(3):930–8.

122. Liu C, Li W, Wu B, et al. 3D fiber tractography with susceptibility tensor imaging. Neuroimage 2012;59(2):1290–8.

123. Henkelman RM, Watts JF, Kucharczyk W. High signal intensity in MR images of calcified brain tissue. Radiology 1991;179(1):199–206.

Imaging of Cerebral Ischemia
From Acute Stroke to Chronic Disorders

May Nour, MD, PhD[a,b], David S. Liebeskind, MD[a],*

KEYWORDS

- Stroke • Ischemia • MRI • CT • Collaterals

KEY POINTS

- Cerebral ischemia spans a temporal continuum from hyperacute presentation and extends into acute, subacute, and chronic phases.
- Serial imaging of patients throughout the dynamic course of ischemia is highly informative.
- Selection of an appropriate imaging modality to answer the clinical question and to complement the clinical examination is crucial.
- Several neuroimaging modalities yield information regarding the integrity of brain parenchyma, changes in tissue demands and metabolism, severity of vascular disease, and neuronal repair over time.
- Taken in the appropriate context, with the correct selection of imaging tests, clinicians can effectively gain insight into disease mechanism, tailor therapeutic decision-making, and monitor patients for progression of disease over time.

INTRODUCTION

Cerebral ischemia spans a temporal continuum from hyperacute presentation into acute, subacute, and chronic phases. Imaging provides detailed information to the clinician that must be evaluated in light of the patient's symptomatic presentation and clinical examination. Imaging results in the context of the patient's examination are valuable in confirming diagnosis, ruling out pathologic conditions, evaluating the degree of disease progression, helping in selection of optimal treatment, and adjusting treatment based on patient response. It also provides invaluable information on patients who may carry the burden of cerebrovascular disease but are clinically asymptomatic. For these patients, findings from imaging will drive a return to the clinical examination and, certainly, affect treatment decision-making. The wide availability of imaging in the current era allows for the possibility of serial evaluations of patients

Disclosures: DSL is a consultant to Stryker, Inc and Covidien, Inc.
[a] Department of Neurology, David Geffen School of Medicine, UCLA Stroke Center, University of California, RNRC, RM 4-126, Los Angeles, CA 90095, USA; [b] Department of Radiology, Division of Interventional Neuroradiology, University of California, Los Angeles, 757 Westwood plaza Suite 2129, Los Angeles, CA 90095, USA
* Corresponding author. UCLA Stroke Center, 710 Westwood Plaza, Los Angeles, CA 90095.
E-mail address: davidliebeskind@yahoo.com

Neurol Clin 32 (2014) 193–209
http://dx.doi.org/10.1016/j.ncl.2013.07.005
0733-8619/14/$ – see front matter © 2014 Elsevier Inc. All rights reserved.

neurologic.theclinics.com

throughout their disease course. This is of particular value in the monitoring of cerebral ischemic disorders, which inherently follow a dynamic course. Irrespective of clinical practice settings, the evolution and refinement of imaging techniques now permit treatment decisions to be made in real time.

REASON FOR CONSULTATION

One may propose that the reason for consultation is perhaps one of the most important guiding aspects in obtaining supportive imaging. Knowing how the specific clinical question can be asked and appropriately answered by a specific imaging modality is fundamental to selecting the appropriate imaging test. Whether the question is related to evaluation of the ischemic core, penumbral tissue, or areas at-risk, a specific vascular lesion or pathologic condition that may culminate in cerebral ischemia, understanding the advantages and limitations of neuroimaging techniques increases the yield of data gathered. In addition, much like a subspecialist consultation, obtaining ancillary imaging in an outpatient clinical setting requires providing a framework for the subspecialty-imaging expert who is analyzing and coordinating the studies. Providing a reason for consultation—whether it is assessing intracranial arterial stenosis in a specific vascular distribution, evaluating a pattern of cerebral ischemia to better understand disease mechanism, or shedding light on ischemic disease progression to modify disease management is essential in providing the evaluating imaging expert with a focus for the study interpretation. This promotes focus on a specific region of interest in the interpretation and it will lead to potential adjustment of the imaging protocol, if needed, to address best the question of interest. Improved patient care, more cost-effective measures, and reduced need for unnecessary repeat imaging will ultimately result. These will augment the clinical examination findings and aid in patient management.

PATHOPHYSIOLOGY OF CEREBRAL ISCHEMIA

The pathophysiology of cerebral ischemia extends beyond the direct effects of anatomic changes in the arterial system leading to brain tissue. Unlike focal ischemia of ischemic stroke, cerebral hypoperfusion or cardiac arrest may lead to global ischemic injury unrestricted to a specific vascular territory. The pathophysiology of ischemia is similar at the tissue and cellular level, involving metabolic dysfunction and cell death due to hypoxia. The regulation of tissue perfusion in the brain is modulated differently from any other organ in the body given that nearly half of cerebrovascular resistance relies on the large arteries at the circle of Willis, in addition to intracranial and extracranial vasculature.[1,2] These arteries and their end arterioles play a primary role in oxygen delivery to the brain parenchyma through their regulation of cerebral blood flow (CBF). Many studies in animals and humans have investigated the threshold below which a reduction in CBF manifests neurologic symptoms and those that correlate to pathologically irreversible neuronal damage.[3–5] Across studies, depending on study design, neurologic symptoms and ischemia have been reported to range in values from below nearly 20 mL/100 mL/min to between 8 and 12 mL/100 mL/min in which tissue oxygenation was no longer sufficient to support the cellular machinery.[5–8] Although conventionally cerebral ischemia was thought to result as a direct consequence of a reduction in CBF, Ostergaard and colleagues[9] recently discussed the concept of capillary transit time heterogeneity and its contribution to the brain's efficacy in extracting oxygen at a given CBF. Regional CBF changes can be demonstrated using CT or MRI (**Fig. 1**). Several fatal outcomes result from the final aftermath of tissue oxygen deprivation that, on a cellular level, includes cell body

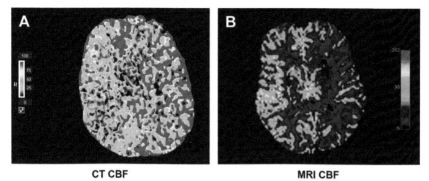

CT CBF   **MRI CBF**

Fig. 1. Regional changes in CBF are shown throughout cerebral parenchyma. (*A*) CT of patient presenting with acute right middle cerebral artery (MCA) stroke with blue demonstrating most severely decreased CBF in ischemic hemisphere. (*B*) MRI of patient presenting with acute left MCA stroke with purple demonstrating most severely decreased CBF in ischemic hemisphere.

shrinkage, chromatin condensation, and nuclear fragmentation, as well as changes to the membrane phospholipid structure.[10-13] It is proposed that phosphatidylethanolamine, one of the members of the phospholipid structure, serves a regulatory role in the blebbing and formation of apoptotic bodies, as well as in mediation of cellular necrosis, because its externalization may contribute, in part, to cytoskeletal organization.[12] In combination, an overwhelming failure of cellular energy resources ensues and results in subsequent cell death.

IMAGING OF ISCHEMIA

The outcomes of cerebral ischemia are not isolated to the acute changes that occur on a tissue, cellular, and molecular level, they also encompass the resultant subacute and chronic lesion evolution. Several imaging modalities may be used to reflect the pathophysiological changes and outcomes of cerebral ischemia at the tissue level. From multiple perspectives, the iterative refinement and versatility of these recent imaging techniques have expanded our understanding of cerebral ischemia as a disorder. This has enabled the use of multiple modalities in the imaging of vascular lesions, blood flow, and many facets of cerebral perfusion, as well as parenchyma changes demonstrating ischemic lesions, stages of evolving ischemia, consequences of ischemic injury, and tissue repair that have been invaluable in advancing therapeutic management of stroke patients. Given that each modality offers specific strengths and limitations, understanding the strengths and weaknesses of these techniques is imperative in choosing the appropriate method of investigation to discern critical mechanisms and to facilitate decision-making for our patients.

IMAGING MODALITIES IN THE ASSESSMENT OF ISCHEMIA

Noncontrast CT was initially one of the only options in assessing cerebral ischemia; however, in recent years, the development of MRI and the application of multimodal techniques with either CT or MRI have provided insight into disease pathogenesis, mechanism, and evolution. Multimodal CT typically includes noncontrast CT, CT angiography (CTA) of the head and neck, and CT perfusion (CTP). Similarly, multimodal MRI also includes several sequences, such as diffusion-weighted imaging (DWI), perfusion-weighted imaging (PWI), fluid-attenuated inversion recovery (FLAIR), gradient recalled echo (GRE) in addition to MR angiography (MRA) of the head and neck. **Fig. 2** highlights the use of multimodal imaging in acute middle cerebral artery (MCA) stroke.

Customization of imaging protocols in patients being evaluated for cerebral ischemia is typically tailored by institution. Multimodal imaging offers a comprehensive view of the patient's condition, including the integrity of brain parenchyma, extent of vascular involvement, and a dynamic view of tissue viability based on status of

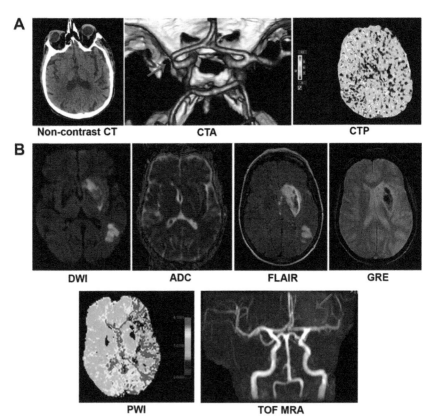

Fig. 2. The informative nature of multimodal imaging using CT and MRI. (A) Multimodal CT of an 88-year-old man with history of heart failure status after pacemaker placement, diabetes, hypertension, hyperlipidemia, and hypothyroidism presenting acutely with left-sided hemiplegia. Initial noncontrast CT with no obvious hypodensity to suggest parenchymal ischemia whereas CTA demonstrates clear right MCA signal cutoff and CTP shows decreased perfusion to the right hemisphere with areas most severely affected represented in red. (B) Multimodal MRI of an 82-year-old woman with history of hypothyroidism later found to have cardiac arrhythmia presenting acutely with right-sided hemiplegia. Ischemic lesion is represented by DWI hyperintensity corresponding with apparent diffusion coefficient (ADC) hypointensity. FLAIR also demonstrates hyperintense signal providing information about the age of the lesion, likely several hours from onset of ischemia. GRE sequence hypointensity represents hemorrhagic transformation with surrounding edema. PWI clearly demonstrates extent of decreased perfusion throughout the left hemisphere, which extends beyond the burden of the ischemic lesion demonstrated on DWI, ADC, and FLAIR, most severely represented by red. Time-of-flight (TOF) MRA demonstrates abrupt cutoff of the distal left M1 segment with decreased number of left M2 branches (*red arrows*).

cerebral perfusion. The choice between CT versus MRI can be tailored to the patient and to the symptoms at presentation. CT becomes the preferred imaging modality in patients unable to undergo MRI, such as in the case of those who have pacemaker devices or implanted metallic objects, and for patients too unstable to sustain placement in a supine position for an extended period. However, in patients who are able to undergo MRI testing, this imaging technique, although relatively more time consuming, offers the unique advantage of providing exquisite detail of brain parenchyma with early sensitivity, which far surpasses CT approaches. Minutes from the onset of neurologic symptoms, and presumably ischemic insult, MRI will display new ischemic lesions as hyperintensities on DWI and corresponding apparent diffusion coefficient (ADC) hypointensity. These lesions, which reflect acute parenchymal cytotoxic edema, are thought to approximate the ischemic core. With resolution of ischemia, it is possible for DWI lesions to become reversible.[14,15] The pattern of distribution of DWI lesions may provide invaluable insight into whether the disease mechanism is thromboembolic in nature, related to a specific vascular territory occlusion, or due to hypoperfusion and border zone ischemia.[16] Mismatch between DWI and FLAIR positivity may reveal temporal facets or the duration of ischemia.[17]

CT has limitations in the detection of very early ischemic injury in the acute setting and is quite restricted in the ability to visualize accurately posterior fossa disease.[18] However, with the wide availability of CT technology, in the community and some institutions, CT scanning continues to prevail as the first-line imaging modality. CTA and CTP, when combined with CT, yield additional insight on early ischemia. In conjunction with patient presentation and clinical examination that are consistent with a vascular event, noncontrast CT may at least be helpful in ruling out cerebral hemorrhage or an existing, nonvascular reason for presentation, such as mass related to infection, malignancy, or other cause. In the cases of suspected cerebral ischemia in which noncontrast CT did not show abnormality, repeat, serial imaging with the evolution of the patient's symptoms is also critical.

The importance of serial imaging and approaching cerebral ischemia as a dynamic condition is best demonstrated by the concept of fogging. In CT, this term has long referred to the temporary loss of visibility of ischemic lesion approximately 2 weeks after the onset of stroke.[19,20] The area of infarction develops a signal intensity similar to the surrounding normal tissue, likely secondary to inflammatory cell infiltration of the lesion. In 2004, O'Brien and colleagues[21] performed an independent, blinded review of serial MRI images for up to 7 weeks from subjects presenting with symptoms of cortical ischemic stroke, assessing for the possible presence of fogging using T2-weighted MRI. On CT imaging, fogging translated into the lesion not being visible at the 2-week interval. On MRI, there was fogging in the images of 50% of subjects (15 subjects), ranging from 6 to 36 days following ischemic event, with a median of 10 days. In these patients with moderately to large infarcts, a reduction in severity of infarct was suggested to lead to an underestimation of the final outcome of stroke and, based on this, it was advised that perhaps final imaging be obtained 7 weeks after ischemic event.[21]

ANGIOGRAPHIC ASSESSMENT OF VASCULAR LESIONS

Indirect features of parenchymal imaging with CT and MRI can be helpful in gleaning information about vascular disease. For example, a large vessel occlusion in the MCA has been described as a hyperdense MCA sign (**Fig. 3**) on noncontrast CT, signifying vascular occlusion. Parallel findings have been described in the setting of internal carotid and posterior cerebral artery occlusion.[22,23] MRI correlates to this

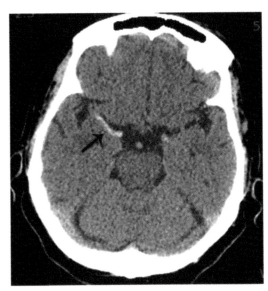

Fig. 3. Hyperdensity sign (*arrow*) of right MCA shown on noncontrast CT signifies vascular occlusion of the artery.

phenomenon of parenchymal imaging shedding light on vascular occlusion. This can be demonstrated on the GRE sequence of MRI when hypointensities in the vessel correlate with clot. Direct evidence of vascular disease can be obtained from the angiographic components of multimodal CT and MRI, which provide vital and detailed information with regard to vascular pathologic changes.

CTA offers multiple advantages because it is performed easily and efficiently following noncontrast CT in an estimated 10-minute window.[24] In the hyperacute presentation of a presumed ischemic event, CTA provides benefit in excluding patients without vascular lesions from acute interventions. For use across the temporal continuum of disease, there are several advantages and potential limitations of CTA technology. This method is advantageous for its remarkable speed and ability to capture the anatomic parameters of the neurovascular tree, including intracranial and extracranial vasculature, in approximately 15 seconds. This decreases the likelihood of motion artifact and lessens the need for large amounts of contrast.[24] Unlike flow-dependent imaging techniques, specifically MRA and ultrasound, CTA has the distinct advantage of providing anatomically accurate information regarding vascular disease, including information regarding degree of calcification, residual lumen dimensions, and length of stenosis.[24] For patients who are critically ill and require support machinery, those who are not able to tolerate lying in a supine position for an extended period, or those for whom MRI in contraindicated, CTA is particularly advantageous. From an outpatient referral standpoint, for patients with a suspected vascular lesion who are able to tolerate CT contrast, CTA is particularly important in quantifying vascular lesion burden. It can easily be used to monitor intracranial or extracranial lesion progression over time in a serial fashion. The limitations of CTA technology include the inability to provide information regarding direction or velocity or direction of flow. Such physiologic and dynamic information is readily provided by MRA or ultrasound. Another disadvantage is related to CT beam hardening in which heavily calcified vascular plaques can alter the precision of image reconstructions.[24] The

CTA portion of multimodal imaging, unlike time-of-flight (TOF) MRA, does necessitate the administration of iodinated contrast material and this may be disadvantageous in some patient populations whether in the inpatient or outpatient settings.[24]

The variations in MRA techniques are numerous. Protocols can be tailored to range from two-dimensional to three-dimensional TOF MRA. Alternatively, contrast may be used to enhance the imaging of vascular disease. TOF MRA is a GRE sequence that relies on radio frequency pulsing of tissue. In terms of two-dimensional versus three-dimensional versions of this technology, the latter offers the advantage of a higher resolution, albeit limited by vascular saturation artifacts. The former is limited by signal loss in areas in which flow turbulence is a component of disease. Another factor that may limit interpretation of TOF MRA is inadequate suppression of background that adds to the artifactual data gathered. Relying on radiofrequency pulsation for artifact suppression may lead to erroneous regions of vascular obscuration or, conversely, false areas of perceived flow because of molecules, such as methemoglobin and fat, that are not easily suppressed.[25] Again, because TOF MRA relies on dynamic flow, it does not deliver a true anatomic representation of vascular occlusion, which can be achieved by CTA. Potential overestimation of degree of stenosis or occlusion is demonstrated in **Fig. 4**, in which both slow flow and no flow cause vascular signal diminution. Phase-contrast MRA, which computes the alteration in transverse magnetization between moving and stationary tissue, may be advantageous compared with TOF MRA. Not only can this technique display the direction of flow, it can also improve on TOF MRA by showing blood that is flowing slowly given that saturation effects can be better avoided using this technique. One limitation that is posed by use of phase contrast MRA is that through its processing their results signal loss around areas of turbulent flow and areas of stenoses.[25] MRA can also be performed in conjunction with gadolinium contrast administration. **Fig. 5** shows an example of contrast-enhanced MRA (CE MRA) in a patient presenting with symptoms of acute stroke. Following a bolus of intravenous gadolinium, this GRE sequence display opacified vessels as T1 hyperintense. The use of contrast allows for shorter acquisition times and hence less likelihood of motion artifact, yet it does have a limitation in that acquisition must be completed in the time window of arterial enhancement and may not be repeated until contrast has cleared.[25]

In patients with a clinical history of trauma or neck manipulation for whom a vascular dissection is suspected, an additional angiography sequence is used, namely fat-saturated axial T1 sequence imaging of the neck, obtained before gadolinium bolus.

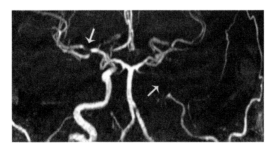

Fig. 4. Relying on flow, rather than anatomic representation of vascular occlusion, TOF MRA may overestimate the degree of vascular stenosis in patients. TOF MRA of a patient presenting with acute infarction involving multiple areas in the left M2 territory with MRA demonstrating occlusion of the posterior left M2 division of MCA with paucity of vessels (*upper arrow*). Imaging also suggests a flow-dependent degree of stenosis in right MCA, which was not clinically symptomatic during presentation (*lower arrow*).

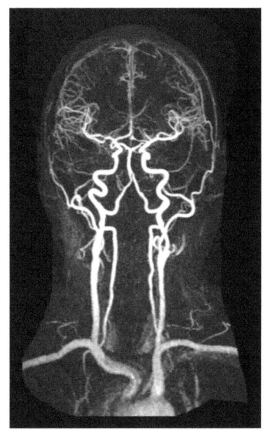

Fig. 5. The clarity of the neurovascular tree imaged using CE MRA. Opacified vessels are T1 hyperintense.

In addition, compared with noncontrast MRA, more anatomic information can be gleaned from contrast-enhanced sequences given that images represent contrast in the lumen of vessels imaged.[25] In patients with a clinical history of trauma or neck manipulation for whom a vascular dissection is suspected, an additional angiography sequence is used, namely fat-saturated axial T1 sequence imaging of the neck, obtained before gadolinium.[25]

In the case of severe vascular stenosis or total occlusion, imaging clues can be helpful in offering likely prognosis and may even predict recanalization. This finding is described as tram tracking, which indicates a minimal degree of flow in occluded lesions.[26] Not only do revascularization and recanalization play a role in the reperfusion of ischemic tissue but collateral circulation is also thought to interplay with the vascular milieu and contribute to the support of tissue perfusion.[27,28]

PERFUSION IMAGING

Perfusion imaging has served an invaluable role in directing therapeutic intervention in stroke patients. Along with DWI, the identification of ischemic core and direct comparison with cerebral perfusion, helps identify vascular territory that is further compromised or at risk (diffusion-perfusion mismatch model). These data not only shed light on diagnosis in terms of better understanding the cause of stroke and providing a dynamic view of tissue integrity, they also influence treatment decisions. For example, based on these data, knowledge of a large territory at risk may support the decision for further revascularization therapy. Perfusion imaging alone is limited because it does not detail changes that may occur in vascular collateral or compensatory changes in circulation.[29] However, with the advent of new technical postprocessing strategies, perfusion maps may be generated from angiographic maps and, in this case, information is yielded from vascular changes and tissue bed perfusion.[30]

Arterial spin labeling, as a noninvasive functional MRI perfusion technique, does not rely on contrast agent administration. This imaging modality captures patterns of CBF and, therefore, perfusion by making use of arterial water as a tracer. It is thought that this offers a repeatedly reliable measure of CBF, spatially and temporally, yet its use has been limited compared with contrast-based perfusion techniques.[31] More recently, investigators have been sharing their positive experience with reproducible and widely applicable results using this perfusion methodology.[32,33]

Routinely, aside from the technique of arterial spin-labeled perfusion MRI, multimodal imaging modalities CT and MRI require contrast agents for visualization of perfusion portion of the study. In CT technology, labeling is achieved by use of iodinated contrast agents whereas MRI relies on a gadolinium-based contrast agent. CBF and blood volume may then be extrapolated based on the anatomic mapping and distribution of contrast flow through vasculature and cerebral tissue beds. With the use of contrast comes the risk of allergic reaction, contrast extravasation, nephrotoxicity, and limited use specifically in patients with compromised renal function but not in patients without concomitant renal disease. Albeit a small risk, there seems to be lower risk and less adverse allergic reaction with gadolinium when compared with iodinated contrast agents.[34] With regard to risk for contrast extravasation, owing to the high volume of material administered and the rapid rate at which it is infused, iodinated contrast is associated with a higher overall probability of occurrence.[34] The controversy of risk for developing contrast material-induced nephropathy (CIN) associated with iodinated contrast agents and nephrogenic systemic fibrosis (NSF) in patients given gadolinium contrast essentially only applies to patients with renal disease. Renal disease exists within a spectrum and patients within this spectrum can be managed based on the following guidelines based on the severity of their disease. In patients with glomerular filtration rate (GFR) values between 30 and 60 mL/min, the recommendation is typically for the administration of gadolinium because their risk for NSF is low and the risk for CIN at this stage of their renal disease exists. In patients not dependent on hemodialysis and with GFR less than 30, the risk for CIN and NSF exists. If the need for contrast material is essential and would change the medical management, whether it be in diagnosis, allowing for prognostication, or in altering the course of therapeutic management, CT with iodinated contrast is preferred. The patient may be prophylactically treated with sodium bicarbonate and N-acetylcysteine and well hydrated before the procedure to decrease the risk of CIN. Additionally, even if CIN occurs in a patient with chronic renal disease, dialysis may be used to treat. In the case of NSF, although it occurs at a frequency of 5% in these patients, the outcome can be lethal.[34] Finally, patients whom are in renal failure and are hemodialysis-dependent, there is a high risk of developing NSF with exposure to gadolinium contrast. In these patients, iodinated contrast is preferred. Given that iodinated contrast administration does not seem to result in worsening renal function, the only risks are volume overload or overhydration. Therefore, in this cohort of patients, there is no restriction on iodinated contrast administration if it is clinically necessary and it need not be coordinated with dialysis schedule.[34]

Patients who are pregnant are also in a high-risk category with contrast administration. Although it is unlikely for gadolinium to harm the fetus or mother, given the theoretical possibility for gadolinium to be retained (not eliminated) and unconjugated, and, therefore, toxic in the amniotic fluid, most academic institutions in the United States recommend against its use. However, the risk of using iodinated contrast material is hypothyroidism for the fetus. This is amenable to therapeutic correction at delivery; therefore, guidelines recommend CT with iodinated contrast in pregnant patients if their medical condition necessitates it.[34]

NUCLEAR NEUROIMAGING

Although no longer logistically a first-line option, particularly in hyperacute presentations of stroke, nuclear imaging provides valuable information with regard to tissue fate. For investigating regional CBF in the early setting, nuclear imaging, including positron emission tomography (PET) and single-photon emission computed tomography (SPECT) have served well as surrogate prognostic markers for patient outcomes.[35–38] Nuclear neuroimaging can be an important tool in imaging of hypoperfused, yet possibly salvageable, ischemic penumbra in acute stroke. This can be evaluated by imaging of perfusion and metabolism, the neuronal integrity, or through hypoxic markers.[39] Oxygen-15 PET has been very effective in simultaneous assessment of perfusion as well as oxygen metabolism taking into account CBF and cerebral metabolic rate of oxygen.[39] Studies have demonstrated the use of SPECT in assessing the ischemic penumbra using tracers such as ^{99m}Tc-hexamethylpropyleneamine oxime and ^{99m}Tc-ethyl cysteinate dimer.[40–42] Imaging neuronal integrity to yield information about the ischemic penumbra has been demonstrated by the use of a central-type benzodiazepine receptor as a marker because changes in the expression of this receptor in the cerebral cortex can serve as a marker of irreversible neuronal damage.[43] In animal models, it was not thought that this receptor was expressed in the cerebellum or in the subcortical parenchyma.[44,45] Hypoxic markers have also been used to follow the active changes in the brain parenchyma following ischemia in acute stroke, specifically ^{18}F-labeled misonidazole in conjunction with PET imaging.[46–48] SPECT, being more widely available, has been suggested as a valuable technique for identifying patients at high risk of reperfusion injury following ischemia. This is extrapolated from studies, such as those performed by Ueda and colleagues,[49,50] which demonstrated the use of SPECT technology to evaluate the risk of hemorrhagic transformation following reperfusion therapy.

IMAGING THE SEQUELAE OF ISCHEMIA: EVOLUTION AND REPAIR

Hemorrhagic transformation as one of the consequences of acute ischemic stroke has been a challenge from an imaging standpoint. This entity is different from primary hemorrhagic stroke, which is not specifically addressed in this article. The transformation of ischemic parenchyma to areas of intracerebral hemorrhage has been described as occurring with and without patient exposure to medical therapy in the form of intravenous tissue plasminogen activator or endovascular intervention.[51] In terms of approaches to imaging, noncontrast CT, for example, has been demonstrated to be unclear in the differentiation between primary hemorrhage and hemorrhagic transformation of an ischemic lesion.[52] Similar to SPECT studies in the case of nuclear neuroimaging, using imaging modalities as a guide for patients who may be at risk for hemorrhagic transformation following reperfusion owing to reperfusion injury will clearly be beneficial in guiding treatment decision-making in the acute setting. Factors that may play a role in the incidence of hemorrhage may include integrity of parenchymal tissue, the severity and extent of ischemia, the level of reperfusion achieved following vascular occlusion, and alterations in serum blood sugar (ie, hyperglycemia). In the setting of MRI assessment, predictors of hemorrhagic transformation include extensive DWI hyperintensity with associated ADC hypointensity and concomitant low CBF,[53–55] and possibly the finding of focal FLAIR hyperintensity in the ischemic lesion.[56] An important predictor of ischemia reperfusion injury is a disturbance in the permeability of the blood-brain barrier. Given the concomitant risk of hemorrhagic transformation following reperfusion, imaging that can identify this finding is very useful in guiding the decision for revascularization.[57–61] These derangements can be demonstrated using either CT or MRI techniques.

Imaging of suspected cerebral ischemia extends far beyond a go or no go-decision during the hyperacute treatment. Special guidance must be used in the interpretation of early serial imaging following contrast-enhanced studies accounting for the phenomenon of contrast retention (**Fig. 6**). In CT imaging, this may translate into hyperdensity whereas, on T1-weighted MRI, this may be visualized as a hyperintensity. This phenomenon on CT imaging may be confounded with possible hemorrhagic transformation. For this reason, clinicians have been evaluating alternative imaging techniques to avoid misinterpretation during serial imaging, one of which is dual-energy CT, which was shown to be sensitive and specific in differentiating between iodinated contrast material staining and hemorrhage following initial ischemia.[62]

A second outcome of ischemia, after reperfusion, may be reperfusion injury in the form of tissue death despite successful recanalization. Recent studies propose that this results from radical free oxide damage, which is shown in multiple models of stroke[12,63–65] and is clinically demonstrated using voxel-based analysis of tissue fate.[66] Diffusion tensor imaging (DTI) is another MRI technique investigated in animal models[65] for its effectiveness in assessing reperfusion injury. It features the changes in brain parenchyma based on the assessment of changes in the diffusion of water molecules, taking into account magnitude and directionality of change, and is exquisitely sensitive, particularly in white matter.[65,67,68]

Serial imaging in the evolution of stroke can yield very valuable information to the outpatient clinician. In combination with the patient's clinical examination, this may

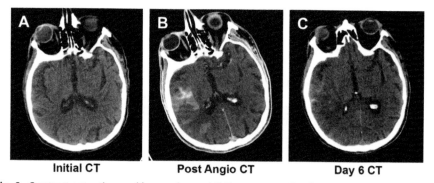

Initial CT   Post Angio CT   Day 6 CT

Fig. 6. Contrast retention and hemorrhage. (*A*) Noncontrast CT of a patient presenting with right MCA stroke. No obvious signs of hypodensity present on initial left hemiplegic presentation at onset of acute ischemia. (*B*) Noncontrast CT following interventional angiography (Post Angio) and mechanical revascularization therapy showing multiple foci of hyperdensity in which it is difficult to differentiate between hemorrhagic transformation versus postprocedural contrast retention. (*C*) Noncontrast CT 6 days following ischemic event showing less burden of hyperdensity than at initial presentation following angiography.

serve to predict and oversee functional recovery while guiding therapeutic management and monitoring for cerebrovascular disease reoccurrence. Functional recovery from deficits related to an ischemic event is thought to stem from a reorganization of brain cells and the strengthening of brain plasticity.[69–72] Repeat imaging taken into context with initial neuroimaging evaluation yields insight into the fate of tissue in the initial peri-infarct zone and ischemic penumbra. MRI images in **Fig. 7** demonstrate the significant evolution of parenchymal findings from initial presentation to 5 days following ischemic stroke in a patient with MCA occlusion.

Capitalizing on the strengths and avoiding the limitations of the available imaging techniques provides incredible insight on the pathophysiology of ischemia and ultimately guides tailored therapeutic approaches.

ISCHEMIC DISORDERS, THE CONTINUUM FROM ACUTE TO CHRONIC

Clinically, cerebral ischemia exists on a continuum ranging from the most acute or hyperacute presentation, as in the case of ischemic stroke with focal hypoperfusion or cardiac arrest leading to a sudden-onset decrease in global cerebral perfusion. Neuroimaging plays a pivotal role in the assessment of ischemic patterns, determining the age of ischemia, understanding disease mechanism, and thereby guiding therapeutic management, response, and longitudinal follow-up. In ischemic stroke, the categories of disease with variable underlying mechanisms include small vessel, large vessel, and thromboembolic disease, as well as cryptogenic, which, although unconfirmed, is likely a permutation of the major mechanisms.

Aside from parenchymal imaging (see previous discussion), angiography can provide crucial information in identifying disease conditions and specific mechanisms. This is of particular importance in the diagnosis of stroke resulting from moyamoya, vasculitis, or fibromuscular dysplasia, as well as stroke resulting from venous

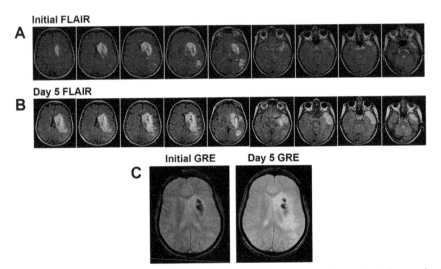

Fig. 7. Serial MRI imaging of stroke evolution. (*A*) FLAIR sequence throughout the cerebral parenchyma at initial presentation of acute ischemic stroke resulting from left MCA occlusion. (*B*) At 5 days following ischemic insult, FLAIR sequences demonstrate the evolution in intensity of lesion burden and the completion of infarction throughout the affected territories. (*C*) GRE hypointensity showing stability of initial hemorrhagic transformation over time.

pathologic conditions such as cerebral venous thrombosis. Moyamoya is a pattern of arterial occlusive disease with an increased incidence in Asian patients and patients with sickle cell disease or neurofibromatosis. This occlusive vasculopathy is progressive in nature and typically begins by affecting the internal carotid artery then evolves to involve the anterior artery and MCA proximally with compensatory dilation in collaterals.[25] The manifestations of this vascular disease in children versus adults are more ischemic in nature in the former, and presents with parenchymal hemorrhage in the latter.[73] **Fig. 8** demonstrates multimodal MRI imaging in an adult diagnosed with moyamoya, presenting with acute hemorrhage. The imaging modality, which is instrumental in making the diagnosis, is MRA, which can demonstrate the vasoocclusive phenomenon as well as the dilation of collaterals.[74,75] Yamada and colleagues,[76] in their evaluation of 26 patients, found this imaging technique to yield 73% sensitivity and 100% specificity in diagnosing the disease. The pattern of collaterals also has been reported to correlate with the onset of subsequent vascular events and, as such, MRA has been instrumental in guiding the treatment of these patients as part of evaluation for revascularization therapy.[25] In the case of vasculitis, which has many causes, parenchymal imaging may reveal ischemic or hemorrhagic lesions and MRA may be clinically useful although less sensitive than digital subtraction angiography imaging.[77] MRA may also serve an important role in delineating the mimicking pathological conditions such as vascular hypoplasia or dissection. A limitation of TOF MRA slice artifacts is that they may be mistaken for alternating stenoses.[25]

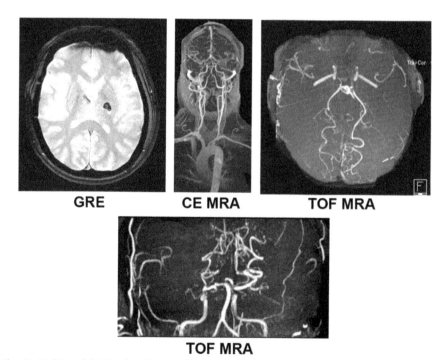

GRE   CE MRA   TOF MRA

TOF MRA

Fig. 8. Multimodal MRI of a 44 year-old woman with history of moyamoya presenting with numbness, tingling, and weakness in the right upper extremity. GRE hypointensity shows left basal ganglia hemorrhage. CE MRA and TOF MRA of the neck and head demonstrate occlusion of bilateral supraclinoid internal carotid arteries with distal reconstitution secondary to vascular collaterals, as well as narrowing of bilateral internal carotid arteries.

REFERENCES

1. Paulson OB, Strandgaard S, Edvinsson L. Cerebral autoregulation. Cerebrovasc Brain Metab Rev 1990;2(2):161–92.
2. Shapiro HM, Stromberg DD, Lee DR, et al. Dynamic pressures in the pial arterial microcirculation. Am J Physiol 1971;221(1):279–83.
3. Finnerty FA, Witkin L, Fazekas JF. Cerebral hemodynamics during cerebral ischemia induced by acute hypotension. J Clin Invest 1954;33(9):1227–32.
4. Jennett WB, Harper AM, Gillespie FC. Measurement of regional cerebral blood-flow during carotid ligation. Lancet 1966;2(7474):1162–3.
5. Astrup J, Siesjö BK, Symon L. Thresholds in cerebral ischemia—the ischemic penumbra. Stroke 1981;12(6):723–5.
6. Marchal G, Beaudouin V, Rioux P, et al. Prolonged persistence of substantial volumes of potentially viable brain tissue after stroke: a correlative PET-CT study with voxel-based data analysis. Stroke 1996;27(4):599–606.
7. Furlan M, Marchal G, Viader F, et al. Spontaneous neurological recovery after stroke and the fate of the ischemic penumbra. Ann Neurol 1996;40(2):216–26.
8. Marchal G, Benali K, Iglesias S, et al. Voxel-based mapping of irreversible ischaemic damage with PET in acute stroke. Brain 1999;122(Pt 12):2387–400.
9. Ostergaard L, Jespersen SN, Mouridsen K, et al. The role of the cerebral capillaries in acute ischemic stroke: the extended penumbra model. J Cereb Blood Flow Metab 2013;33(5):635–48.
10. Taylor RC, Cullen SP, Martin SJ. Apoptosis: controlled demolition at the cellular level. Nat Rev Mol Cell Biol 2008;9(3):231–41.
11. Balasubramanian K, Schroit AJ. Aminophospholipid asymmetry: a matter of life and death. Annu Rev Physiol 2003;65:701–34.
12. Zhang Y, Stevenson GD, Barber C, et al. Imaging of rat cerebral ischemia-reperfusion injury using (99m)Tc-labeled duramycin. Nucl Med Biol 2013; 40(1):80–8.
13. Broughton BR, Reutens DC, Sobey CG. Apoptotic mechanisms after cerebral ischemia. Stroke 2009;40(5):e331–9.
14. Kidwell CS, Saver JL, Mattiello J, et al. Thrombolytic reversal of acute human cerebral ischemic injury shown by diffusion/perfusion magnetic resonance imaging. Ann Neurol 2000;47(4):462–9.
15. Fiehler J, Foth M, Kucinski T, et al. Severe ADC decreases do not predict irreversible tissue damage in humans. Stroke 2002;33(1):79–86.
16. Caplan LR, Wong KS, Gao S, et al. Is hypoperfusion an important cause of strokes? If so, how? Cerebrovasc Dis 2006;21(3):145–53. http://dx.doi.org/10.1159/000090791.
17. Thomalla G, Cheng B, Ebinger M, et al. DWI-FLAIR mismatch for the identification of patients with acute ischaemic stroke within 4·5 h of symptom onset (PRE-FLAIR): a multicentre observational study. Lancet Neurol 2011;10(11):978–86.
18. Selco SL, Liebeskind DS. Hyperacute imaging of ischemic stroke: role in therapeutic management. Curr Cardiol Rep 2005;7(1):10–5.
19. Becker H, Desch H, Hacker H, et al. CT fogging effect with ischemic cerebral infarcts. Neuroradiology 1979;18(4):185–92.
20. Skriver EB, Olsen TS. Transient disappearance of cerebral infarcts on CT scan, the so-called fogging effect. Neuroradiology 1981;22(2):61–5.
21. O'Brien P, Sellar RJ, Wardlaw JM. Fogging on T2-weighted MR after acute ischaemic stroke: how often might this occur and what are the implications? Neuroradiology 2004;46(8):635–41.

22. Ozdemir O, Leung A, Bussiére M, et al. Hyperdense internal carotid artery sign: a CT sign of acute ischemia. Stroke 2008;39(7):2011–6.
23. Krings T, Noelchen D, Mull M, et al. The hyperdense posterior cerebral artery sign: a computed tomography marker of acute ischemia in the posterior cerebral artery territory. Stroke 2006;37(2):399–403.
24. Josser E, Delgado Almandoz JE, Kamalian S, et al. Acute ischemic stroke. In: González RG, Hirsch JA, Lev MH, et al, editors. Acute Ischemic Stroke. Imaging and Intervention. Berlin: Springer Berlin Heidelberg; 2011. p. 57–82.
25. Kim AC, Vu D, Gilberto González R, et al. Acute ischemic stroke. In: González RG, Hirsch JA, Lev MH, et al, editors. Acute Ischemic Stroke. Imaging and Intervention. Berlin: Springer Berlin Heidelberg; 2011. p. 123–44.
26. Otsuka Y, Waki R, Yamauchi H, et al. Angiographic demarcation of an occlusive lesion may predict recanalization after intra-arterial thrombolysis in patients with acute middle cerebral artery occlusion. J Neuroimaging 2008;18(4):422–7.
27. Liebeskind DS. Collateral perfusion: time for novel paradigms in cerebral ischemia. Int J Stroke 2012;7(4):309–10.
28. Liebeskind DS. Reperfusion for acute ischemic stroke: arterial revascularization and collateral therapeutics. Curr Opin Neurol 2010;23(1):36–45.
29. Liebeskind DS. Imaging the future of stroke: I. Ischemia. Ann Neurol 2009;66(5): 574–90.
30. Liebeskind DS, Black SE. Abstract - Perfusion angiography: a novel technique for characterization of perfusion in cerebral ischemia. Available at: http://research.baycrest.org/publication/view/id/7917. Accessed March 19, 2013.
31. Borogovac A, Asllani I. Arterial Spin Labeling (ASL) fMRI: advantages, theoretical constrains, and experimental challenges in neurosciences. Int J Biomed Imaging 2012;2012:818456.
32. Hendrikse J, Petersen ET, Golay X. Vascular disorders: insights from arterial spin labeling. Neuroimaging Clin N Am 2012;22(2):259–69, x–xi.
33. Deibler AR, Pollock JM, Kraft RA, et al. Arterial spin-labeling in routine clinical practice, part 3: hyperperfusion patterns. AJNR Am J Neuroradiol 2008;29(8): 1428–35.
34. Halvorsen RA. Which study when? Iodinated contrast-enhanced CT versus gadolinium-enhanced MR imaging. Radiology 2008;249(1):9–15.
35. Friedman PJ, Davis G, Allen B. Semi-quantitative SPECT scanning in acute ischaemic stroke. Scand J Rehabil Med 1993;25(3):99–105.
36. Marchal G, Bouvard G, Iglesias S, et al. Predictive value of (99m)Tc-HMPAO-SPECT for neurological outcome/recovery at the acute stage of stroke. Cerebrovasc Dis 2000;10(1):8–17.
37. Alexandrov AV, Bladin CF, Ehrlich LE, et al. Noninvasive assessment of intracranial perfusion in acute cerebral ischemia. J Neuroimaging 1995;5(2):76–82.
38. Giubilei F, Lenzi GL, Di Piero V, et al. Predictive value of brain perfusion single-photon emission computed tomography in acute ischemic stroke. Stroke 1990; 21(6):895–900.
39. Oku N, Kashiwagi T, Hatazawa J. Nuclear neuroimaging in acute and subacute ischemic stroke. Ann Nucl Med 2010;24(9):629–38.
40. Mahagne MH, David O, Darcourt J, et al. Voxel-based mapping of cortical ischemic damage using Tc 99m L, L-ethyl cysteinate dimer SPECT in acute stroke. J Neuroimaging 2004;14(1):23–32.
41. Hatazawa J, Shimosegawa E, Toyoshima H, et al. Cerebral blood volume in acute brain infarction: a combined study with dynamic susceptibility contrast MRI and 99mTc-HMPAO-SPECT. Stroke 1999;30(4):800–6.

42. Watanabe Y, Takagi H, Aoki S, et al. Prediction of cerebral infarct sizes by cerebral blood flow SPECT performed in the early acute stage. Ann Nucl Med 1999; 13(4):205–10.

43. Sette G, Baron JC, Young AR, et al. In vivo mapping of brain benzodiazepine receptor changes by positron emission tomography after focal ischemia in the anesthetized baboon. Stroke 1993;24(12):2046–57 [discussion: 2057–8].

44. d'Argy R, Persson A, Sedvall G. A quantitative cerebral and whole body autoradiographic study of a intravenously administered benzodiazepine antagonist 3H-Ro 15-1788 in mice. Psychopharmacology 1987;92(1):8–13.

45. Hantraye P, Kaijima M, Prenant C, et al. Central type benzodiazepine binding sites: a positron emission tomography study in the baboon's brain. Neurosci Lett 1984;48(2):115–20.

46. Markus R, Reutens DC, Kazui S, et al. Topography and temporal evolution of hypoxic viable tissue identified by 18F-fluoromisonidazole positron emission tomography in humans after ischemic stroke. Stroke 2003;34(11):2646–52.

47. Read SJ, Hirano T, Abbott DF, et al. The fate of hypoxic tissue on 18F-fluoromisonidazole positron emission tomography after ischemic stroke. Ann Neurol 2000;48(2):228–35.

48. Read SJ, Hirano T, Abbott DF, et al. Identifying hypoxic tissue after acute ischemic stroke using PET and 18F-fluoromisonidazole. Neurology 1998;51(6): 1617–21.

49. Ueda T, Sakaki S, Yuh WT, et al. Outcome in acute stroke with successful intraarterial thrombolysis and predictive value of initial single-photon emission-computed tomography. J Cereb Blood Flow Metab 1999;19(1):99–108.

50. Ueda T, Hatakeyama T, Kumon Y, et al. Evaluation of risk of hemorrhagic transformation in local intra-arterial thrombolysis in acute ischemic stroke by initial SPECT. Stroke 1994;25(2):298–303.

51. Khatri P, Wechsler LR, Broderick JP. Intracranial hemorrhage associated with revascularization therapies. Stroke 2007;38(2):431–40.

52. Lovelock CE, Anslow P, Molyneux AJ, et al. Substantial observer variability in the differentiation between primary intracerebral hemorrhage and hemorrhagic transformation of infarction on CT brain imaging. Stroke 2009;40(12):3763–7.

53. Campbell BC, Christensen S, Butcher KS, et al. Regional very low cerebral blood volume predicts hemorrhagic transformation better than diffusion-weighted imaging volume and thresholded apparent diffusion coefficient in acute ischemic stroke. Stroke 2010;41(1):82–8.

54. Lee SH, Kim BJ, Ryu WS, et al. White matter lesions and poor outcome after intracerebral hemorrhage: a nationwide cohort study. Neurology 2010;74(19): 1502–10.

55. Singer OC, Humpich MC, Fiehler J, et al. Risk for symptomatic intracerebral hemorrhage after thrombolysis assessed by diffusion-weighted magnetic resonance imaging. Ann Neurol 2008;63(1):52–60.

56. Cho AH, Kim JS, Kim SJ, et al. Focal fluid-attenuated inversion recovery hyperintensity within acute diffusion-weighted imaging lesions is associated with symptomatic intracerebral hemorrhage after thrombolysis. Stroke 2008;39(12): 3424–6.

57. Aviv RI, d'Esterre CD, Murphy BD, et al. Hemorrhagic transformation of ischemic stroke: prediction with CT perfusion. Radiology 2009;250(3):867–77.

58. Bang OY, Saver JL, Alger JR, et al. Patterns and predictors of blood-brain barrier permeability derangements in acute ischemic stroke. Stroke 2009; 40(2):454–61. http://dx.doi.org/10.1161/STROKEAHA.108.522847.

59. Fiehler J, Remmele C, Kucinski T, et al. Reperfusion after severe local perfusion deficit precedes hemorrhagic transformation: an MRI study in acute stroke patients. Cerebrovasc Dis 2005;19(2):117–24.

60. Hom J, Dankbaar JW, Soares BP, et al. Blood-brain barrier permeability assessed by perfusion CT predicts symptomatic hemorrhagic transformation and malignant edema in acute ischemic stroke. AJNR Am J Neuroradiol 2011;32(1):41–8.

61. Kassner A, Thornhill R. Measuring the integrity of the human blood-brain barrier using magnetic resonance imaging. Methods Mol Biol 2011;686:229–45.

62. Gupta R, Phan CM, Leidecker C, et al. Evaluation of dual-energy CT for differentiating intracerebral hemorrhage from iodinated contrast material staining. Radiology 2010;257(1):205–11.

63. Bolaños JP, Almeida A. Roles of nitric oxide in brain hypoxia-ischemia. Biochim Biophys Acta 1999;1411(2–3):415–36.

64. Yang GY, Betz AL. Reperfusion-induced injury to the blood-brain barrier after middle cerebral artery occlusion in rats. Stroke 1994;25(8):1658–64 [discussion: 1664–5].

65. Guo J, Zheng HB, Duan JC, et al. Diffusion tensor MRI for the assessment of cerebral ischemia/reperfusion injury in the penumbra of non-human primate stroke model. Neurol Res 2011;33(1):108–12.

66. Nour M, Scalzo F, Liebeskind DS. Insight into human ischemia reperfusion injury in acute stroke: voxel-based MRI analysis of tissue fate. Int J Stroke 2013;44: Abstract TP56.

67. Granziera C, Ay H, Koniak SP, et al. Diffusion tensor imaging shows structural remodeling of stroke mirror region: results from a pilot study. Eur Neurol 2012; 67(6):370–6.

68. Pierpaoli C, Basser PJ. Toward a quantitative assessment of diffusion anisotropy. Magn Reson Med 1996;36(6):893–906.

69. Lee RG, Van Donkelaar P. Mechanisms underlying functional recovery following stroke. Can J Neurol Sci 1995;22(4):257–63.

70. Steinberg BA, Augustine JR. Behavioral, anatomical, and physiological aspects of recovery of motor function following stroke. Brain Res Brain Res Rev 1997; 25(1):125–32.

71. Johansson BB. Brain plasticity and stroke rehabilitation. The Willis lecture. Stroke 2000;31(1):223–30.

72. Seil FJ. Recovery and repair issues after stroke from the scientific perspective. Curr Opin Neurol 1997;10(1):49–51.

73. Scott RM, Smith ER. Moyamoya disease and moyamoya syndrome. N Engl J Med 2009;360(12):1226–37.

74. Yamada I, Matsushima Y, Suzuki S. Moyamoya disease: diagnosis with three-dimensional time-of-flight MR angiography. Radiology 1992;184(3):773–8.

75. Yamada I, Nakagawa T, Matsushima Y, et al. High-resolution turbo magnetic resonance angiography for diagnosis of moyamoya disease. Stroke 2001; 32(8):1825–31.

76. Yamada I, Suzuki S, Matsushima Y. Moyamoya disease: comparison of assessment with MR angiography and MR imaging versus conventional angiography. Radiology 1995;196(1):211–8.

77. Demaerel P, De Ruyter N, Maes F, et al. Magnetic resonance angiography in suspected cerebral vasculitis. Eur Radiol 2004;14(6):1005–12.

Imaging and Decision-Making in Neurocritical Care

Paul M. Vespa, MD

KEYWORDS

- Traumatic brain injury • Imaging modalities • Central nervous system

KEY POINTS

- There are several central nervous system–based neurocritical care disorders that are highly dependent on advanced imaging.
- Imaging modalities are very important in the diagnosis and treatment of traumatic brain injury.
- In contrast to conventional magnetic resonance imaging, proton-magnetic resonance spectroscopy documents evolutionary metabolic and neurochemical dysfunction after traumatic brain injury.
- Subarachnoid hemorrhage affects about 30,000 patients per year in the United States and even more worldwide.
- Intracerebral hemorrhage is a common disease with a substantial need for imaging.

INTRODUCTION

Critically ill neurologic patients are common in the hospital practice of neurology and are often in extreme states requiring accurate and specific information. Imaging, especially using advanced imaging techniques, can provide an important means of garnering this information. The reasons for this are many but do involve the lack of a clinical examination and the necessity to select treatments that are high risk but also high reward. This article focuses on the clinical utilization of selective imaging methods that are commonly used in critically ill neurologic patients to render diagnoses, to monitor effects of treatment, or have contributed to a better understanding of pathophysiology in the intensive care unit (ICU). The discussion focuses on clinical decision-making using neuroimaging and outlines the pitfalls and controversies of these techniques.

NEUROCRITICAL CARE DISORDERS

There are several central nervous system–based neurocritical care disorders that are highly dependent on advanced imaging. These disorders include traumatic brain

David Geffen School of Medicine at UCLA, 757 Westwood Boulevard, Room 6236A, Los Angeles, CA 90095, USA
E-mail address: Pvespa@mednet.ucla.edu

Neurol Clin 32 (2014) 211–224
http://dx.doi.org/10.1016/j.ncl.2013.07.010
0733-8619/14/$ – see front matter © 2014 Elsevier Inc. All rights reserved.

injury, stroke, intracerebral hemorrhage (ICH), subarachnoid hemorrhage (SAH), status epilepticus, spinal cord injury, hypoxic-iscuemic coma, and hepatic coma. Most of these disorders share a common theme of a primary insult at the moment of injury or stroke followed by a progressive illness that rapidly worsens over a short period of time. During this progressive illness, cerebral edema, metabolic dysfunction, and ischemia may occur and this results in a secondary injury. The time course of secondary insults is many days if not weeks after the original injury. If the combination of the primary and secondary injuries is severe enough, long-term neurologic outcome will be poor. Therefore, the goals of neurocritical care are to forestall the secondary injuries and provide an opportunity for stabilization and recovery of function. These critical illnesses typically affect the brain in a heterogeneous fashion and hence imaging-based assessments of brain function are important, because imaging is capable of distinguishing regional brain structure and function.

A common theme in comatose patients is the evolution of pathophysiology over several days. This pathophysiology typically involves early ischemia followed by evolving brain edema, cell death, and/or hydrocephalus. This evolving brain pathologic condition is difficult to monitor in the absence of neuroimaging and hence creates a requirement for serial imaging and strategic timed imaging. The timing of imaging is outlined on a disease-by-disease basis in the following text.

IMAGING MODALITIES—RELEVANCE TO THE SPECIFIC DISORDERS
Traumatic Brain Injury

Brain trauma is a very common neurocritical care illness, with over 500,000 patients affected each year, and at least 200,000 hospitalized with moderate-to-severe injuries. Imaging modalities are very important in the diagnosis and treatment of traumatic brain injury (TBI). Principal among these are magnetic resonance imaging (MRI), magnetic resonance spectroscopy (MRS), computed tomography (CT), and positron emission tomography (PET) imaging. CT scanning is commonly used to screen patients for moderate to severe injury and to triage patients to surgery rapidly. Noncontrast CT is best used for serial imaging in TBI. The purpose of CT in TBI is to detect surgical lesions and cerebral edema. **Fig. 1** outlines several important lesion types in acute TBI. CT is typically performed on an emergency basis and is then repeated periodically during the ICU stay to detect brain edema. **Table 1** outlines the use of CT, including the timing and potential adjustments in clinical care that ensues. Cerebral edema can be evaluated and medical treatment can be titrated based on the CT findings. Special attention to midline shift, compression of the cisterns, and mass effect from hemorrhages can be helpful to the intensivist and can guide treatment. For example, an increase in hemorrhage volume, as shown in **Fig. 2**, could be used to make a decision about intracranial pressure monitoring or decompressive surgery. Clinical prognostication using the Marshall grading system has become commonplace and is an important component of the Project-Impact prognostic scoring system.[1] It is recognized that there is variability in interpretation of these scans, and the clinician is advised to review these scans personally for evolution of brain edema, using the Marshall grading scale (**Table 2**).

MRI

The important MRI sequences for the assessment of TBI include gradient echo recall, signal-weighted intensity, fluid attenuation inversion recovery, and diffusion tensor imaging (DTI). Using MRI, permanent injuries have been widely documented: (1) MRI is able to detect an increased number of subcortical injuries that are not apparent on conventional computerized tomography.[2–5] (2) Diffuse shear injuries occur but are

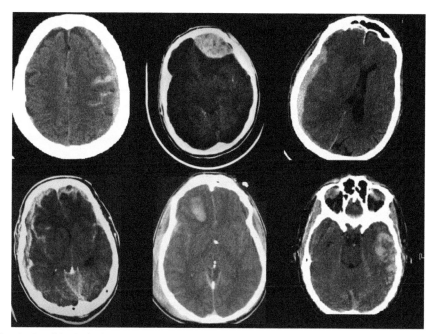

Fig. 1. CT of brain lesions.

not uniformly hemorrhagic.[2] (3) Many areas of the brain appear quite normal without evidence of edema or structural change.[6–8] (4) The location and number of deep shearing injuries are correlated with poor outcome, with lesions of the corpus callosum and dorsal brainstem having particularly negative influence on outcome.[2,6,9] The

Table 1			
Imaging clinical protocol in traumatic brain injury in the ICU			
Imaging Test	**Frequency**	**Interpretative Queries**	**ICU Treatment Decision**
Noncontrast CT	PIH 1, 6, 12	Surgical lesion Progressive edema Elevated ICP	Surgical decompression ICP/EVD monitor Osmolar therapy
Noncontrast CT	PIH 72 or 96	Progressive edema Hydrocephalus	Surgical decompression Osmolar therapy Tapering EVD
CTA	PIH 6 and clinical suspicion	Vascular injury	Endovascular or surgical treatment of vascular injury
MRI	PID 1–7	Lesion location and total lesion burden	Prognostic assessment Osmolar therapy Treat ongoing ischemia
MRS	PID 1–7	Metabolic function of the brain	Prognostic assessment
PET	PID 1–7	Metabolic function of the brain	Research tool at present; glucose control and CO_2 control

Abbreviations: EVD, external ventricular drain; ICP, intracranial pressure; PID, post injury day; PIH, post injury hour.

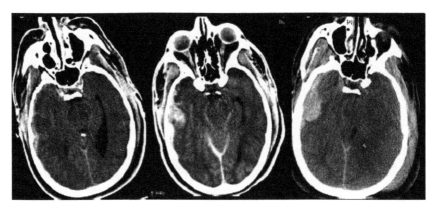

Fig. 2. Evolution and expansion of traumatic brain hemorrhage.

extent of these acute brain lesions suggests that a small portion of the brain has some element of injury because of the deep shear lesions or brain edema, whereas many regions on MRI demonstrate no apparent injury at all. Special sequences such as the susceptibility weighted image provide enhanced detection of magnetic field inhomogeneity, which results in increased signal attenuation in regions of brain hemorrhage and is useful for detecting microhemorrhages that are caused by traumatic axonal injury. **Fig. 3** demonstrates the typical appearance of many small traumatic hemorrhages in a patient with severe TBI.

DTI

DTI is widely being applied to acute stroke for the determination of early stroke location and vascular anatomy definitions and is covered elsewhere in this issue. DTI is also being applied to patients with hypoxic ischemic injury (HIE), and TBI. In HIE, there are early diffuse signs of cortical and subcortical diffusion restriction that can make the diagnosis of ischemic brain injury. In TBI, DTI in the form of tractography and fractional

Table 2
Major CT imaging designation using the Marshall classification

Marshall Class	Finding	Clinical Significance
Diffuse injury type 1	No visible lesion	Low likelihood of ICP
Diffuse injury type II	Cisterns present Midline shift 0–5 mm No high density lesion >25 mL	Moderate likelihood of ICP
Diffuse injury type III	Cisterns compressed or absent with midline shift 0–5 mm No high-density or mixed-density lesion >25 mL	High likelihood of ICP Deeper coma
Diffuse injury type IV	Cistersn compressed Midline shift >5 mm High-density or mixed-density lesion >25 mL	High likelihood of ICP Deeper coma
Nonevacuated mass lesion	Mass lesion remains	High likelihood of ICP Deeper coma
Evacuated mass lesion	Mass lesion removed	Variable ICP

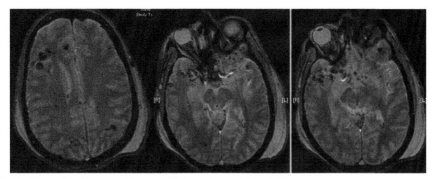

Fig. 3. Example of traumatic axonal injury detected by MRI.

anisotropy (FA) is being used to evaluate mild TBI and can be useful in moderate and severe TBI. However, the use of DTI in TBI is somewhat less applicable to clinical practice at this time. Recently, DTI imaging has been used for the description of white matter injuries. The main measure is that of FA. FA is typically reduced after TBI, due to tissue edema in white matter or to traumatic axonal injury, resulting in subtle findings on visible MRI. Quantitative measures are required to detect reductions in FA. Three-dimensional imaging transforms DTI measures into visible tractography through a variety of methods, many of which are automated in clinical MRI instruments. **Fig. 4** demonstrates an example of tractogram image in severe TBI. With severe brain injury, the white matter tracts are disrupted and loss of vector-related tracts can be seen.

MRS
In contrast to conventional MRI, proton-magnetic resonance spectroscopy (H-MRS) documents evolutionary metabolic and neurochemical dysfunction after TBI. H-MRS has the ability to detect concentrations of several metabolites that become reversibly abnormal after TBI. The abnormal metabolic profile includes a reduction in levels of NAA (*n*-acetyl-aspartate), NAA/Cho (NAA/choline) and NAA/Cr levels (NAA/creatine). In nontraumatized normal adults, the normal values are as follows: NAA 10 mmol/L $\pm$ 0.9, Cr 6.0 $\pm$ 1.3, Cho 1.6 $\pm$ 0.3, and for ratios normal values are NAA/Cr >4, NAA/Cho >3, and Cho/Cr >1.5.[10-13] There is some age-related decrease in NAA with a lower limit of normal 7 $\pm$ 0.6 in patients greater than 70 years. Values are reduced after TBI in both normal-appearing white matter and pericontusional tissue and these reductions persist for weeks to months. Most changes are related to a

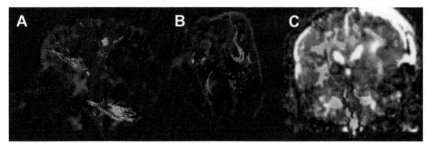

Fig. 4. Diffusion tensor tractography in acute brain injury. (*A*) Sagittal image showing long fiber tracts, (*B*) Axial image showing white matter connecting fiber tracts, (*C*) Coronal image showing crossing and long fiber tracts.

primary reduction in NAA and increase in Cho without significant change in Cr levels. NAA reductions in mild TBI have been used to document metabolic dysfunction in the normal-appearing white matter despite a lack of structural MRI findings. MRS NAA levels have been correlated with 6-month outcome after mild to moderate TBI.[14–16] The MRS neurochemical abnormalities are in part reversible and exhibit a predictable time course of resolution. A limited number of studies have combined early imaging (<8 hours after injury) with subacute scans. Reversible changes in NAA and lactate have been documented,[17] indicating a gradual improvement in brain metabolism with time after the injury. However, others have documented permanent reduction in NAA.[16,18] The reduction in NAA can occur in regions remote from the primary injury site,[19] may be partially reversible at 6 months, or may be long-lasting.[18] Thus changes in NAA are uniformly seen after TBI in areas that are not primarily injured yet display metabolic dysfunction.

NAA is a marker of mitochondrial dysfunction: despite the robust changes in NAA after experimental and human TBI, the metabolic factors underlying reduction in NAA have not been identified. NAA is located almost exclusively in neurons,[20–24] although small amounts have been found in oligodendroglia. NAA synthesis depends on mitochondrial function.[25] NAA is made from aspartate and N-acetyl-CoA by L-aspartate-N-acetyltransferase, or by cleavage of N-aspartylglutamate by N-acety-lated-α-linked-aminopeptidase. Both processes are attributed to neuronal function and depend on mitochondrial function. NAA is hydrolyzed by amidohydrolase located primarily in oligodendrocytes. NAA can serve as an osmolyte and as a metabolic inter-mediate in protein synthesis serving as an acetyl group donor.[26] Reduction in NAA was initially thought to reflect neuronal loss, but recently, reversibility of NAA reduc-tions have been documented with return of both NAA and ATP with moderate TBI.[19,27] Reductions in NAA can be transient in mild brain injury with the extent and duration of the reductions related to the injury severity of the model. NAA reduction is independent of cell loss and has a time course of recovery that correlates with the recovery of glucose metabolism and mitochondrial α-glycerophosphate dehydro-genase activity in the rodent diffuse axonal injury model.[28] The reduction in NAA is correlated with a reduction in ATP and is correlated with impaired function of the mito-chondria.[27] This correlation attests to the potential reversibility of NAA changes that may occur in acute neurocritical care when conditions of brain injury, metabolic crisis, or ischemia occur. **Fig. 5** demonstrates alterations of H-MRS NAA in areas of TBI.

PET

Human metabolic studies in brain injury using PET have documented impaired oxida-tive metabolism and altered glucose metabolism.[29–33] Oxidative metabolism is reduced by 50% as long as weeks after the insult.[34–38] Increased glucose metabolism (eg, hyperglycolysis) is found in 60% of severely brain-injured adults in the absence of cerebral ischemia but in the presence of reduced oxidative metabolism. Reduction in cerebral blood flow and $CMRO_2$ without ischemia has been independently demon-strated by PET.[35,39] The burden of ischemic brain tissue has been debated in the liter-ature with recent reports suggesting that less than 10% of the brain is ischemic, but wide regions of the brain have impaired $CMRO_2$ with reduced CBF.[34] Most recently, the author has documented that reduced $CMRO_2$ is reduced and is the most profound independent factor in clinical outcome,[40] even when the initial severity of injury is factored in. Thus the reduction in $CMRO_2$ may be a persistent and modifiable factor that affects outcome. Preliminary studies have indicated a modest ability to alter the rate of oxidative metabolism through augmentation of cerebral perfusion pressure[37] but it is not clear that such interventions will result in improved outcome. Longterm

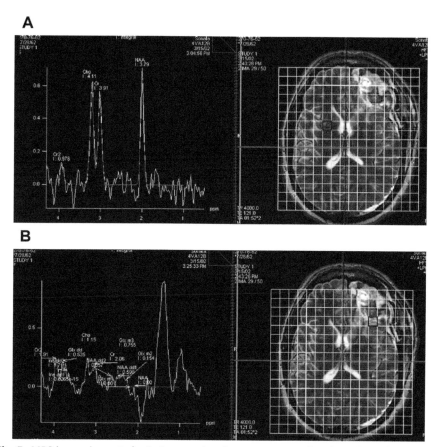

Fig. 5. MRS image in acute brain trauma showing spectroscopy in selected voxels (*outlined in blue squares*). (*A*) Normal spectra in a normal appearing matter area, contralateral to the left frontal contusion. (*B*) Abnormal spectra showing near complete loss of N-acetyl-aspartate in a tissue that is adjacent to the left frontal contusion.

clinical outcome seems to be related to the extent of early metabolic distress, as seen on PET imaging.[33] PET can be used to adjust serum glucose and to determine the proper metabolic state for the patient **Fig. 5**.[41] Similarly, alteration of ventilation strategies can be assessed by measuring sequential changes in oxygen PET imaging.[34] Excessive hyperventilation may lead to brain ischemia. Progressive loss of tissue and long-term atrophy can be determined by PET imaging.[33,42] In summary, brain metabolism is impaired because of poor mitochondrial function resulting in an increased reliance on glucose metabolism and a lack of energy supply, or energy crisis.

SAH

SAH affects about 30,000 patients per year in the United States and even more worldwide. SAH has a temporal course that requires the use of neuroimaging in a repeated fashion over the course of 2 to 3 weeks. Conventionally, conventional CT imaging and invasive 4-vessel angiography have been the mainstay methods to diagnose and treat SAH. Computed tomographic angiography (CTA) is very useful for diagnosis of the

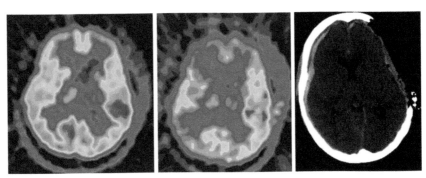

Fig. 6. PET image during ICU of severe TBI.

intracranial aneurysm and planning for surgery or coiling. In the past, conventional angiography was mandatory for aneurysm treatment, but new guidelines[43] recommend the use of CTA for aneurysm detection and diagnosis because CTA has the ability to detect very small aneurysms as the source of the SAH with a high degree of reliability.[44] However, CTA and computed tomographic perfusion (CTP) have been reported to have significant clinical impact on patient care. CTA and CTP have been used to detect vasospasm, with vascular narrowing being seen in the former and

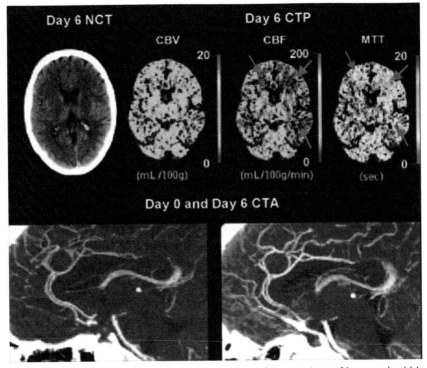

Fig. 7. CTA and CTP in vasospasm after SAH. *Arrows* indicate regions of low cerebral blood flow associated angiographic vasospasm. (*Adapted from* Dankbaar JW, Rijsdijk M, van der Schaaf IC, et al. Relationship between vasospasm, cerebral perfusion, and delayed cerebral ischemia after aneurysmal SAH. Neuroradiology 2009;51:813–9; with permission.)

reduction tissue cerebral blood flow seen in the latter. The overall sensitivity and specificity of CTA and CTP for vasospasm have been studied, and preliminary findings indicate a positive predictive value of 0.88 for CTP and 0.7 for CTA.[45–48] **Figs. 6** and **7** show an example of vasospasm-related reduction in cerebral blood flow on a diagnostic CTP and CTA study.[49,50] MRI and MR angiography are somewhat less useful in this condition given the lack of time-of-flight MR angiography to detect small aneurysms, and the difficulty in detecting subarachnoid blood with MRI. MRI however is useful in detecting small strokes after the onset of SAH and/or during the subacute period.[51]

HIE

HIE is a common neurocritical care disorder affecting about 175,000 patients per year. HIE is a global insult leading to coma. The American Heart Association has recommended therapeutic hypothermia treatment for HIE after cardiac arrest.

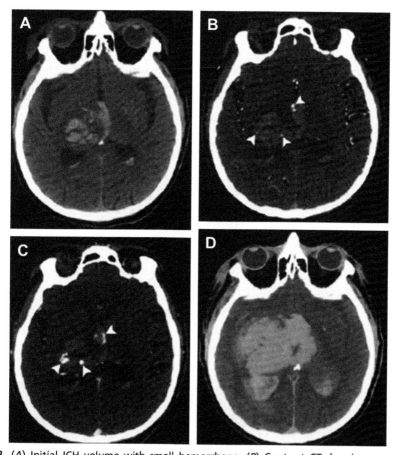

Fig. 8. (*A*) Initial ICH volume with small hemorrhage, (*B*) Contrast CT showing spot signs (*arrowheads*), (*C*) Delayed ICH with greater volume and spot signs (*arrowheads*), (*D*) Later ICH with large expansion of hematoma. (*From* Almandoz JE, Yoo AJ, Stone MJ, et al. Systematic characterization of the computed tomography angiography spot sign in primary intracerebral hemorrhage identifies patients at highest risk for hematoma expansion: the spot sign score. Stroke 2009;40:2994–3000; with permission.)

Neurologists are becoming increasingly involved in the treatment of these patients. Imaging to assessment prognosis remains an important topic.

In HIE, CT imaging may look normal or show diffuse edema. Hence, CT is often not helpful. MRI DTI has great potential to show ischemic injury in cortical and subcortical regions.[52] Typically, cortical and subcortical lesions are seen early on in those patients with the worst prognosis. Recently, the MRI feature of bilateral hippocampal hyperintensities on fluid attenuation inversion recovery imaging has been associated with poor functional outcome after cardiac arrest.[53–55] This finding can be appreciated on standardized MRI using diffusion-weighted imaging. Abnormal DTI and perfusion MRI are also useful in prognosis.[56] Functional MRI has been used in a limited number of studies in the early phase after HIE.[57] During the initial week after HIE, patients who were destined to survive at 3 months had a greater BOLD (blood oxygen level detection) signal in the somatosensory cortex contralateral to a sensory stimulation.

ICH

ICH is a common disease with a substantial need for imaging. ICH is most routinely diagnosed by noncontrast CT. However, MRI using the gradient recall echo sequence is very good at detecting ICH. Imaging yields several important features about ICH that affect diagnosis and treatment, including: (1) the location of the ICH, (2) the size of the ICH, (3) the degree of brain edema and midline shift, (4) the occurrence of obstructive hydrocephalus, (5) the extent of brain edema, (6) the ability to detect the propensity for

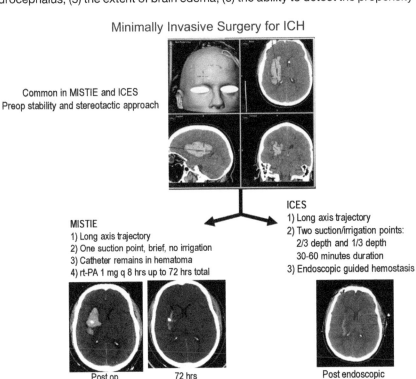

Fig. 9. Minimally invasive surgery imaging. (*Adapted from* Vespa PM, Martin N, Zuccarello M, et al. Surgical trials in intracerebral hemorrhage. Stroke 2013;44(6 Suppl 1):S79–82; with permission.)

hemorrhagic expansion through the use of the "spot sign."[58–65] The spot sign is region of contrast extravasation along the wall of a hematoma.

CT is also used for the purpose of stereotactic surgery for intracerebral hemorrhage. Stereotactic surgery make uses of high-resolution CT scans of the brain, which involves contiguous 1-mm cuts of a CT scan, and reconstruction of the scan into a usable map of the brain. The image is then incorporated into a navigation system that facilitates the surgeon to access the ICH. This method has been used in randomized controlled trials of minimally invasive surgery for ICH.[32,66] **Figs. 8** and **9** show the fundamental approach to this minimally invasive surgery.

REFERENCES

1. Maas AIR. IMPACT. Available at: http://www.tbi-impact.org/.
2. Gentry LR. Imaging of closed head injury. Radiology 1994;191(1):1–17.
3. Sklar EM, Quencer RM, Bowen BC, et al. Magnetic resonance applications in cerebral injury. Radiol Clin North Am 1992;30(2):353–66.
4. Taylor DL, Davies SE, Obrenovitch TP, et al. Investigation into the role of N-acetylaspartate in cerebral osmoregulation. J Neurochem 1995;65(1):275–81.
5. Vespa P, McArthur DL, Alger J, et al. Regional heterogeneity of post-traumatic brain metabolism as studied by microdialysis, magnetic resonance spectroscopy and positron emission tomography. Brain Pathol 2004;14:210–4.
6. Kampfl A, Franz G, Aichner F, et al. The persistent vegetative state after closed head injury: clinical and magnetic resonance imaging findings in 42 patients. J Neurosurg 1998;88(5):809–16.
7. Ashwal S, Holshouser B, Tong K, et al. Proton spectroscopy detected myoinositol in children with traumatic brain injury. Pediatr Res 2004;56(4):630–8. Epub 2004 Aug 4.
8. Babikian T, Freier MC, Ashwal S, et al. MR spectroscopy: predicting long-term neuropsychological outcome following pediatric TBI. J Magn Reson Imaging 2006;24(4):801–11.
9. Firsching R, Woischneck D, Klein S, et al. Classification of severe head injury based on magnetic resonance imaging. Acta Neurochir (Wien) 2001;143(3): 263–71.
10. Gonen O, Viswanathan AK, Catalaa I, et al. Total brain N-acetylaspartate concentration in normal, age-grouped females: quantitation with non-echo proton NMR spectroscopy. Magn Reson Med 1998;40:684–9.
11. Gonen O, Grossman RI. The accuracy of whole brain N-acetylaspartate quantification. Magn Reson Imaging 2000;18(10):1255–8.
12. Parnetti L, Tarducci R, Presciutti O, et al. Proton magnetic resonance spectroscopy can differentiate Alzheimer's disease from normal aging. Mech Ageing Dev 1997;97:9–14.
13. Rutgers DR, van Osch MJ, Kappelle LJ, et al. Cerebral hemodynamics and metabolism in patients with symptomatic occlusion of the internal carotid artery. Stroke 2003;34:648–52.
14. Friedman SD, Brooks WM, Jung RE, et al. Quantitative proton MRS predicts outcome after traumatic brain injury. Neurology 1999;52(7):1384–91.
15. Ross BD, Ernst T, Kreis R, et al. 1H MRS in acute traumatic brain injury. J Magn Reson Imaging 1998;8(4):829–40.
16. Sinson G, Bagley LJ, Cecil KM, et al. Magnetization transfer imaging and proton MR spectroscopy in the evaluation of axonal injury: correlation with clinical outcome after traumatic brain injury. AJNR Am J Neuroradiol 2001;22:143–51.

17. Condon B, Oluoch-Olunya D, Hadley D, et al. Early 1H magnetic resonance spectroscopy of acute head injury: four cases. J Neurotrauma 1998;15(8): 563–71.

18. Ariza M, Junque C, Mataro M, et al. Neuropsychological correlates of basal ganglia and medial temporal lobe NAA/Cho reductions in traumatic brain injury. Arch Neurol 2004;61(4):541–4.

19. Brooks WM, Friedman SD, Gasparovic C. Magnetic resonance spectroscopy in traumatic brain injury. J Head Trauma Rehabil 2001;16(2):149–64.

20. Birken DL, Oldendorf WH. N-acetyl-L-aspartic acid: a literature review of a compound prominent in 1H spectroscopic studies of brain. Neurosci Biobehav Rev 1989;13(1):23–31.

21. Chun KA, Manley GT, Stiver SI, et al. Interobserver variability in the assessment of CT imaging features of traumatic brain injury. J Neurotrauma 2010;27: 325–30.

22. Moffett JR, Namboodiri MA, Cangro CB, et al. Immunohistochemical localization of N acetylaspartate in rat brain. Neuroreport 1991;2(3):131–4.

23. Nael K, Villablanca JP, Mossaz L, et al. 3-T contrast-enhanced MR angiography in evaluation of suspected intracranial aneurysm: comparison with MDCT angiography. AJR Am J Roentgenol 2008;190:389–95.

24. Obrist WD, Wilkinson WE. Regional cerebral blood flow measurement in humans by xenon-133 clearance. Cerebrovasc Brain Metab Rev 1990;2:283–327.

25. Bates TE, Strangward M, Keelan J, et al. Inhibition of N-acetylaspartate production: implications for 1H MRS studies in vivo. Neuroreport 1996;7(8):1397–400.

26. Taylor DL, Davies SE, Obrenovitch TP, et al. Investigation into the role of N-acetylaspartate in cerebral osmoregulation. J Neurochem 1995;65(1):275–81.

27. Signoretti S, Marmarou A, Tavazzi B, et al. N-Acetylaspartate reduction as a measure of injury severity and mitochondrial dysfunction following diffuse traumatic brain injury. J Neurotrauma 2001;18(10):977–91.

28. Gasparovic C, Arfai N, Smid N, et al. Decrease and recovery of N-acetylaspartate/creatine in rat brain remote from focal injury. J Neurotrauma 2001;18(3): 241–6.

29. Bergsneider MA, Hovda DA, Shalmon E, et al. Cerebral hyperglycolysis following severe human traumatic brain injury: a positron emission tomography study. J Neurosurg 1997;86:241–51.

30. Bergsneider M, Hovda DA, Lee SM, et al. Dissociation of cerebral glucose metabolism and level of consciousness during the period of metabolic depression following human traumatic brain injury. J Neurotrauma 2000;17: 389–401.

31. Bergsneider M, Hovda DA, McArthur DL, et al. Metabolic recovery following human traumatic brain injury based on FDG-PET: time course and relationship to neurological disability. J Head Trauma Rehabil 2001;16:135–48.

32. Vespa P, McArthur D, Miller C, et al. Frameless stereotactic aspiration and thrombolysis of deep intracerebral hemorrhage is associated with reduction of hemorrhage volume and neurological improvement. Neurocrit Care 2005;2(3): 274–81.

33. Xu Y, McArthur DL, Alger JR, et al. Early nonischemic oxidative metabolic dysfunction leads to chronic brain atrophy in traumatic brain injury. J Cereb Blood Flow Metab 2010;30(4):883–94.

34. Coles JP, Fryer TD, Smielewski P, et al. Defining ischemic burden after traumatic brain injury using 15O PET imaging of cerebral physiology. J Cereb Blood Flow Metab 2004;24:191–201.

35. Diringer MN, Videen TO, Yundt K, et al. Regional cerebrovascular and metabolic effects of hyperventilation after severe traumatic brain injury. J Neurosurg 2002; 96(1):1038.

36. Eisenberg HM, Gary HE Jr, Aldrich EF, et al. Initial CT findings in 753 patients with severe head injury. A report from the NIH traumatic coma data bank. J Neurosurg 1990;73:688–98.

37. Johnston AJ, Steiner LA, Coles JP, et al. Effect of cerebral perfusion pressure augmentation on regional oxygenation and metabolism after head injury. Crit Care Med 2005;33:18895.

38. Miller C, Vespa P, Saver J, et al. Image guided endoscopic evacuation of spontaneous intracerebral hemorrhage. Surg Neurol 2008;69(5):441–6.

39. Hutchinson PJ, Gupta AK, Fryer TF, et al. Correlation between cerebral blood flow, substrate delivery, and metabolism in head injury: a combined microdialysis and triple oxygen positron emission tomography study. J Cereb Blood Flow Metab 2002;22:735–45.

40. Glenn TC, Kelly DF, Boscardin WJ, et al. Energy dysfunction as a predictor of outcome after moderate or severe head injury: Indices of oxygen, glucose and lactate metabolism. J Cereb Blood Flow Metab 2003;23:1239–50.

41. Vespa P, McArthur DL, Stein N, et al. Tight Glycemic Control Increases Metabolic Distress in Traumatic Brain Injury: A Randomized Controlled Within-subjects Trial. Critical Care Med 2012;40:1923–9.

42. Wu HM, Huang SC, Vespa P, et al. Redefining the pericontusional penumbra following traumatic brain injury: evidence of deteriorating metabolic derangements based on positron emission tomography. J Neurotrauma 2013;30(5):352–60.

43. Connolly ES Jr, Rabinstein AA, Carhuapoma JR, et al. Guidelines for the management of aneurysmal subarachnoid hemorrhage: a guideline for healthcare professionals from the American Heart Association/american Stroke Association American Heart Association Stroke Council; Council on Cardiovascular Radiology and Intervention; Council on Cardiovascular Nursing; Council on Cardiovascular Surgery and Anesthesia; Council on Clinical Cardiology. Stroke 2012; 43(6):1711–37. Epub 2012 May 3.

44. Villablanca JP, Jahan R, Hooshi P, et al. Detection and characterization of very small cerebral aneurysms by using 2D and 3D helical CT angiography. AJNR Am J Neuroradiol 2002;23(7):1187–98.

45. Greenberg ED, Gold R, Reichman M, et al. Diagnostic accuracy of CT angiography and CT perfusion for cerebral vasospasm: a meta-analysis. AJNR Am J Neuroradiol 2010;31:1853–60.

46. Greenberg ED, Gobin YP, Riina H, et al. Role of CT perfusion imaging in the diagnosis and treatment of vasospasm. Imaging Med 2011;1(3):287–97.

47. Sanelli PC, Ugorec I, Johnson CE, et al. Using quantitative CT perfusion for evaluation of delayed cerebral ischemia following aneurysmal subarachnoid hemorrhage. AJNR Am J Neuroradiol 2011;32:2047–53.

48. Dankbaar. 2010.

49. Dankbaar JW, Rijsdijk M, van der Schaaf IC, et al. Relationship between vasospasm, cerebral perfusion, and delayed cerebral ischemia after aneurysmal subarachnoid hemorrhage. Neuroradiology 2009;51:813–9.

50. Delgado Almandoz JE, Yoo AJ, Stone MJ, et al. The spot sign score in primary intracerebral hemorrhage identifies patients at highest risk of in-hospital mortality and poor outcome among survivors. Stroke 2010;41(1):54–60.

51. Nael K, Meshksar A, Liebeskind DS, et al. UCLA Stroke investigators. Periprocedural arterial spin labeling and dynamic susceptibility contrast perfusion in

detection of cerebral blood flow in patients with acute ischemic syndrome. Stroke 2013;44(3):664–70.

52. Greer D, Scripko P, Bartscher J, et al. Serial MRI changes in comatose cardiac arrest patients. Neurocrit Care 2011;14(1):61–7.

53. Greer DM, Scripko PD, Wu O, et al. Hippocampal magnetic resonance imaging abnormalities in cardiac arrest are associated with poor outcome. J Stroke Cerebrovasc Dis 2013;22:899–905.

54. Holshouser BA, Ashwal S, Luh GY, et al. Proton MR spectroscopy after acute central nervous system injury: outcome prediction in neonates, infants, and children. Radiology 1997;202:487–96.

55. Holshouser BA, Ashwal S, Shu S, et al. Proton MR spectroscopy in children with acute brain injury: comparison of short and long echo time acquisitions. J Magn Reson Imaging 2000;11:9–19.

56. Järnum H, Knutsson L, Rundgren M, et al. Diffusion and perfusion MRI of the brain in comatose patients treated with mild hypothermia after cardiac arrest: a prospective observational study. Resuscitation 2009;80:425–30.

57. Gofton TE, Chouinard PA, Young GB, et al. Functional MRI study of the primary somatosensory cortex in comatose survivors of cardiac arrest. Exp Neurol 2009; 217(2):320–7.

58. Delgado Almandoz JE, Kelly HR, Schaefer PW, et al. CT angiography spot sign predicts in-hospital mortality in patients with secondary intracerebral hemorrhage. J Neurointerv Surg 2012;4:442–7.

59. Demchuk AM, Dowlatshahi D, Rodriguez-Luna D, et al, PREDICT/Sunnybrook ICH CTA Study Group. Prediction of haematoma growth and outcome in patients with intracerebral haemorrhage using the CT-angiography spot sign (PREDICT): a prospective observational study. Lancet Neurol 2012;11:307–14.

60. Huynh TJ, Demchuk AM, Dowlatshahi D, et al, on behalf of the PREDICT/Sunnybrook ICH CTA Study Group. Spot sign number is the most important spot sign characteristic for predicting hematoma expansion using first-pass computed tomography angiography: analysis from the PREDICT study. Stroke 2013; 44(4):972–7.

61. Ionita CC, Graffagnino C, Alexander MJ, et al. The value of CT angiography and transcranial doppler sonography in triaging suspected cerebral vasospasm in SAH prior to endovascular therapy. Neurocrit Care 2008;9:8–12.

62. Wada R, Aviv RI, Fox AJ, et al. CT angiography "spot sign" predicts hematoma expansion in acute intracerebral hemorrhage. Stroke 2007;38(4):1257–62.

63. Wintermark M, Ko NU, Smith WS, et al. Vasospasm after subarachnoid hemorrhage: utility of perfusion CT and CT angiography on diagnosis and management. AJNR Am J Neuroradiol 2006;27:26–34.

64. Wu HM, Huang SC, Vespa P, et al. Redefining the pericontusional penumbra following traumatic brain injury: evidence of deteriorating metabolic derangements based on positron emission tomography. J Neurotrauma 2013;30:352–60.

65. Xu Y, McArthur DL, Alger JR, et al. Early nonischemic oxidative metabolic dysfunction leads to chronic brain atrophy in traumatic brain injury. J Cereb Blood Flow Metab 2010;30:883–94.

66. Miller CM, Vespa PM, McArthur DL, et al. Frameless stereotactic aspiration and thrombolysis of deep intracerebral hemorrhage is associated with reduced levels of extracellular cerebral glutamate and unchanged lactate pyruvate ratios. Neurocrit Care 2007;6:22–9.

Novel Multimodality Imaging Techniques for Diagnosis and Evaluation of Arteriovenous Malformations

Maxim Mokin, MD, PhD, Travis M. Dumont, MD,
Elad I. Levy, MD, MBA*

KEYWORDS

- Arteriovenous malformation • Digital subtraction angiography
- Computed tomography • Perfusion • Magnetic resonance imaging

KEY POINTS

- Dynamic time-resolved computed tomography (CT) or magnetic resonance angiography can visualize important hemodynamic features of arteriovenous malformations (AVMs), such as feeding arteries or early venous drainage.
- CT perfusion can help identify local pathologic phenomena, such as arterial steal and venous congestion, that can cause ischemic or hemorrhagic complications.
- Digital subtraction angiography (catheter angiography) remains the gold standard in AVM evaluation.
- In parametric imaging, an entire digital subtraction angiographic image sequence (arterial, capillary, and venous phases of radiographic contrast filling) is converted into a single composite color image.
- Both invasive and noninvasive intraoperative imaging techniques are available to determine the presence of a residual AVM during open surgical resection.

Financial relationships/potential conflicts of interest: Dr Dumont has no conflicts to disclose. Dr Levy receives research grant support, other research support (devices), and honoraria from Boston Scientific Corporation; receives research support from Codman & Shurtleff, Inc. and ev3/Covidien; has ownership interests in Intratech Medical Ltd. and Mynx/AccessClosure, Inc.; is a consultant for Codman & Shurtleff, Inc., ev3/Covidien, and TheraSyn Sensors, Inc.; and receives fees for carotid stent training from Abbott Vascular and ev3/Covidien. Dr Mokin has received an educational grant from Toshiba Medical Systems Corporation.
Department of Neurosurgery, Gates Vascular Institute-Kaleida Health, University at Buffalo, State University of New York, 100 High Street, Suite B4, Buffalo, NY 14203, USA
* Corresponding author.
E-mail address: elevy@ubns.com

INTRODUCTION

Brain arteriovenous malformations (AVMs) are abnormal communications between cerebral arterial supply and venous drainage that form a nidus. Their defining hallmark is shunting of blood flow from brain arteries to large veins, noted radiographically by early venous drainage. Diagnostic imaging is of chief importance for managing brain AVMs. Estimation of risk for rupture and hemorrhage and determination of treatment strategy (surgical, radiosurgical, endovascular, or a combination of these) rely on an understanding of the location and angioarchitecture of a patient's AVM.

Traditionally, AVM was diagnosed using basic noninvasive studies, such as noncontrast computed tomography (CT) and magnetic resonance (MR) imaging, followed by CT or MR angiography, to differentiate AVMs from developmental venous anomalies, intracranial aneurysms, or other vascular lesions. Catheter-based digital subtraction angiography was then performed to confirm the diagnosis and characterize the hemodynamic properties of the AVM.

Over the past decade, several novel CT- and MR-based noninvasive imaging modalities have emerged, allowing more detailed evaluation of these complex lesions and providing hemodynamic profiles of abnormal vessels (feeding pedicles, draining veins) that could not be detected previously. This article reviews these modern imaging techniques and discusses their application in various clinical settings. The current role of catheter angiography in the diagnosis and treatment of AVMs is also reviewed, and grading scales that are used to characterize rupture and assess perioperative risk are compared. Finally, novel intraoperative imaging approaches used for AVM treatment are discussed.

INCIDENCE AND NATURAL HISTORY

The incidence of brain AVMs remains unclear[1,2] but has been estimated to be as high as 0.5% based on autopsy data.[3] AVMs typically present with neurologic symptoms but may be diagnosed incidentally. They generally cause symptoms such as hemorrhage or seizure, but also may have clinical manifestations from mass effect and ischemia. Ruptured vascular malformations are generally treated because of the risk of rerupture,[4,5] which is highest during the 5 years after the first presentation with hemorrhage. The annual rupture risk in patients with symptomatic but untreated AVMs has been reported to be between 2% and 4%,[5,6] and treatment of unruptured AVMs is frequently offered to avoid perceived risk of future hemorrhage. Treatment is also sought for unruptured but symptomatic AVMs to abate symptomatology, including seizure, mass effect from hydrocephalus,[7,8] cranial neuropathy,[9,10] and ischemia.[11]

NOVEL IMAGING MODALITIES
Whole-Brain CT Angiography and Perfusion Imaging

Whole-brain CT angiography and perfusion imaging for evaluating patients with AVMs became available after the introduction of a 320-detector row CT scanner capable of evaluating the whole brain. It combines dynamic time-resolved 3-dimensional CT angiography (thus called *4-dimensional [4D] CT angiography*) of the brain with whole-brain CT perfusion imaging that can be performed simultaneously.[12] This technique provides excellent spatial resolution and allows recognition of important AVM properties, including identifying feeding arteries and distinguishing them from normal arteries, and showing arteriovenous shunting and early venous filling.[13,14]

Because of its noninvasive nature, whole-brain CT angiography in combination with perfusion imaging is now widely used to evaluate patients with suspected AVMs (eg, in cases with intracranial hemorrhage when clinical presentation is suspicious for an underlying AVM or other vascular lesions with altered blood flow) or as an imaging technique to monitor progression of a known AVM (eg, to evaluate changes in AVM hemodynamics after embolization). **Fig. 1** shows a giant AVM studied with 4D CT angiography during preprocedural evaluation to assess hemodynamic properties of the lesion.

Given its noninvasive nature, wide availability, and straightforward use in emergent situations, whole-brain angiography in combination with perfusion imaging currently serves as one of the best available techniques for AVM evaluation. However, in particularly complex lesions, this technique is inferior to catheter angiography, which allows selective catheterization and microexploration of each individual feeder to determine its contribution to the AVM nidus.

Normal brain parenchyma that is adjacent to the AVM nidus can exhibit different pathologic phenomena because of proximity of a high-flow abnormal AVM area. Two processes that have been studied most extensively include the arterial steal phenomenon (which can lead to focal ischemia causing neurologic deficits) and venous congestion (which can lead to hemorrhage).[15] Recognition of those phenomena is critically important for the treatment of AVMs to avoid ischemic or hemorrhagic complications. Whole-brain perfusion can directly visualize these patterns of perfusion anomalies (**Fig. 2**) and guide clinicians in the decision-making process.[16]

Dynamic MR Angiography

Dynamic MR angiography, similar to dynamic CT angiography, is based on separation of the arterial, capillary, and venous phases of contrast passage to identify abnormal filling of the feeding arteries, nidus, and draining vessels of the AVM during the arterial phase. To overcome the suboptimal resolution of dynamic MR angiography, which limits its application in a clinical setting, newer imaging protocols such as time-resolved angiography with interleaved stochastic trajectories, time-resolved imaging of contrast kinetics, and contrast-enhanced timing-robust angiography have been developed,[17–20] allowing improved spatial and temporal resolution of the AVM components (**Fig. 3**). Obvious advantages of MR angiography over CT-based studies are avoidance of radiation exposure and use of iodinated contrast material. Multiple devices (such as pacemakers) that are not MR-compatible and certain

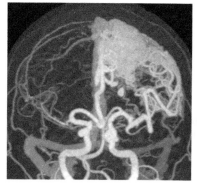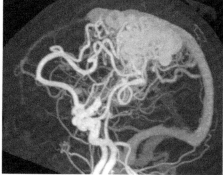

Fig. 1. In a patient with a giant left parietal AVM, the arterial phase of 4D CT angiography (*left*, coronal view; *right*, sagittal view) shows prominent abnormally dilated arterial feeders originating from the anterior and middle cerebral arteries. Venous outflow from the nidus is directed into the superior sagittal sinus.

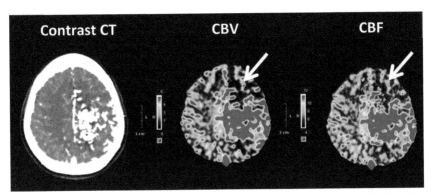

Fig. 2. In a patient with a large frontal AVM, CT perfusion maps (*center* and *right*) show a focal area of decreased cerebral blood volume (CBV, *arrow*) and cerebral blood flow (CBF, *arrow*) indicating an arterial steal phenomenon.

surgical hardware limit the use of this modality in clinical practice, especially in the emergency setting.

Digital Subtraction Angiography

Digital subtraction angiography remains the gold standard for brain AVM imaging. This modality allows for time-based assessment of blood flow, enabling assessment of early venous drainage to correctly distinguish abnormal veins from normal vasculature in even the smallest lesions or large complex lesions, which often cannot be accurately depicted using noninvasive imaging approaches. Detailed assessment of arterial pedicles is required for consideration of endovascular treatment, and is best performed with angiography. Angiography affords superior assessment of arterial pedicle number, caliber, and distribution.

Angiography provides additional diagnostic data on angioarchitectural components that are usually not available with noninvasive imaging, such as determination of the geometric type of arterial pedicle. Geographic subtypes of arterial pedicles are direct (or terminal) and indirect (or en passage) vessels. Direct arterial pedicles contribute supply to the AVM nidus but not to normal brain tissue, whereas indirect arterial pedicles supply both the AVM nidus and normal brain tissue.

Selective angiography is performed with catheterization of an individual arterial pedicle proximal to the AVM nidus. Each AVM may have multiple arterial pedicles, and multiple selective angiographic runs may be required to understand the geographic subtype of each pedicle. Selective angiography enables direct visualization of a single arterial pedicle, which is important for planning the optimal therapeutic approach.

Angioarchitectural components that may be hidden when a standard angiographic injection is performed are more likely to be visualized with microangiography. Microangiography may be performed as a diagnostic test or as a prelude to endovascular embolization.

Parametric imaging

Parametric imaging provides a novel approach to displaying an entire digital subtraction angiographic image sequence (arterial, capillary, and venous phases of radiographic contrast filling) as a single composite image. **Fig. 4** illustrates an example of an AVM embolization case in which parametric imaging was applied to measure

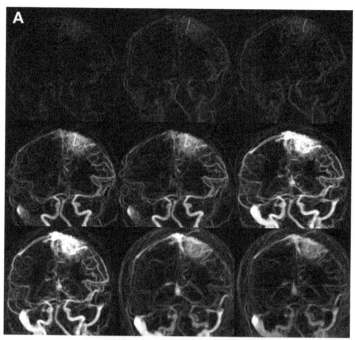

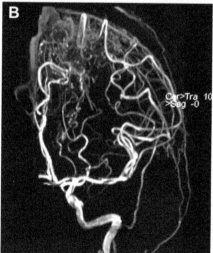

Fig. 3. (A) In a patient with a complex left frontoparietal AVM, dynamic time-resolved MR angiography (time-resolved angiography with interleaved stochastic trajectories sequence shows sequential arterial, capillary, and venous phases starting from top left image) shows that the AVM is supplied by feeders originating from the left anterior cerebral and middle cerebral arteries, and contribution to the nidus from the recurrent artery of Heubner. (B) For comparison, on a static MR angiogram image of the same AVM, the exact location and size of the nidus can be easily observed; however, the exact origin and number of arterial feeders and their contribution to the blood supply of the nidus are difficult to appreciate.

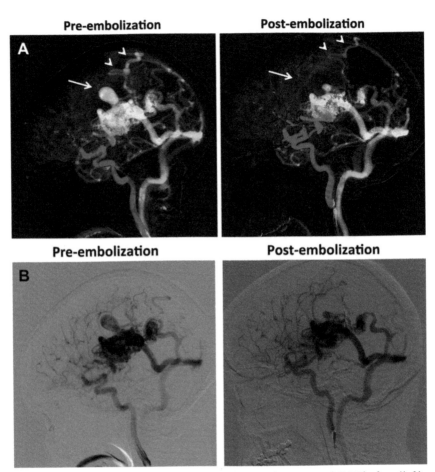

Fig. 4. (A) Single composite parametric images of a complex temporal AVM before (*left*) and immediately after (*right*) embolization of a single pedicle show changes in the hemodynamic properties of the AVM. Postembolization, a venous varix is no longer observed (*arrow*), and attenuation of flow within a large draining vein is seen (*arrowheads*). Preserved venous output within the transverse and sagittal sinuses is also seen. (B) For comparison, single images from the capillary phase of the digital subtraction angiography runs from the same case pre-embolization (*left*) and postembolization (*right*) are shown. Although the nidus is clearly recognized, the origin of the arterial feeders or the venous outflow is difficult to appreciate on these images.

immediate response to intervention. Parametric imaging technique relies on calculation of contrast intensity in each pixel in the sequential images. The calculated parameters are somewhat analogous to CT perfusion maps, and are designed to demonstrate hemodynamic properties of the AVM that otherwise would not be as accurately appreciated on the standard digital subtraction angiography images. Early experience with parametric imaging suggests that this technique is especially useful in evaluating AVMs with a complex flow pattern, such as those with multiple pedicles, to distinguish abnormal feeders from normal arteries and veins.[21] Comparison of parametric imaging maps before and after AVM treatment can help the interventionist elucidate changes in AVM hemodynamics immediately after embolization, and potentially estimate risk for complications, such as hemorrhage or focal ischemia, which is critical for guiding the decision-making process for treating these complex lesions.

Potential limitations of this technique include susceptibility to artifacts because of variations in contrast injection rate, and dependence of cardiac output. This approach to imaging and evaluation of AVMs has not been studied as extensively as other imaging modalities, and it will be interesting to see whether parametric imaging evolves into a major tool for AVM evaluation.

ASSESSMENT OF RUPTURE RISK

Key AVM features that the authors use for directing treatment decisions are summarized in **Box 1**. Macroscopic and microscopic components should be considered separately. Macroscopic components include nidus size or volume, drainage pattern, and location. When present, these features generally increase the risk associated with treatment.[22–24] Microscopic components include direct fistulous components, prenidal aneurysm, and venous varix. High-risk microscopic components, when present, generally have no bearing on risk associated with treatment but may be associated with greater likelihood of hemorrhage.[5,25–28] Treatment risk is frequently summarized with AVM classification systems. The 3 grading schemes the authors consider most relevant when estimating risks of AVM treatment are specific for the 3 modalities of treatment. Patients are offered the treatment modality associated with the greatest likelihood of success and the lowest risk of complications.

The Spetzler-Martin grading scheme[23] is used for estimating risk with AVM resection. Its 3 components are AVM size, AVM location, and venous drainage pattern. This grading scheme[23] (and its 3-tiered simplification[24]) is summarized in **Table 1**. Nidus size may be estimated with either noninvasive imaging or digital subtraction angiography. The authors typically favor estimation with MR imaging, because angiographic projections may be misleading. Eloquent location is best assessed with MR imaging. The venous drainage pattern may be best understood with dynamic MR

Box 1
Principal AVM features considered for treatment decisions

Macroscopic high-risk features (presence would portend greater risk with treatment)

- Large nidus size: applies primarily to surgical and radiosurgical treatment
- Location within functional brain tissue: applies to all treatment modalities
- Deep location: applies primarily to surgical treatment
- Functional distribution of arterial pedicles: applies primarily to endovascular treatment
- Large number of arterial pedicles: applies primarily to endovascular treatment
- Small diameter of arterial pedicles: applies primarily to endovascular treatment

Microscopic high-risk features (angioarchitectural components of high risk for hemorrhage[5,25–28])

- Direct fistulous component
- Prenidal aneurysm
- Exclusively deep venous drainage
- Venous varix

Table 1
Spetzler-Martin operative grading scheme and its 3-tiered simplification

Graded Feature	Points Assigned
Size of AVM	
<3 cm	1
3–6 cm	2
>6 cm	3
Eloquence of adjacent brain	
Noneloquent	0
Eloquent	1
Venous drainage	
Superficial only	0
Any deep drainage	1
AVM grade = [size] + [eloquence] + [drainage]	

Three-tiered AVM grade: class A = grade 1 or 2; class B = grade 3; class C = grade 4 or 5.
Data from Spetzler RF, Martin NA. A proposed grading system for arteriovenous malformations. J Neurosurg 1986;65:476–83; and Spetzler RF, Ponce FA. A 3-tier classification of cerebral arteriovenous malformations. Clinical article. J Neurosurg 2011;114:842–9.

imaging or CT angiography; however, because those modalities have not been extensively validated clinically, the authors currently prefer to assess this pattern with digital subtraction angiography. A grade IV or V[23] (class C[24]) AVM is more likely to have complications associated with surgical resection.

The Pollock-Flickinger grading scheme (**Table 2**) is used to estimate risk associated with radiosurgical treatment of AVMs.[22] This grading scheme has been validated as a relevant predictor of obliteration rates and complication incidence associated with treatment of AVMs with radiosurgery. The radiographic components of the score include nidus volume and location. These factors are best assessed with thin-slice MR imaging. An AVM with a higher score is less likely to have an excellent and uncomplicated outcome.

No consensus scheme exists for estimation of risk with endovascular treatment. The authors favor the Buffalo classification (**Table 3**), which they devised and internally validated for its ability to predict complication incidence after endovascular treatment. The components are number and diameter of arterial pedicles and functional distribution of vessels. Although functional distribution of vessels may be estimated with MR

Table 2
Pollock-Flickinger radiosurgery grading scale

Graded Feature	Points Assigned
AVM volume	in mL
Patient age	in years
Location	
Hemispheric/corpus callosum/cerebellar	0
Basal ganglia/brainstem	1
AVM score = 0.1 × [volume] + 0.02 × [age] + 0.3 × [location]	

Data from Pollock BE, Flickinger JC. Modification of the radiosurgery-based arteriovenous malformation grading system. Neurosurgery 2008;63:239–43.

Table 3 Buffalo endovascular treatment grading scale	
Graded Feature	**Points Assigned**
Number of arterial pedicles	
1 or 2	1
3 or 4	2
5 or more	3
Diameter of arterial pedicles	
Most >1 mm	0
Most ≤1 mm	1
Location	
Nonfunctional tissue	0
Functional tissue	1
AVM grade = [number] + [diameter] + [location]	

imaging (according to the same definition as the Spetzler-Martin classification[23]), digital subtraction angiography allows assessment of geographic subtype of the arterial pedicle, and superselective Wada testing allows superior assessment of the functional distribution of an arterial pedicle.[29] Because these features are not routinely assessed in full until an embolization procedure is performed, the authors favor using the eloquent brain location of an AVM nidus as a preoperative predictive variable of risk with endovascular treatment. Arterial pedicle number and size are best estimated with angiography. Complications related to endovascular embolization are more likely to occur in an AVM with a higher score (Dumont TM, Kan P, Snyder KV, et al, personal communication, 2012).

INTRAOPERATIVE IMAGING

Intraoperative angiography is of chief importance in detecting the presence of unsuspected residual immediately after open resection of an AVM, which is estimated to be 10% in large series.[30–33] Given the relatively high incidence of unexpected residual AVMs reported in these series, the value of intraoperative angiography is clear but must be weighed against the risk of complications of this approach.[34] Smaller AVMs are unlikely to have an unexpected residual nidus, and therefore intraoperative angiography has a greater yield for larger AVMs.[34]

With the complication profile of intraoperative angiography,[34] less-invasive intraoperative imaging approaches are desirable. Neuronavigation, ultrasonography, and indocyanine green video angiography (ICG-VA) may be useful adjuncts to intraoperative imaging of AVM.

Neuronavigation is a frameless stereotaxy technique that incorporates a previously acquired thin-slice CT or MR image to locate an intracranial target. In this technique, the image is referenced with the patient's surface anatomy (surface scalp anatomy or adhesive fiducial scalp markers) with a software interface. For AVM resection, the principal use of neuronavigation is for localizing the lesion to precisely position the planned craniotomy and locate deeply seated AVM components.[35] Limitations in accuracy because of brain shifts from surgery are expected[36–38] but not typically debilitating to the overall utility of this technique.

Ultrasonography enables dynamic visualization of flow, which assists the operator in identifying arterial pedicles and venous outflow.[39] Its strength is in real-time assessment of blood flow through the AVM. Its principal limitation is poor resolution compared with other intraoperative imaging modalities.

ICG-VA is another noninvasive intraoperative imaging technique that is a useful adjunct for microsurgical resection of an AVM.[40,41] Indocyanine green is an intravenously administered agent that enables real-time visualization of blood flow within the exposed vascular anatomy in the surgical field, which can also be recorded for reviewing. ICG-VA may be applied to garner a better understanding of superficial arterial pedicles and venous outflow of an AVM. With ICG-VA, vascular structures are generally not visualized through brain tissue or a hematoma, limiting its utility for deeply seated or ruptured AVMs.

SUMMARY

Modern noninvasive imaging approaches, such as dynamic 4D CT and MR angiography, allow excellent visualization of hemodynamic properties of AVMs, which previously could be achieved exclusively with catheter angiography. Whole-brain perfusion can help clinicians recognize certain pathologic phenomena associated with AVMs, such as arterial steal and venous congestion. Digital subtraction angiography remains the gold standard for evaluating AVMs, and microcatheter injections provide critical information about each individual pedicle. Several classification systems exist to estimate risk associated with treatment of AVMs. Advances in invasive and noninvasive intraoperative imaging techniques now allow immediate detection of a residual AVM during surgical resection.

REFERENCES

1. Berman MF, Sciacca RR, Pile-Spellman J, et al. The epidemiology of brain arteriovenous malformations. Neurosurgery 2000;47:389–97.
2. Stapf C, Mohr JP, Pile-Spellman J, et al. Epidemiology and natural history of arteriovenous malformations. Neurosurg Focus 2001;11:e1.
3. McCormick WF. Pathology of vascular malformations of the brain. In: Wilson CB, Stein BM, editors. Intracranial arteriovenous malformations: current neurosurgical practice. Baltimore (MD): Williams & Wilkins; 1984. p. 44–63.
4. Halim AX, Johnston SC, Singh V, et al. Longitudinal risk of intracranial hemorrhage in patients with arteriovenous malformation of the brain within a defined population. Stroke 2004;35:1697–702.
5. Hernesniemi JA, Dashti R, Juvela S, et al. Natural history of brain arteriovenous malformations: a long-term follow-up study of risk of hemorrhage in 238 patients. Neurosurgery 2008;63:823–31.
6. Ondra SL, Troupp H, George ED, et al. The natural history of symptomatic arteriovenous malformations of the brain: a 24-year follow-up assessment. J Neurosurg 1990;73:387–91.
7. Pribil S, Boone SC, Waley R. Obstructive hydrocephalus at the anterior third ventricle caused by dilated veins from an arteriovenous malformation. Surg Neurol 1983;20:487–92.
8. U HS, Kerber C. Ventricular obstruction secondary to vascular malformations. Neurosurgery 1983;12:572–5.
9. Lesley WS. Resolution of trigeminal neuralgia following cerebellar AVM embolization with Onyx. Cephalalgia 2009;29:980–5.
10. Simon SD, Yao TL, Rosenbaum BP, et al. Resolution of trigeminal neuralgia after palliative embolization of a cerebellopontine angle arteriovenous malformation. Cent Eur Neurosurg 2009;70:161–3.

11. Mast H, Mohr JP, Osipov A, et al. 'Steal' is an unestablished mechanism for the clinical presentation of cerebral arteriovenous malformations. Stroke 1995;26:1215–20.
12. Orrison WW Jr, Snyder KV, Hopkins LN, et al. Whole-brain dynamic CT angiography and perfusion imaging. Clin Radiol 2011;66:566–74.
13. Siebert E, Bohner G, Dewey M, et al. 320-slice CT neuroimaging: initial clinical experience and image quality evaluation. Br J Radiol 2009;82:561–70.
14. Willems PW, Taeshineetanakul P, Schenk B, et al. The use of 4D-CTA in the diagnostic work-up of brain arteriovenous malformations. Neuroradiology 2012;54: 123–31.
15. Moftakhar P, Hauptman JS, Malkasian D, et al. Cerebral arteriovenous malformations. Part 2: physiology. Neurosurg Focus 2009;26:E11.
16. Kim DJ, Krings T. Whole-brain perfusion CT patterns of brain arteriovenous malformations: a pilot study in 18 patients. AJNR Am J Neuroradiol 2011;32:2061–6.
17. Hadizadeh DR, von Falkenhausen M, Gieseke J, et al. Cerebral arteriovenous malformation: Spetzler-Martin classification at subsecond-temporal-resolution four-dimensional MR angiography compared with that at DSA. Radiology 2008; 246:205–13.
18. Nogueira RG, Bayrlee A, Hirsch JA, et al. Dynamic contrast-enhanced MRA at 1.5 T for detection of arteriovenous shunting before and after onyx embolization of cerebral arteriovenous malformations. J Neuroimaging 2013. [Epub ahead of print].
19. Petkova M, Gauvrit JY, Trystram D, et al. Three-dimensional dynamic time-resolved contrast-enhanced MRA using parallel imaging and a variable rate k-space sampling strategy in intracranial arteriovenous malformations. J Magn Reson Imaging 2009;29:7–12.
20. Yu S, Yan L, Yao Y, et al. Noncontrast dynamic MRA in intracranial arteriovenous malformation (AVM), comparison with time of flight (TOF) and digital subtraction angiography (DSA). Magn Reson Imaging 2012;30:869–77.
21. Strother CM, Bender F, Deuerling-Zheng Y, et al. Parametric color coding of digital subtraction angiography. AJNR Am J Neuroradiol 2010;31:919–24.
22. Pollock BE, Flickinger JC. Modification of the radiosurgery-based arteriovenous malformation grading system. Neurosurgery 2008;63:239–43.
23. Spetzler RF, Martin NA. A proposed grading system for arteriovenous malformations. J Neurosurg 1986;65:476–83.
24. Spetzler RF, Ponce FA. A 3-tier classification of cerebral arteriovenous malformations. Clinical article. J Neurosurg 2011;114:842–9.
25. Kader A, Young WL, Pile-Spellman J, et al. The influence of hemodynamic and anatomic factors on hemorrhage from cerebral arteriovenous malformations. Neurosurgery 1994;34:801–8.
26. Lv X, Wu Z, Jiang C, et al. Angioarchitectural characteristics of brain arteriovenous malformations with and without hemorrhage. World Neurosurg 2011;76:95–9.
27. Stapf C, Mast H, Sciacca RR, et al. Predictors of hemorrhage in patients with untreated brain arteriovenous malformation. Neurology 2006;66:1350–5.
28. Stefani MA, Porter PJ, terBrugge KG, et al. Large and deep brain arteriovenous malformations are associated with risk of future hemorrhage. Stroke 2002;33: 1220–4.
29. Tawk RG, Tummala RP, Memon MZ, et al. Utility of pharmacologic provocative neurological testing before embolization of occipital lobe arteriovenous malformations. World Neurosurg 2011;76:276–81.
30. Barrow DL, Boyer KL, Joseph GJ. Intraoperative angiography in the management of neurovascular disorders. Neurosurgery 1992;30:153–9.

31. Martin NA, Bentson J, Vinuela F, et al. Intraoperative digital subtraction angiography and the surgical treatment of intracranial aneurysms and vascular malformations. J Neurosurg 1990;73:526–33.
32. Vitaz TW, Gaskill-Shipley M, Tomsick T, et al. Utility, safety, and accuracy of intraoperative angiography in the surgical treatment of aneurysms and arteriovenous malformations. AJNR Am J Neuroradiol 1999;20:1457–61.
33. Yuan G, Zhao JZ, Wang S, et al. Intraoperative angiography in the surgery of brain arteriovenous malformations. Beijing Da Xue Xue Bao 2007;39:412–5.
34. Chalouhi N, Theofanis T, Jabbour P, et al. Safety and efficacy of intraoperative angiography in craniotomies for cerebral aneurysms and arteriovenous malformations: a review of 1093 consecutive cases. Neurosurgery 2012;71:1162–9.
35. Akdemir H, Oktem S, Menku A, et al. Image-guided microneurosurgical management of small arteriovenous malformation: role of neuronavigation and intraoperative Doppler sonography. Minim Invasive Neurosurg 2007;50:163–9.
36. Dorward NL, Alberti O, Velani B, et al. Postimaging brain distortion: magnitude, correlates, and impact on neuronavigation. J Neurosurg 1998;88:656–62.
37. Hill DL, Maurer CR Jr, Maciunas RJ, et al. Measurement of intraoperative brain surface deformation under a craniotomy. Neurosurgery 1998;43:514–28.
38. Roberts DW, Hartov A, Kennedy FE, et al. Intraoperative brain shift and deformation: a quantitative analysis of cortical displacement in 28 cases. Neurosurgery 1998;43:749–60.
39. Woydt M, Vince GH, Krauss J, et al. New ultrasound techniques and their application in neurosurgical intra-operative sonography. Neurol Res 2001;23:697–705.
40. Raabe A, Beck J, Gerlach R, et al. Near-infrared indocyanine green video angiography: a new method for intraoperative assessment of vascular flow. Neurosurgery 2003;52:132–9.
41. Raabe A, Beck J, Seifert V. Technique and image quality of intraoperative indocyanine green angiography during aneurysm surgery using surgical microscope integrated near-infrared video technology. Zentralbl Neurochir 2005;66:1–8.

Neurologic Applications of Whole-Brain Volumetric Multidetector Computed Tomography

Kenneth V. Snyder, MD, PhD[a],*, Maxim Mokin, MD, PhD[a],
Vernice E. Bates, MD[b]

KEYWORDS

- 320-detector row CT scanner • CT perfusion • 4D-CTA • Carotid occlusion
- Cerebrovascular reserve

KEY POINTS

- Imaging with 320-slice volumetric multimodal computed tomography (CT) is able to visualize dynamic changes in the blood flow of the entire brain because of its 16-cm z-axis coverage.
- Whole-brain perfusion allows direct visualization of the posterior circulation (brainstem, cerebellum) as well as anatomic areas close to the vertex (distal anterior cerebral artery territories).
- Dynamic four-dimensional CT angiography combines whole-brain CT perfusion with time-resolved three-dimensional angiography and can differentiate between anterograde flow in cases with a partially occluded artery versus retrograde collateral flow.
- Dynamic CT angiography can assist in differentiating between extracranial chronic internal carotid occlusion versus acute pseudo-occlusion.
- Combining CT perfusion with acetazolamide challenge provides a powerful insight into the brain's hemodynamic status by evaluating its cerebrovascular reserve.

INTRODUCTION

The introduction of computed tomography (CT) scanning in 1973 as a clinical tool revolutionized the way in which neurologists and neurosurgeons could diagnose

Financial Relationships/Conflicts of Interest: Dr Bates, nil. Dr Mokin, educational grant from Toshiba Medical System Corporation. Dr Snyder, consultant/speakers' bureau/honoraria from Toshiba; speakers' bureau/honoraria from ev3/Covidien, The Stroke Group.
[a] Department of Neurosurgery, Gates Vascular Institute, Kaleida Health, School of Medicine and Biomedical Sciences, University at Buffalo, State University of New York, 100 High Street, Suite B4, Buffalo, NY 14203, USA; [b] Dent Stroke/TIA Clinic, Dent Neurological Institute, 3980 Sheridan Drive, Amherst, NY 14226, USA
* Corresponding author.
E-mail address: ksnyder@ubns.com

and treat ischemic stroke, hemorrhagic stroke, and other causes of stroke syndrome. However, early scanners were slow, requiring several minutes for a single tomographic slice, were associated with a high radiation dose, and had prominent susceptibility to metallic artifacts. Several methods to reduce radiation dose were developed and are listed in **Table 1** and shown graphically in **Fig. 1**. Metal artifact can be reduced by several means, as listed in **Table 2**. This suppression of metallic artifact is particularly helpful in visualizing flow within vessels previously treated with metallic stents and coil material. Several technological advances have significantly reduced scan time and are listed in **Table 3**. Key developments in this regard include slip ring gantry and multidetector technology. A recently developed 320-slice (detector) CT scanner acquires a thin-slice volumetric study of the whole brain in less than a second. The introduction of whole-brain volumetric multimodal CT scanners has given clinicians a powerful tool to visualize dynamic changes in hemodynamic parameters of the brain and its vasculature. This information can be used to manage patients with acute ischemic stroke caused by large vessel arterial occlusion and assess hemodynamic reserve, and it plays an important role in the evaluation of patients with other neurologic conditions, such as moyamoya disease, venous sinus thrombosis, or arteriovenous malformations. This new CT technology fundamentally changes the way treatment options for certain cerebrovascular disorders can be conceptualized. This article presents case examples of how volumetric multimodal CT data is used in diagnosing and managing these various cerebrovascular conditions.

Table 1 CT dose reduction techniques		
	Dose Reduction Technique	**How It Helps**
1	Optimize technique with lower input current	Trade SNR and penetration for dose
2	Detector material	Less technique required for same detector light output
3	Filtering	Noise removal via postprocessing
4	4 slice	Fewer rotations required, therefore less radiation overlap
5	Tube modulation	Technique adapts to requirements at each axial level
6	16 slice	Fewer rotations required, therefore less radiation overlap
7	64 slice, ECG modulation	Fewer rotations, full dose applied only during image acquisition (eg, during diastole)
8	Filtering	Improvements in postprocessing
9	Dynamic sampling methods	For perfusion or dynamic CT angiography, full dose is not required for all temporal samples; reduced temporal sampling during steady state periods (eg, washout phase)
10	Volume acquisition	Single rotation, no overlapping radiation, dynamic scans require no table movement
11	Active collimation	Radiation profile optimized
12	Reconstruction processing	Improved cone beam processing and noise filtering
13	Iterative reconstruction	Statistical processing that uses information about system noise characteristics to maximize SNR

Abbreviations: ECG, electrocardiogram; SNR, signal/noise ratio.

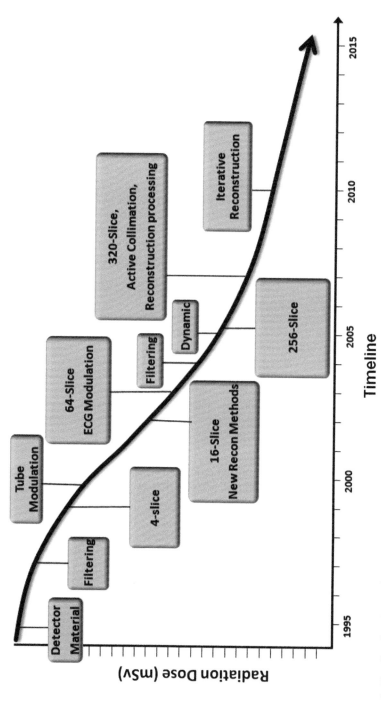

Fig. 1. Timeline for the evolution of CT dose reduction techniques.

Table 2
Metal artifact reduction techniques

	Metal Artifacts	Artifact Suppression Methods
1	Conventional stents	Thin slices
2	Pipeline stents (additional metal)	Collimation
3	Spine fusion materials	Image filtering
4	Calcification	Reconstruction processing, multienergy

ISCHEMIC STROKE

Despite progress in prevention and treatment, stroke remains the number 1 cause of long-term disability, and approximately 795,000 people experience a new or recurrent stroke in the United States each year.[1] Timely brain imaging is critical in management of acute ischemic stroke. With advances in CT perfusion technology, it is now possible to visualize the extent of tissue at risk during a stroke as well as assess the tissue viability. This ability allows the clinician to differentiate acute from chronic ischemia and understand patterns of intracranial circulation including presence and extent of collateral flow; information that is critical for the evaluation of patients with acute stroke. It helps determine whether acute intervention is necessary as well as which type of treatment strategy is appropriate.

CT Perfusion in Stroke

The introduction of brain perfusion imaging has allowed the dynamic mapping of brain ischemia with anatomic accuracy.[2] Such perfusion studies are commonly used in the emergent evaluation of patients with suspected acute ischemic stroke caused by large vessel occlusion with the goal of determining the extent of irreversibly infarcted brain tissue (core) as well as potentially salvageable hypoperfused tissue at risk (ischemic penumbra). From a review of the literature, infarct core and ischemic penumbra volumes may be significant predictors of clinical outcome and could be used to select patients for intravenous thrombolysis beyond the established strict time window or for intra-arterial endovascular therapies.[3]

Perfusion maps

These neuroimaging predictors of outcome are based on quantitative and qualitative analysis of perfusion parameters (**Box 1**) that are derived from time-resolved

Table 3
Recent improvements in CT scan times

Speed of Scan	Slices Per Second	Temporal Resolution(s) of Dynamic Volume Acquisition
1 s per rotation	1	320
0.5 s per rotation	2	160
0.3 s per rotation	3	96
4 slice	13	24
16 slice	64	6
64 slice	213	2
256 slice	853	0.4
320 slice	1067	0.3
320 with partial rotation	—	0.18

Box 1
Computed tomographic perfusion parameters and definitions

- Cerebral blood volume (CBV): describes volume of blood flow within a given volume of brain tissue. Measured in mL/100 g.

- Cerebral blood flow (CBF): describes blood flow over a certain period of time. Measured in mL/100 g/min.

- Mean transit time (MTT): calculated based on time of contrast material flow from the arterial to the venous states. Measured in seconds.

- Time to peak (TTP): describes time required to reach maximum intensity of contrast within a particular region of the brain tissue. Measured in seconds.

- Relationship between CBV, CBF, and MTT: CBF = CBV/MTT

- Ischemic core: area of irreversible brain damage, defined by significantly decreased blood volume

- Ischemic penumbra: potentially salvageable brain tissue, defined as mismatch between CBF or MTT and CBV (decreased CBF, increased MTT, and preserved CBV).

---

tissue-density curves from the brain parenchyma.[4] Cerebral blood volume (CBV, measured as milliliters per 100 g) describes the volume of blood flow within a given volume of brain tissue, whereas cerebral blood flow (CBF, measured as milliliters per 100 g per minute) calculates blood flow over a certain period of time. Mean transit time (MTT) is based on time of contrast flow from the arterial to the venous states, and time to peak (TTP) describes the time required for maximum intensity of contrast within a particular region of brain tissue. These maps focus on small vessel flow to brain tissue. Large vessels are removed from the calculation.

Whole-brain perfusion

A disadvantage of limited brain coverage encountered in the era of 16-detector, 32-detector, or 64-detector row CT scanners was that a decision needed to be made ahead of time regarding the region of brain to analyze, leaving a large section of brain uncovered. This usually resulted in poor evaluation of posterior circulation structures, such as the brainstem and cerebellum. Unless posterior circulation ischemia is suspected clinically and the perfusion window is manually adjusted to include relevant brainstem structures, a diagnosis of posterior circulation stroke could be missed and the areas not provided by the scan would be left to the observer's interpretation.[5,6] Cortical areas close to the vertex, such as distal anterior cerebral artery territories, similarly are typically not visualized by CT perfusion scanners with a limited area width (**Fig. 2**).

Although less frequent, even when evaluating patients with suspected middle cerebral artery infarction, perfusion maps generated with 32-detector or 64-detector row CT scanners can miss areas of ischemia, necessitating repeat contrast injection until the proper diagnosis is made or applying a toggling-table technique by alternating the position of the table in relation to the scanning area.[5,7,8] Although shifting the CT table doubles the amount of brain that is imaged, it reduces temporal resolution and is difficult to standardize. Additional contrast injection can be harmful because of increase contrast load, especially in patients with impaired renal function.

Such limitations can be overcome by extending the perfusion scan area to whole-brain perfusion. Clinical data show that even increasing the scan coverage from 2 cm to 9.6 cm adds clinically important information that assists in the evaluation of patients with suspected acute stroke.[9]

A

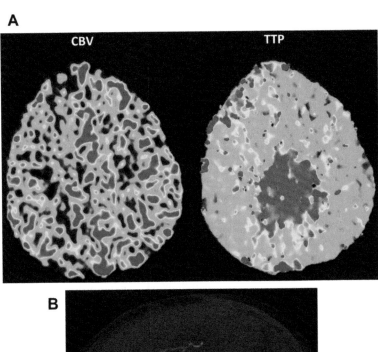

B

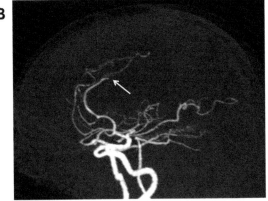

Fig. 2. Anterior cerebral artery stroke. (*A*) A patient with acute-onset bilateral leg weakness presented to the emergency room. Although a diagnosis of spinal cord ischemia was suspected, initial neurologic evaluation revealed subtle confusion and difficulty following commands, raising the possibility of cortical ischemia as a differential diagnosis. Whole-brain perfusion revealed a perfusion abnormality in the distribution of the distal anterior cerebral arteries bilaterally. (*B*) Suspecting that the location of arterial occlusion was within the anterior cerebral artery territory, careful analysis of CT angiography detected a single anterior cerebral artery supplying both hemispheres with occlusion at the pericallosal segment (*arrow*). The patient was successfully treated with intravenous thrombolysis.

The improvement in technology has also reduced the radiation dose to the patient. The methodology of perfusion calculations on scanners with fewer than 320 detectors can be as high as 5 noncontrast CT scan equivalents. The current dose using the Aquilion ONE Perfusion algorithm and adaptive-dose reduction algorithm (Toshiba Medical Systems, Nasu, Japan)[10] is equivalent to that of 1.5 noncontrast CT scans.

Dynamic Three-Dimensional Angiography

Time-resolved dynamic CT angiography is sometimes called four-dimensional (4D) angiography because, in addition to obtaining three-dimensional (3D) evaluation of intracranial vasculature, it allows visualization of contrast flow from its arterial to venous phases (time being the fourth dimension that is evaluated). This powerful technique provides an opportunity to visualize leptomeningeal collaterals and noninvasively differentiate between anterograde flow, in cases with a partially occluded intracranial artery, versus retrograde collateral flow.[11] In a study using whole-brain perfusion evaluation, 4D-CT angiography showed superior diagnostic accuracy compared with single-phase (conventional) CT angiography.[12]

By evaluating the hemodynamic properties of the occluded segment, 4D-CT angiography has the potential to serve as an important predictor of response to intravenous thrombolysis and other available treatments, thus guiding clinicians when evaluating patients with acute stroke (**Fig. 3**). **Figs.** 2 and 3 show clinical scenarios

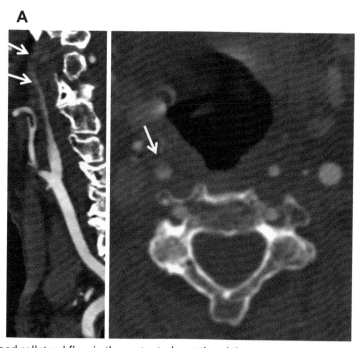

Fig. 3. Good collateral flow in the acute stroke setting. (A) In a patient with the acute onset of right hemiparesis and neglect, sagittal (*left*) and axial (*right*) views using single-phase CT angiography show acute right internal carotid artery occlusion extending from the distal cervical segment intracranially, suspicious for a fresh thrombus. There is a partial filling defect (*arrows*) within the cervical carotid artery segment, which becomes a complete occlusion on higher intracranial sections (not shown here). (B) Review of perfusion maps showed preserved CBF and CBV. There was only mild increase in MTT in the right hemisphere, and the major increase in TTP was seen predominantly in watershed right anterior cerebral to middle cerebral and middle cerebral to posterior cerebral territories (*arrows*). (C) Dynamic time-resolved 4D angiography reconstructions showed delayed but preserved supply to the right hemisphere from the left internal carotid artery via the anterior communicating artery. Note the filling of the right hemisphere in delayed fashion in the arterial (4–5.9 seconds) and venous (12.1–16 seconds) phases. Decision was made not to pursue intra-arterial endovascular revascularization considering the high risk for dislodging a thrombus and causing distal embolic complications. Instead, the patient was treated with aggressive hydration, intravenous heparin, and intravenous pressors, which resulted in clinical improvement of the original neurologic deficit.

in which information obtained using dynamic CT angiography was a critical step in guiding the treatment of patients with acute ischemic stroke. This modality also plays a significant role in helping differentiate carotid occlusion from pseudo-occlusion.

CAROTID ARTERY OCCLUSION

Near-complete occlusion (also called pseudo-occlusion) of the internal carotid artery can be mistaken for a chronic internal carotid artery occlusion when only a snapshot in time is used to generate a CT angiogram. Differentiation between the two can be critical when evaluating patients with acute stroke. Patients with pseudo-occlusion can benefit from emergent revascularization, such as carotid artery stenting, whereas patients with chronic occlusion might be treated with medical therapy or bypass surgery.[13] Although the diagnosis of pseudo-occlusion can be made by CT angiography

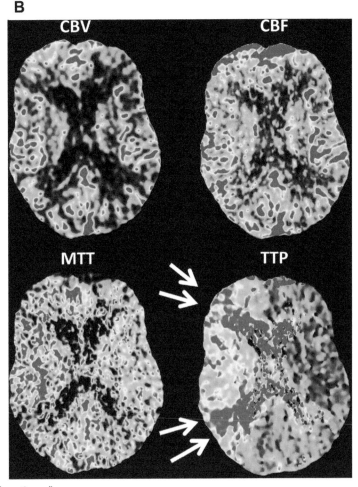

Fig. 3. (continued)

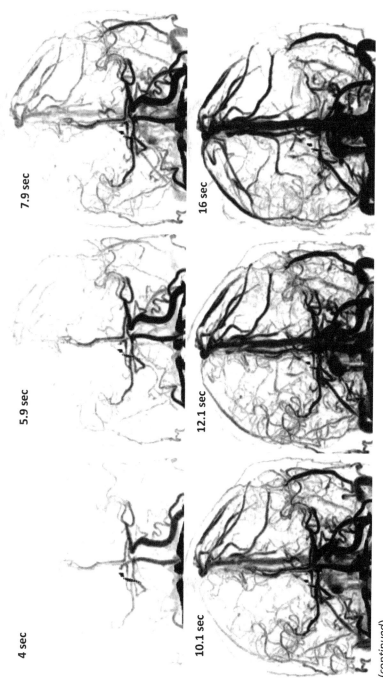

4 sec

5.9 sec

7.9 sec

10.1 sec

12.1 sec

16 sec

C

Fig. 3. (continued)

by identifying subtle angiographic findings, such as the string sign, it is sometimes difficult to differentiate between the two conditions.[13,14] Dynamic 3D-angiography can be of additional value in those situations; delayed anterograde filling of the internal carotid artery further supports the diagnosis of pseudo-occlusion, whereas in chronic occlusion either retrograde or no flow within the internal carotid artery is often observed, even in the delayed venous phase (**Figs. 4** and **5**).

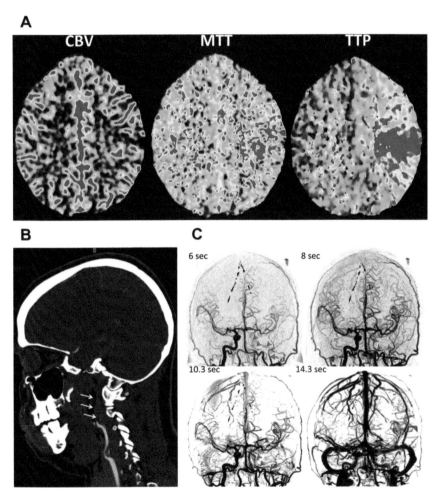

Fig. 4. Pseudo-occlusion. (A) Diagnostic evaluation in a patient with acute onset of mild right hemiparesis with fluctuating degree of weakness revealed a perfusion deficit within the left frontal. (B) On CT angiography, the left internal carotid artery was not visualized. It was difficult to determine whether the observed string sign (*arrows*) was caused by pseudo-occlusion of the left internal carotid artery versus a small branch of the left external carotid artery. (C) Dynamic 4D angiography showed delayed but anterograde filling of the left internal carotid artery, supporting the initial diagnosis of pseudo-occlusion. The course of the left internal carotid artery intracranially (*arrowheads*) is faint in the arterial phase but becomes more evident in the later venous phase. The patient underwent successful emergent stenting of the left internal carotid artery.

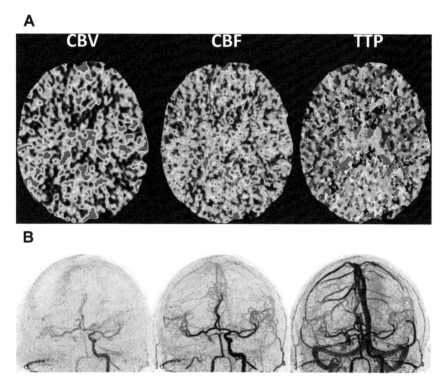

Fig. 5. Chronic occlusion. (*A*) In a patient with transient left-sided weakness, CT angiography failed to visualize the right internal carotid artery (not shown). Symmetric perfusion maps argued against the acute onset of occlusion, indicating that this condition was chronic. (*B*) The chronic nature of the right internal carotid artery occlusion was further supported by review of dynamic CT angiography, in which simultaneous filling of both cerebral hemispheres was observed during the arterial phase. Throughout the phase of contrast injection, no flow was observed within the right internal carotid artery.

Dynamic 3D-angiography is also becoming more widely used in the evaluation of other neurologic conditions, including brain tumors such as meningiomas (to depict hemodynamic properties of the tumor and surrounding normal vasculature), arteriovenous malformations, and fistulas (to differentiate between abnormal arterial feeders and draining veins vs normal arteries and veins).[14] The application of dynamic 3D-angiography in the evaluation and management of arteriovenous malformations is discussed by Mokin and colleagues elsewhere in this issue.

EVALUATION OF CEREBROVASCULAR RESERVE

Acetazolamide is a carbonic anhydrase inhibitor that dilates the vasculature by increasing carbon dioxide levels within the bloodstream.[15] This property can be used to provide insight into the brain's hemodynamic status. In a healthy response, acetazolamide-induced vasodilation causes an increase in CBF and CBV. In a pathologic state, such as in patients with chronic ischemia caused by intracranial stenosis, if the vasculature is already maximally dilated it does not show a further augmentation of CBV with the expected increase in CBF. Using this principle, acetazolamide provides a means of determining cerebrovascular reserve and helps estimate the risk for future ischemic events. In the past, this was measured using single-photon emission CT (SPECT). More recently, the degree of cerebrovascular reserve has been determined with acetazolamide challenge using CT perfusion, which is a more readily accessible imaging method compared with SPECT. Measuring whole-brain response to acetazolamide allows more accurate measurement of cerebral reserve (**Fig. 6**).

Moyamoya Disease

Acetazolamide challenge testing is often combined with CT perfusion imaging in patients with moyamoya disease.[15] This condition has unique hemodynamic properties because progressive stenosis of the distal internal carotid and proximal middle

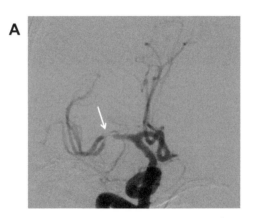

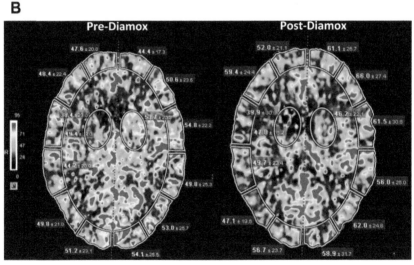

Fig. 6. Cerebrovascular reserve. (*A*) A patient with recurrent left facial droop and left arm weakness had severe right middle cerebral artery stenosis at the M1 bifurcation segment (*arrow*). (*B*) CT perfusion with acetazolamide challenge showed increased CBF (CBF measurements are provided for comparison before and after acetazolamide administration) in the unaffected (*left*) hemisphere, indicating that the patient was responsive to the medication. Increase in CBF within the affected territory of the right hemisphere indicated presence of good vascular reserve. The patient was treated with appropriate medical therapy. Despite the high degree of stenosis, the presence of good reserve argued against surgical intervention, such as angioplasty.

cerebral arteries causes dramatic revascularization, and changes in CBF correlate well with the degree of stenosis seen on angiography. Additional information on the degree of cerebrovascular reserve in patients with moyamoya helps in preoperative evaluation and postoperative follow-up.

In-stent Stenosis

Intracranial stenting can be used for treatment of various cerebrovascular diseases, such as in the treatment of aneurysms with stent-assisted coiling or as a single modality with a special type of stents known as flow diverters. Suboptimal stent deployment with kinking or twisting of the stent can occur during the procedure, which can result in the development of in-stent stenosis leading to ischemic complications. CT angiography can be applied in surveillance of in-stent stenosis; however, it can miss as many as 15% of in-stent stenoses compared with catheter angiography.[16] CT perfusion can assist in diagnosing in-stent stenosis by detecting a perfusion deficit in the territory of the stented vessel, providing important additional information in cases with equivocal findings on CT angiography (**Fig. 7**).

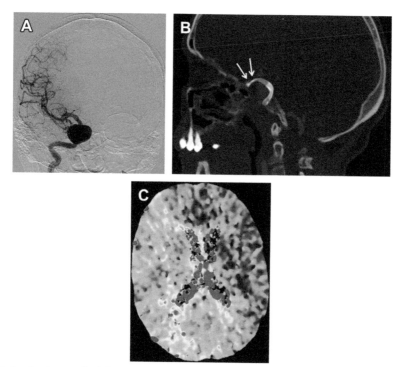

Fig. 7. In-stent stenosis. (*A*) A patient with a giant intracranial carotid artery aneurysm underwent treatment with a flow diversion device to reconstruct the vessel and redirect blood flow away from the aneurysm. The preoperative digital subtraction angiogram showed a giant right internal carotid artery aneurysm. (*B*) Follow-up postoperative CT angiogram raised suspicion for in-stent kinking and development of in-stent stenosis (*arrows*); however, the degree of stenosis did not appear critical. (*C*) A CT perfusion study was done and showed a perfusion deficit within the right internal carotid artery territory, suggesting that the degree of stenosis was hemodynamically significant. The patient was scheduled for angiography and underwent balloon angioplasty, with successful reopening of the stenotic segment within the stent.

SUMMARY

Modern advances in volumetric multimodal CT imaging allow perfusion parameter measurements of the brain while simultaneously delivering 4D angiography at a lower radiation dose than previous CT systems. Whole-brain CT perfusion has been successfully used in various clinical settings, such as evaluation of acute ischemic stroke and assessment of cerebrovascular reserve.

REFERENCES

1. Go AS, Mozaffarian D, Roger VL, et al. Executive summary: heart disease and stroke statistics–2013 update: a report from the American Heart Association. Circulation 2013;127:143–52.
2. Latchaw RE. Cerebral perfusion imaging in acute stroke. J Vasc Interv Radiol 2004;15:S29–46.
3. Latchaw RE, Alberts MJ, Lev MH, et al. Recommendations for imaging of acute ischemic stroke: a scientific statement from the American Heart Association. Stroke 2009;40:3646–78.
4. Konstas AA, Goldmakher GV, Lee TY, et al. Theoretic basis and technical implementations of CT perfusion in acute ischemic stroke, part 1: theoretic basis. AJNR Am J Neuroradiol 2009;30:662–8.
5. Roberts HC, Roberts TP, Smith WS, et al. Multisection dynamic CT perfusion for acute cerebral ischemia: the "toggling-table" technique. AJNR Am J Neuroradiol 2001;22:1077–80.
6. Rother J, Jonetz-Mentzel L, Fiala A, et al. Hemodynamic assessment of acute stroke using dynamic single-slice computed tomographic perfusion imaging. Arch Neurol 2000;57:1161–6.
7. Konstas AA, Goldmakher GV, Lee TY, et al. Theoretic basis and technical implementations of CT perfusion in acute ischemic stroke, part 2: technical implementations. AJNR Am J Neuroradiol 2009;30:885–92.
8. Schaefer PW, Barak ER, Kamalian S, et al. Quantitative assessment of core/penumbra mismatch in acute stroke: CT and MR perfusion imaging are strongly correlated when sufficient brain volume is imaged. Stroke 2008;39:2986–92.
9. Morhard D, Wirth CD, Fesl G, et al. Advantages of extended brain perfusion computed tomography: 9.6 cm coverage with time resolved computed tomography-angiography in comparison to standard stroke-computed tomography. Invest Radiol 2010;45:363–9.
10. Orrison WW Jr, Snyder KV, Hopkins LN, et al. Whole-brain dynamic CT angiography and perfusion imaging. Clin Radiol 2011;66:566–74.
11. Menon BK, O'Brien B, Bivard A, et al. Assessment of leptomeningeal collaterals using dynamic CT angiography in patients with acute ischemic stroke. J Cereb Blood Flow Metab 2013;33:365–71.
12. Frolich AM, Psychogios MN, Klotz E, et al. Antegrade flow across incomplete vessel occlusions can be distinguished from retrograde collateral flow using 4-dimensional computed tomographic angiography. Stroke 2012;43:2974–9.
13. Terada T, Tsuura M, Matsumoto H, et al. Endovascular treatment for pseudo-occlusion of the internal carotid artery. Neurosurgery 2006;59:301–9.
14. Matsumoto M, Kodama N, Endo Y, et al. Dynamic 3D-CT angiography. AJNR Am J Neuroradiol 2007;28:299–304.
15. Kang KH, Kim HS, Kim SY. Quantitative cerebrovascular reserve measured by acetazolamide-challenged dynamic CT perfusion in ischemic adult Moyamoya

disease: initial experience with angiographic correlation. AJNR Am J Neuroradiol 2008;29:1487–93.

16. Golshani B, Lazzaro MA, Raslau F, et al. Surveillance imaging after intracranial stent implantation: non-invasive imaging compared with digital subtraction angiography. J Neurointerv Surg 2013;5(4):361–5.

Magnetic Resonance–Guided Focused Ultrasound

A New Technology for Clinical Neurosciences

Ferenc A. Jolesz, MD[a],*, Nathan J. McDannold, PhD[b]

KEYWORDS

- Magnetic resonance imaging • Focused ultrasound • Neurosurgery • Brain tumor
- Targeted drug delivery • Chemotherapy • Neuromodulation • Blood-brain-barrier

KEY POINTS

- Transcranial MRI-guided focused ultrasound (TcMRgFUS) is an old idea but a new technology that may change the entire clinical field of the neurosciences.
- TcMRgFUS has no cumulative effect, and it is applicable for repeatable treatments, controlled by real-time dosimetry, and capable of immediate tissue destruction.
- Most importantly, it has extremely accurate targeting and constant monitoring.
- It is potentially more precise than proton beam therapy and definitely more cost effective.
- Neuro-oncology may be the most promising area of future TcMRgFUS applications.

INTRODUCTION

Diseases of the central nervous system (CNS) account for more hospitalizations and a greater need for long-term care than most other clinical areas. Most currently available therapeutic interventions are suboptimal. Surgery, radiation therapy, and drug delivery all have significant limitations; therefore, completely new approaches and technologies are desperately needed.

Over the past 2 decades, the authors and other investigators have developed the fundamentals of TcMRgFUS, a noninvasive technology that, according those who

Funding Acknowledgments: NIH grants P41 EB015898 (previously U41RR019703), P01CA067165 (primary investigator F.A. Jolesz), R01EB003268, R33EB000705, RC2NS69413.
Financial Disclosure and Conflict of Interest: The authors have nothing to disclose.
[a] Division of MRI, National Center for Image-Guided Therapy, Department of Radiology, Brigham and Women's Hospital, Harvard Medical School, 75 Francis Street, Boston, MA 02115, USA; [b] Focused Ultrasound Laboratory, National Center for Image-Guided Therapy, Department of Radiology, Brigham and Women's Hospital, Harvard Medical School, 221 Longwood Avenue, Room 521, Boston, MA 02115, USA
* Corresponding author.
E-mail address: jolesz@bwh.harvard.edu

are familiar with it, will have a profound impact on all aspects of the clinical neurosciences.[1-7] TcMRgFUS is a disruptive technology that can improve on or replace existing treatments and enable therapies that are not possible today. It is a radical departure from current treatment methods and involves expertise from multiple disciplines. Although the full potential that focused ultrasound (FUS) can have for disorders of the CNS is not widely known, the transformational process has already begun.

As described in this article, FUS has the ability to precisely focus acoustic energy to anatomically and functionally targeted locations in the brain and noninvasively induce a broad range of bioeffects that can be utilized to develop new diagnostic and therapeutic methods. Despite this great promise, this new enabling technology has several critical hurdles to overcome before widespread clinical translation is possible; a large-scale concentrated multidisciplinary effort is necessary. Currently, a diverse team of physicists, neuroscientists, engineers, and clinicians is working to advance FUS in clinical applications with the greatest impact. This review is based on innovations made by the authors' group and other investigators who have demonstrated the promise of TcMRgFUS. There are only a few prior examples of any other technology that has the same disruptive and transformative potential in any other field of medicine. If translated into everyday clinical practice, this enabling technology will change all aspects of clinical neuroscience.

FUS is uniquely capable of producing changes that can be used for the treatment of a potentially extensive range of CNS diseases and disorders. It is a completely noninvasive, targeted, and repeatable method that can be integrated with MRI to enable the necessary precise anatomic and functional guidance and control of energy deposition.[8,9] MRgFUS has been applied to treat benign and malignant tumors, such as uterine fibroids, breast tumors, prostate and liver cancer, and bone metastases.[8-10] The capabilities of FUS include the ability not only to noninvasively ablate tissue volumes (potentially replacing neurosurgery and radiosurgery) but also to deliver drugs to targeted brain regions through a temporary disruption of the blood-brain barrier (BBB).[11] This FUS-mediated method can revolutionize both neuro-oncology and neuropharmacology. In addition, FUS can reversibly modulate neuronal function (providing a tool that can be used in diagnosis and treatment in basic or clinical neuroscience).[12-14]

In recent years, with the development of a commercial TcMRgFUS device that is capable of FUS through the human skull, the feasibility of the technology was proved in humans in brain tumor ablation and functional neurosurgical applications.[7,15] Also, through a large number of preclinical studies that have been published recently, it has become clear that this technique has matured and is ready to be translated into clinical practice. This translation will be difficult however, because, to most clinicians, the therapeutic use of ultrasound in the brain is a radical concept. Therefore, significant work is needed to prove that FUS can be applied safely. Progress has been slow, with the feasibility of TcMRgFUS thermal ablation in humans reported only within the past few years.[7,15]

HISTORY OF BRAIN FUS

FUS has been investigated for more than 50 years, primarily for noninvasive ablation in the brain as a potential alternative to surgical resection, functional neurosurgery, and radiosurgery.[16-21] The enormous benefits of applying FUS as a noninvasive method for treating brain tumors, epilepsy, and movement disorders have been understood for many years, but the need for a craniotomy and the absence of imaging technologies delayed its development. Until recently, clinical tests of the method have required the removal of a section of the skull[22] to allow for ultrasound propagation into the brain due to high ultrasound absorption and heating of the skull bone and beam phase aberration caused by the skull's irregular shape and thickness and its large acoustic impedance.

The acoustic energy deposited in the focal region can be utilized in many ways and has fascinated neuroscientists for more than 60 years.[16–21,23] In the past 10 to 15 years, significant technologic developments made by the authors' group and other investigators have made the use of FUS in the brain a reality. The creation of devices that can safely and precisely focus high-intensity ultrasound beams through the intact human skull[2,3] and the integration of these devices to high-field MRI[4–6] have made it realistic to expect that technology will reach its potential in multiple clinical applications. Initial human trials with these devices are ongoing,[7,15] and the research community investment in FUS technology is growing exponentially. Although MRgFUS technology has great potential for targets throughout the body, its greatest potential, in the authors' view, is in the brain because of the lack of invasiveness. TcMRgFUS can overcome significant limitations of current therapies because it can spare normal structures adjacent to the therapeutic target. The potential of FUS for noninvasive brain tumor treatment and functional neurosurgery was recognized in the 1950s and several investigators have tried to develop a clinically applicable device.[18–22,24–31] Several technical problems, however, have prevented the use of FUS in humans. Among those problems are the issues of penetration of the acoustic beam through the intact skull and localization of both the target and the focus. The need for large craniotomies to create sufficient acoustic windows and the lack of tumor definition and temperature-sensitive imaging were the main reasons that brain FUS was not developed.

The solutions for these problems surfaced in the early 1990s. MRI was integrated with FUS and used for target definition and for the control of energy deposition by MRI-based temperature-sensitive imaging.[32,33] To transfer a sufficient amount of acoustic energy, many phased array transducer elements were applied, and the difficulty of focusing through the irregular skull was resolved by using x-ray CT to measure skull sickness at each transducer elements and to correct phase aberrations.[2,4–6,34,35] As a result, the world's first TcMRgFUS system (ExAblate 2000) was developed by InSightec (Haifa, Israel). Currently, an updated 1000-element version (ExAblate 4000) at 650 kHz is used for initial human clinical trials for brain tumors and functional neurosurgical applications at multiple academic sites (**Fig. 1**).

The TcMRgFUS systems reduce skull heating through active cooling of the scalp and have a transducer design with a large aperture to distribute the ultrasound energy over a large skull region. Furthermore, using a complex phased array transducer design, they correct for phase aberrations. When combined with methods that use acoustic simulation based on CT scans of the skull bone to determine the phase and amplitude corrections for the phased array and magnetic resonance temperature imaging to monitor the heating, a completely noninvasive alternative to surgical resection in the brain becomes possible.

The potential applications of TcMRgFUS are wide ranging.[20] The ExAblate Neuro system is under evaluation for clinical safety and efficacy in functional neurosurgery[15] and tumor ablation.[7] In these early implementations, the imaging of the thermal focus and the safety of skull heating have been demonstrated.

In functional neurosurgical trials to date, more than 50 patients have been treated for movement disorders (essential tremor and Parkinson disease) and more than 20 for neuropathic pain. The Essential Tremor Phase I trial was completed.[36] Multisite pivotal studies are under development. It can be concluded that MRI-based temperature monitoring provides accurate targeting and safe energy deposition during

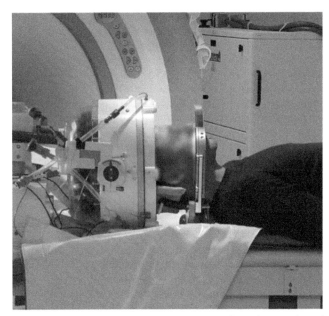

Fig. 1. Brain treatment system (Exablate 4000). (*Courtesy of* InSightec, Ltd, Haifa, Israel; with permission.)

thalamotomies. Other CNS diseases that can be treated with TcMRgFUS in the future are epilepsy, obsessive-compulsive disorders, and trigeminal neuralgia.

The major issues that have hindered the use of FUS in the brain in the past have been solved, and there is no longer any question that the technique can be delivered through the intact skull in humans. With these hurdles surpassed, efforts should be dedicated to bringing novel, innovative FUS therapies beyond thermal ablation to the clinical fields of neuroscience. These novel nonthermal techniques, achieved through the combination of FUS and injections of preformed microbubbles, have the potential to greatly expand the abilities of FUS in the brain. Although significant work has already been done by the authors' team and numerous other research groups, significant issues remain to be resolved before they can be translated to the clinical practice.

TCMRGFUS OF BRAIN TUMORS

Despite progress in drug development, radiation therapy, and radiosurgery, the standard of care for many patients with CNS tumors remains complete or incomplete (debulking) surgical resection, which is an invasive and risky procedure. Despite advances in therapy, malignant brain tumors remain an extraordinary challenge. Due to the inherent risks associated with surgical resection and radiation therapy, combined with the aggressiveness of many CNS tumors and the difficulties of drug delivery in the brain, the prognosis for patients with many types of CNS tumors remains grim. New and less-invasive alternatives are desperately needed. Technologies that can precisely ablate tumors while sparing surrounding critical structures would be a huge benefit to brain tumor patients. Thermal ablation has been pursued as a less-invasive alternative to surgery for tumor therapy in several targets,[37,38] including the brain.[39–41] FUS has been investigated for noninvasive ablation in the brain as a potential alternative to surgical resection and radiosurgery.[20,21,42–44] Until recently, clinical tests of the method required removing a section of the skull for ultrasound propagation into the brain,[22,43–48] given that there is high ultrasound absorption and heating of the skull bone and beam aberration caused by the skull's irregular shape and large acoustic impedance.

In the past decade, FUS thermal ablation systems have been developed that overcome these obstacles produced by the skull.[49–51] As discussed previously, they reduce skull heating through active cooling of the scalp and a transducer design with a large aperture to distribute the ultrasound energy over a large skull region, and, importantly, they correct for beam aberrations using a phased array transducer design. When combined with methods that use acoustic simulation based on CT scans of the skull bone to determine the phase and amplitude corrections for the phased array[2,3] and MR-based temperature imaging to monitor the heating,[52–54] a completely noninvasive alternative to surgical resection in the brain becomes possible. These systems have been tested in animals[4,55] and in initial human trials.[5,15] Such systems may also be useful for ultrasound-based targeted drug delivery methods in the brain[11] and for the treatment of stroke.[56]

TcMRgFUS offers clear, unambiguous advantages over other current treatment modalities (surgery, radiation therapy, and probe-delivered thermal ablations, such as interstitial laser therapy), because it is noninvasive (ie, incisionless, scarless, and bloodless) and does not involve ionizing radiation. Therefore, complications, such as bleeding and infection, are minimized and the MRI-guided targeting collateral damage to nontargeted tissue is almost nonexistent. The goal of ideal brain tumor surgery is complete removal of the entire tumor volume of the target lesion with functional and structural preservation of the surrounding tissue, including sparing of the tissue in the surgical path. An invasive or even minimally invasive surgical procedure is only an approximation of the ideal surgery. The ideal therapeutic modality, TcMRgFUS, is noninvasive and targeted at the point of acoustic convergence, thereby sparing the overlying tissue and it deposits sufficient thermal energy to ablate even deep-seated tumors.

Certain primary malignant brain tumors, in particular gliomas, invade and infiltrate the normal brain and, therefore, they cannot be completely removed or ablated without associated injury of normal tissue and related functional damage. In most patients with these tumors, tumor debulking by surgery to decrease tumor volume can be considered a satisfactory outcome. Benign tumors and most metastases, alternatively, demonstrate more confined and often well-defined borders, in which case complete destruction of tumor volume would be deemed adequate treatment. Whether in gross total or total resection, however, MRgFUS unmistakably maintains anatomic and functional preservation of the surrounding brain parenchyma. Furthermore, in cases of debulking surgery, specifically in glioblastoma, where recurrence invariably occurs, FUS allows for unlimited retreatment sessions, an option not present in surgery or radiation therapy. The ability to repeat unlimited treatment sessions coupled with the presence of real-time intraprocedural feedback (closed-loop control of the deposited thermal dose) provides a personalized treatment, especially when confronted with geometrically asymmetric or noncircular target lesions that are difficult to cover with probe-delivered ablations. Secondary tumor formation, caused by radiosurgery and radiotherapy, does not occur with FUS therapy. Furthermore, because the thermal gradients of FUS are much narrower than the dose curves in radiotherapy, FUS is more precise and causes less thermal damage to adjacent tissues.

Brain surgeries at the skull base, in particular, even for benign tumors, are particularly difficult due to their location and proximity to critical nerve and vascular structures.[57] Although skull base surgical approaches are used for vascular disease, congenital anomalies, and some non-neoplastic bony disorders, difficulties for surgical management remain and are related to the presence of critical structures: cranial nerves, blood vessels, and the brainstem. Access is also limited by bony structures and the presence of air-containing paranasal sinuses. Radiosurgery can also be challenging to use without damaging these critical structures. Although extraordinary advances have been made in neurosurgical techniques that permit better surgical access to these challenging regions in the brain, surgery near the skull base has remained a traumatic, time-consuming procedure that poses significant risk to patients who are often poor candidates for surgery. Surgical resection of recurrence can also be a challenge. In recent years, the field of skull base surgery has been revolutionized by multidisciplinary improvements in anesthetic and surgical techniques. The development of brain-exposing osteotomies, neuro-endoscopic surgery, and infection prevention methods (eg, galeal, frontalis, and myofascial flaps) and improved techniques for reconstruction has allowed surgeons to perform biopsies and resections on many skull base masses. In addition, radiosurgery with Gamma Knife or a linear accelerator (LINAC) has become a highly useful tool in treating pathologic conditions at the skull base. As expertise with surgical approaches to the skull base has grown, the optimal application of these methods in combination with adjuvant therapies has become the focus of skull base neurosurgery, which is invasive even using the best surgical approaches. Nevertheless, many skull base tumors, even benign ones, are not operable because the danger of vision loss or of other essential functions because of cranial nerve injury.

TcMRgFUS provides alternatives to surgical resection and radiosurgery that can remotely target tissue volumes in the brain, even at the skull base, while sparing the surrounding tissues. As described later, FUS has the potential to provide new "surgical" options for patients who fail after surgery or radiosurgery. Ultimately, with enough research to prove its safety and efficacy, it may ultimately replace them. The technology of TcMRgFUS can greatly extend FUS brain surgery, making it possible throughout the brain.

The effects of FUS can be enhanced by combining sonications with microbubble agents. These agents, which are available as ultrasound imaging contrast agents, consist of semirigid lipid or albumin shells that encapsulate a gas, typically a perfluorocarbon. They range in size from approximately 1 μm to 10 μm and are constrained to the vasculature. The presence of the preformed microbubbles that make up the contrast agent circulating in the vasculature concentrates the ultrasound effects to the microvasculature and greatly reduces the FUS exposure levels needed to produce bioeffects. Thus, with these microbubbles FUS can be applied transcranially without significant skull heating or distortion of the ultrasound beam. When microbubbles interact with an ultrasound beam, a range of biologic effects has been observed. Depending on their size, the bubbles can oscillate within the ultrasound field, growing in size via rectified diffusion. At high enough acoustic pressures, they can collapse during the positive-pressure cycle, a phenomenon known as inertial cavitation, producing shock waves and high-velocity jets,[58] free radicals,[59] and high local temperatures.[60,61] In addition, the medium surrounding the bubbles undergoes acoustic streaming,[62] which may be associated with large shear stresses. Furthermore, a radiation force on the bubbles is produced along the direction of the ultrasound beam.[58] The preformed microbubbles used in ultrasound contrast agents presumably can exhibit these behaviors, either with their shells intact or after being broken apart by the ultrasound beam and their gas contents released.

A current limitation of TcMRgFUS is that thermal ablation is restricted to brain targets that are distant from the skull bone. If the focal point is placed in peripheral regions, the incidence angle between large portions of the skull bone and ultrasound wave front becomes more oblique. As this angle increases, less of the ultrasound beam penetrates the skull and, at extreme angles, the beam is totally reflected. As a result, fewer elements in the array can be effectively utilized when peripheral regions are targeted, increasing the peak energy density and the heating on the skull surface. Shear mode conversion also increases as this angle increases, further increasing the heating due to the higher absorption coefficient of the shear mode. This limitation was evident in analysis of magnetic resonance temperature measurements in the focal region and on the brain surface in the first patient treatments with a TcMRgFUS system.[5] Placing the focal point near the skull base adds an additional challenge, as the beam in the far field (ie, beyond the focal point) heats the bone and could damage nearby brain, nerve, and vascular structures. Large myelinated nerves may be at particular risk due to their lower vascularity and perfusion that prevent the heat from being drawn away. To target peripheral areas and targets near the skull base with TcMRgFUS, new methods are needed.

One way to increase the focal heating without increasing the time-averaged acoustic power deposition (which determines the degree of skull heating) is to use microbubble-enhanced heating.[63,64] By using ultrasound bursts with peak pressure amplitudes above the cavitation threshold, microbubbles are generated from gas nuclei within fluid in the tissue. These microbubbles can locally enhance the heating in the focal zone through viscous heating, absorption of bubble acoustic emission, and other factors.[63] If the ultrasound bursts are delivered with a low duty cycle, the time averaged intensity on the skull can potentially be largely reduced. Although this approach can expand the targetable areas for TcMRgFUS, it does not permit ablation of targets directly adjacent to the skull bone. To target such areas, a more radical decrease in the time averaged acoustic power is necessary. A way to achieve this reduction is to combine FUS with an intravenously injected microbubble-based ultrasound contrast agent.

At slightly higher exposure levels, the microbubbles collapse violently, leading to vascular destruction and tissue death in the focal region. This method of nonthermal ablation, which can be applied without overheating the skull, can greatly expand the areas of the brain that can be targeted compared with thermal ablation, providing a noninvasive alternative to surgery and radiosurgery. The current standard of care for many primary brain tumors and brain metastases includes radiation therapy. Although it is effective and improves outcomes, its effectiveness is limited. Most importantly, it cannot be repeated in cases of recurrence, which occur frequently, and at which time a patient's options are limited or nonexistent. In radiation therapy and radiosurgery (Gamma Knife, LINAC, proton beam, and so forth), the radiation dose is statistically set based on accumulated prior experience, and, because of their toxic cumulative effects, lend themselves to only a single treatment session (irrelevant of the treatment success). Alternatively, FUS is nontoxic, allowing for unlimited treatments in a single session and unlimited repeated sessions over a period of time, which is a feature of particular importance when a tumor recurs. In addition, unlike radiosurgery, FUS effects can be performed under image guidance with high-field MRI, which provides outstanding anatomic definition of the target site, real-time guidance and monitoring during therapy, and immediate post-treatment confirmation of the treatment effects. For FUS thermal ablation, magnetic resonance thermometry[33,34,53] in FUS therapy permits accurate real-time noninvasive intraprocedural monitoring.

There is a need to develop methods to provide similar feedback during microbubble-enhanced FUS applications to evaluate whether radiation-induced changes to the tissue have an effect on the safety and efficacy of these FUS/microbubble techniques. Radiation induces changes to the vasculature, which may make it more or less sensitive to the mechanical effects induced by FUS and microbubbles. Other changes to the tissue may change its response to the therapy, such as altering drug penetration after BBB disruption. Before patients who have had radiation are treated with FUS and microbubbles, it must be established that it can be done safely and how radiation can change the outcome of the therapy must be understood. Combining microbubble-enhanced FUS with high-resolution MRI offers a means to noninvasively and precisely target tumors or other regions anywhere in the brain, including the skull base. FUS produces immediate ablation. It is repeatable and can be applied without general anesthesia. No other technology is available that can achieve this result. The authors and other investigators have spent the past decade developing FUS and MRI technologies that have allowed clinical trials of thermal ablation.[7,15] In contrast, research combining FUS with microbubbles for ablation in the brain is only just beginning, and substantial work is needed to apply it reliably in a controlled manner and to understand and optimize the ablation process.

Recent work has demonstrated that the method is ready for such intense testing and has the potential to have a large impact as a replacement for surgery and radiosurgery. The authors tested the ability to ablate targets at the skull base in rats next to the optic chiasm and optic tract without having an impact on nerve function. Before FUS, MRI compatible electrodes were placed bilaterally on the dura above the primary visual cortex, and visual evoked potential (VEP) measurements were acquired. These measurements were repeated weekly after a sonication on or adjacent to the optic tract or chiasm to determine whether visual function was intact. The authors found that this was possible and that histology showed that the fibers in the tract were mostly intact, even when the lesion was directly adjacent to it, and no significant changes were observed in the VEP measurements.

The authors have also evaluated the feasibility of ablating brain structures adjacent to the optic nerve in nonhuman primates with the low-frequency TcMRgFUS system. In rhesus macaques, the authors found that discrete lesions were produced at the targets that were consistent with prior experience in rats. Based on histology and observation after the monkeys recovered from anesthesia, the optic tract seemed only minimally effected. These results are highly encouraging and demonstrate that noninvasive ablation can be achieved with this TcMRgFUS system, even at the skull base, without overheating the bone and damaging surrounding structures.

These results would not be possible with any existing radiosurgery technology, including proton beam therapy. Using this method, there is a sharp demarcation between treated and untreated areas. The TcMRgFUS system not only has a great targeting accuracy but also can be monitored in real time and with subthreshold energy levels that cause no irreversible tissue damage. The lesion location can be identified before irreversible lesions are made. To get this method to patients, the authors have developed a plan to optimize the exposures, monitor the effect in real time, and test the safety of the method in nonhuman primates.

TARGETED DRUG DELIVERY

Most systemically administered therapeutic agents are not effective in the CNS because they are blocked by the BBB. The BBB restricts the passage of substances except for small (molecular weight less than approximately 400 Da), hydrophobic molecules, preventing most small-molecule drugs and essentially all large-molecule drugs from reaching the brain interstitial space.[65] It is the primary hurdle to the development and use of drugs in the CNS. As many as one-third of the population is expected to experience a CNS disorder in their lifetime, but the global pharmaceutical market for CNS-related drugs would have to increase by a factor of 5 to equal that for cardiovascular disease. Most methods that have been tested to circumvent the BBB are invasive, are nontargeted, or require the expense of developing new drug carriers that use endogenous transport mechanisms.[65] Because of the BBB, most chemotherapies have not been effective treatments for malignant brain tumors. Although the vessels in most brain tumors do not have a fully intact BBB and can be permeable, infiltrating cancer cells and small metastatic seeds are disseminated in the normal brain, where the normal brain blood vessels and the BBB prevent drug extravasation.[66] Furthermore, it is known that tumor vasculature permeability is heterogeneous and that there are additional barriers to drug delivery, such as increased interstitial pressures[67] and efflux pumps.[68,69] Major efforts have thus been undertaken to develop pharmaceuticals that circumvent the BBB, such as designing more lipid-soluble drugs, designing water-soluble drugs with high affinities for natural carriers at the BBB, or through the use of vectors, such as amino acids and peptide carriers.[70–72] Other investigators have diffusely and reversibly disrupted the BBB by introducing a catheter into an arterial branch within the brain and applying an infusion of hyperosmotic solution or other substances.[73] The only current method to deliver drugs to selected regions of the brain is directly to inject agents or to use implanted delivery systems.[74,75] A method to disrupt the BBB noninvasively and reversibly at targeted locations would have a major impact on clinical neuroscience. The National Institutes of Health Brain Tumor Progress Review Group recently recognized the need for such targeted drug delivery.[76]

The combination of FUS with circulating microbubbles, which directs the acoustic effects to the vasculature and reduces the energy needed to produce bioeffects, can greatly expand brain applications of FUS beyond thermal ablation. At low exposure levels, a combination of FUS and microbubbles induces a temporary permeabilization of the blood vessels in the brain and in brain tumors, leading to a targeted way to get drugs past the BBB. The combination of FUS and circulating microbubble agents has the potential to revolutionize drug delivery to the brain. This technology enables the crossing of drugs across the BBB, to deliver drugs to a preferred target and to do it noninvasively so it can be readily repeated to match a patient's drug schedule. Today, even when drugs that have maximal efficiency preferentially at the target tissue are applied, systemic toxicity can still occur and limit the dose. With MRgFUS, preferred targeting can occur even with systemic administration because the BBB is disrupted only in the desired location. Ultimately, this can be extended because the drugs can be designed for FUS-triggered release through encapsulation in gas-containing bubbles, liposomes, nanoparticles, or other carriers before being administered systemically.

Microbubble-induced opening of the BBB is transient and reversible. No permanent histologic damage is seen, and the function of BBB is preserved after a few hours. The increased permeability for larger molecules is most likely explained by the acoustic-mechanical effect of ultrasound on the tight junctions.[11,76–84] Transfer of various size molecules has been demonstrated after FUS-induced BBB disruption. That included antibodies[85]; chemotherapies, like Herceptin (Trastuzumab)[86] and doxorubicin[87–89]; and DNA.[90]

The increased BBB permeability and the improved delivery of chemotherapies were tested in animal experimental tumor models. Tumor growth and survival rates were monitored via MRI for 7 weeks after sonication. HER 2/neu–positive breast cancer metastasis models were treated with trastuzumab and, in almost half of the animals, the tumor seemed completely resolved in MRI, an outcome not observed in control groups.[91] Similar results were seen with Herceptin treatments. 9L gliosarcoma of rats was treated with liposomal doxorubicin. Post-treatment MRI showed that after FUS-mediated BBB opening, doxorubicin reduced tumor growth compared with controls without FUS treatment.[88] There was a modest but significant increase in median survival time after a single FUS plus doxorubicin treatment, whereas neither doxorubicin nor FUS had any significant impact on survival on its own. These results suggest that combined ultrasound-mediated BBB disruption may significantly increase the antineoplastic efficacy of liposomal doxorubicin in the brain.

The use of FUS to temporarily disrupt the BBB overcomes the greatest single hurdle to the development of therapies for CNS disorders. Being able to modify this barrier and allow drugs to reach the brain and to be able to do so only in the locations where the drugs are needed will revolutionize drug therapies in the brain. It is important that this can be done safely and in a controlled way.

The presence of the BBB is the primary hurdle to the development and use of drugs in the CNS. As many as one-third of the population is expected to experience a CNS disorder in their lifetime, but the global pharmaceutical market for CNS-related drugs would have to increase by a factor of 5 to equal that for cardiovascular disease. The opportunity that FUS technology presents is to overcome these restrictions. Enabling in the brain the full arsenal of drugs and removing limitations that currently hinder drug development for CNS disease would lead to long-term improvements and growth in research, enterprise, public health, and health care delivery.

Although most brain disorders may benefit from this approach, the first obvious target for this technology is to deliver anticancer drugs to brain tumors and the surrounding brain that may be infiltrated. Although primary brain tumors may be good targets for this technology, a more immediate target could be brain metastases from non-CNS tumors. The authors expect that brain metastases will be the best application for initial clinical tests because brain tumor patients lack treatment options, and there are existing approved agents that are known to be effective with extracranial disease.

The authors recently completed in preparation for clinical work a safety study of the technique in nonhuman primates using a commercially available TcMRgFUS system[92] and have tested this device in 40 sessions in 10 rhesus macaques. After sonicating more than 200 discrete loci or relatively large volumes in the brain, the authors found that the BBB disruption can be achieved safely with no evidence for either histologic or functional damage. This result was true even when the same brain target was sonicated repeatedly 5 or more times over several weeks.

The ability of FUS-induced oscillations of circulating microbubbles to permeabilize vascular barriers, such as the BBB, holds great promise for noninvasive targeted drug delivery. A major issue has been a lack of control over the procedure to ensure safe and effective treatment. Passively recorded acoustic emissions may achieve this control. An acoustic emissions monitoring system was constructed and integrated into a clinical TcMRgFUS[93] to control FUS-induced BBB disruption. The authors found that this monitoring system provides signatures that can predict both BBB disruption and the small vessel damage that occurs with overexposure. Overall, this study demonstrated that the method can be applied safely, reliably, and in a controlled manner using a commercial TcMRgFUS system that is already available for patient use.

Such promising results along with the growing body of literature on this technique demonstrate its safety and effectiveness and are supportive of its translating to patients.

NEUROMODULATION

In the past decade, neuroscience has been revolutionized by the ability to noninvasively map brain function and, to a lesser extent, modulate regional brain activity in a controlled manner. Applications of neuromodulation range from functional testing to the treatment of diverse neurologic or neuropsychiatric disorders. Subdural and epidural cortical stimulation as well as deep brain stimulation are finding increasing acceptance in neurotherapeutics. Transcranial magnetic stimulation (TMS) and transcranial direct current stimulation offer noninvasive alternatives but lack spatial specificity and have limited depth of penetration. The ability of these technologies to image and modulate neuronal function has led to an explosion of studies that are providing a deeper understanding of brain function and potential therapies for CNS disorders.

The authors believe that such abilities are just the tip of the iceberg of what can be achieved with TcMRgFUS, which offers capabilities that are not possible with any other technology. It has been known for decades that FUS can stimulate the brain[12,13,94] and can block nerve conduction.[95] FUS can modulate brain function by itself, which is a completely new way to diagnose and treat a range of CNS disorders and to study brain function. A deeper understanding of how to use FUS to modulate brain function that can be translated to clinical tests is needed. Transient modulation of brain function using image-guided and anatomically targeted FUS would enable the investigation of functional connectivity between brain regions and eventually lead to a better understanding of localized brain functions. It is anticipated that the use of this technology will have an impact on brain research and may offer novel therapeutic interventions in various neurologic conditions and psychiatric disorders.

The mechanism by which FUS achieves neuromodulation is not known, but it is thought that it could be related to transient changes in cell membrane permeability.[14] With devices that can precisely focus an ultrasound beam through the intact human skull, small volumes deep in the brain can be noninvasively targeted, greatly improving on the capabilities of TMS. FUS-induced neuromodulation can be combined with simultaneous functional imaging, providing real-time evaluation of the effects of suppression and stimulation of neural circuits. These technologies can be combined for complex experimental designs involving different stimuli, tasks, and mapping of functional activity throughout the brain.

In rabbits, the authors demonstrated that the pulsed application of low-intensity FUS bursts (ie, lower than the intensity approved for diagnostic ultrasound imaging) can modulate neural tissue excitability through nonthermal mechanisms.[14] The authors have also reduced chemically induced epileptic states in rats[96] and have demonstrated that FUS can modulate the extracellular level of dopamine and serotonin when applied to the rat thalamus.

In addition to the potential of using FUS alone for neuromodulation, FUS-induced BBB disruption can be used to deliver neuroactive agents to targeted specific locations in the brain, which is an ability that opens exciting new opportunities for neuromodulation. Translating this technology to clinics will be more challenging than the other FUS applications that aim to provide new and less-invasive treatments to desperately sick patients with brain tumors. Although it has potential application in neurosurgical planning, especially for functional neurosurgery, the authors think its main potential lies in other areas, such as those in which TMS or other methods for stimulation are used (movement and psychiatric disorders, for example) and in healthy subjects for neuroscience research.

If the safety of the method is established and its technical challenges worked out, an unparalleled research opportunity for the study of brain function noninvasively will be provided. Being able to noninvasively and repeatedly modulate the levels of neuroactive agents opens the door to new investigations that exploit specific molecular pathways. In addition to neurotransmitters, targeting the delivery of other substances, such as neurosteroids or neuropeptides (perhaps encapsulated to allow for systemic application), that induce specific effects on different neuronal populations can be envisioned. Being able to do such experiments in alert animals with simultaneous functional MRI would be a powerful tool in understanding brain function and potentially for developing new methods to diagnose and treat disorders of the CNS.

SUMMARY

TcMRgFUS is an old idea but a new technology that may change the entire clinical field of the neurosciences. In neurosurgery it provides an excisionless, scarless, and noninvasive way to treat malignant and benign brain tumors and produce accurate lesions for functional neurosurgical applications. It eventually can replace most of the ionizing radiation-based radiosurgeries. TcMRgFUS has no cumulative effect, and it is applicable for repeatable treatments, controlled by real-time dosimetry, and capable of immediate tissue destruction. Most importantly, it has extremely accurate targeting and constant monitoring. It is potentially more precise than proton beam therapy and definitely more cost effective. Neuro-oncology may be the most promising area of future TcMRgFUS applications. It can deliver targeted chemotherapy through open BBB using drugs of any size; therefore, it most likely will change the entire field of neuropharmacology and have a profound effect on the pharmacology industry. It can be applied to gene therapy and stem cell–based therapy. TcMRgFUS can be used for the treatment of thrombotic and hemorrhagic stroke. Finally, neuromodulation is an exciting new application that can replace TMS and other modalities, apply neurotransmitters in a targeted way, and localize epileptic foci. The treatments possible with TcMRgFUS, applied alone or in combination, can completely change current clinical practice and open up entirely new directions in the treatment of CNS diseases. Although the investigation of therapeutic applications of FUS in brain is not new, clinical translation of this technology has been hampered by its novelty, the large expense needed for clinical translation of new treatments for CNS disease, and the perceived high risks involved in developing and applying new technologies for brain treatments, particularly for nononcologic applications like functional neurosurgery. This need to demonstrate safety creates a dilemma. Early trials likely will be done with the sickest of patients; in these trials, patient accrual, industry support, and the ability to improve outcomes may be limited. These trials are needed, however, before moving to a broad patient group, the impact on whom this technology can have its greatest impact. TcMRgFUS is a potentially game-changing revolutionary technology. Preclinical data are largely mature, and a clinical device to begin these tests is now available commercially. The need to move FUS forward is substantial and requires resources. Compared with the enormous clinical potential, however, the investment needed to demonstrate that these uses of FUS are possible is small. FUS is a classic high-risk, high-reward, and truly transformative technology for which the reward is uniquely high. This technology has been evaluated for decades but only now are there the devices, image guidance, and monitoring or control methods to deliver treatments safely and effectively. So far, all supporting data demonstrate its clinical feasibility and broad applicability.

REFERENCES

1. Jagannathan J, Sanghvi NT, Crum LA, et al. High-intensity focused ultrasound surgery of the brain: part 1–A historical perspective with modern applications. Neurosurgery 2009;64:201–10.
2. Clement GT, Hynynen K. A non-invasive method for focusing ultrasound through the human skull. Phys Med Biol 2002;47:1219–36.
3. Aubry JF, Tanter M, Pernot M, et al. Experimental demonstration of non-invasive transskull adaptive focusing based on prior computed tomography scans. J Acoust Soc Am 2003;113:84–93.
4. Hynynen K, Clement GT, McDannold N, et al. 500-element ultrasound phased array system for non-invasive focal surgery of the brain: a preliminary rabbit study with ex vivo human skulls. Magn Reson Med 2004;52:100–7.
5. Hynynen K, McDannold N, Clement G, et al. Pre-clinical testing of a phased array ultrasound system for MRI-guided non-invasive surgery of the brain-A primate study. Eur J Radiol 2006;59:149–56.
6. Clement GT, White PJ, King RL, et al. A magnetic resonance imaging-compatible, large-scale array for trans-skull ultrasound surgery and therapy. J Ultrasound Med 2005;24:1117.
7. McDannold N, Clement GT, Black P, et al. Transcranial magnetic resonance imaging-guided focused ultrasound surgery of brain tumors: initial findings in 3 patients. Neurosurgery 2010;66:323–32.
8. Jolesz FA. MRI-guided focused ultrasound surgery. Annu Rev Med 2009;60: 417–30.
9. Tempany CM, McDannold NJ, Hynynen K, et al. Focused ultrasound surgery in oncology: overview and principles. Radiology 2011;259(1):39–56.
10. Jolesz FA, McDannold N. Current status and future potential of MRI-guided focused ultrasound surgery. J Magn Reson Imaging 2008;27(2):391–9.
11. Hynynen K, McDannold N, Vykhodtseva N, et al. Non-invasive MR imaging-guided focal opening of the blood-brain barrier in rabbits. Radiology 2001; 220:640–6.
12. Gavrilov LR, Tsirulnikov EM, Davies IA. Application of focused ultrasound for the stimulation of neural structures. Ultrasound Med Biol 1996;22:179–92.
13. Tufail Y, Matyushov A, Baldwin N, et al. Transcranial pulsed ultrasound stimulates intact brain circuits. Neuron 2010;66:681–94.
14. Yoo SS, Bystritsky A, Lee JH, et al. Focused ultrasound modulates region-specific brain activity. Neuroimage 2011;56:1267–75.
15. Martin E, Jeanmonod D, Morel A, et al. High-intensity focused ultrasound for non-invasive functional neurosurgery. Ann Neurol 2009;66:858–61.
16. Lynn JG, Zwemer RL, Chick AJ, et al. A new method for the generation and use of focused ultrasound in experimental biology. J Gen Physiol 1942;26: 179–93.
17. Fry WJ. Intense ultrasound in investigations of the central nervous system. Adv Biol Med Phys 1958;6:281–348.
18. Ballantine HT, Bell E, Manlapaz J. Progress and problems in the neurological applications of focused ultrasound. J Neurosurg 1960;17:858–76.
19. Lele PP. Effects of ultrasound on "solid" mammalian tissues and tumors in vivo. In: Repacholi MH, Grondolfo M, Rindi A, editors. Ultrasound: medical

applications, biological effects and hazard potential. New York: Plenum Pub. Corp; 1987. p. 275–306.

20. Colen RR, Jolesz FA. Future potential of MRI-guided focused ultrasound brain surgery. Neuroimaging Clin N Am 2010;20(3):355–66.

21. Medel R, Monteith SJ, Elias WJ, et al. Magnetic resonance-guided focused ultrasound surgery: part 2: a review of current and future applications. Neurosurgery 2012;71(4):755–63.

22. Ram Z, Cohen ZR, Harnof S, et al. Magnetic resonance imaging-guided, high-intensity focused ultrasound for brain tumor therapy. Neurosurgery 2006;59: 949–55.

23. Vykhodtseva NI, Hynynen K, Damianou C. Histologic effects of high intensity pulsed ultrasound exposure with subharmonic emission in rabbit brain in vivo. Ultrasound Med Biol 1995;21:969–79.

24. Fry WJ, Barnard JW, Fry FJ, et al. Ultrasonic lesions in the mammalian central nervous system. Science 1955;122:517–8.

25. Fry WJ, Barnard JW, Fry FJ. Ultrasonically produced localized selective lesions in the central nervous system. Am J Phys Med 1955;34:413–23.

26. Barnard JW, Fry WJ, Fry FJ, et al. Small localized ultrasonic lesions in the white and gray matter of the cat brain. AMA Arch Neurol Psychiatry 1956; 75:15–35.

27. Fry WJ, Brennan JF, Barnard JW. Histological study of changes produced by ultrasound in the gray and white matter of the central nervous system. Ultrasound Med Biol 1957;3:110–30.

28. Lele PP. A simple method for production of trackless focal lesions with focused ultrasound: physical factors. J Physiol 1962;160:494–512.

29. Basauri L, Lele PP. A simple method for production of trackless focal lesions with focused ultrasound: statistical evaluation of the effects of irradiation on the central nervous system of the cat. J Physiol 1962;160:513–34.

30. Lele PP. Production of deep focal lesions by focused ultrasound–current status. Ultrasonics 1967;5:105–12.

31. Lele PP, Pierce AD. The thermal hypothesis of the mechanism of ultrasonic focal destruction in organized tissues. Interaction of ultrasound and biological tissues. Washington, DC: Bureau of Radiological Health; 1973.

32. McDannold NJ, King RL, Jolesz FA, et al. Usefulness of MR imaging-derived thermometry and dosimetry in determining the threshold for tissue damage induced by thermal surgery in rabbits. Radiology 2000;216:517–23.

33. Chung AH, Jolesz FA, Hynynen K. Thermal dosimetry of a focused ultrasound beam in vivo by magnetic resonance imaging. Med Phys 1999;26:2017–26.

34. Hynynen K, Chung A, Fjield T, et al. Feasibility of using ultrasound phased arrays for MRI monitored non-invasive surgery. IEEE Trans Ultrason Ferroelectrics Freq Contr 1996;43:1043.

35. Hynynen K, Jolesz FA. Demonstration of potential non-invasive ultrasound brain therapy through an intact skull. Ultrasound Med Biol 1998;24:275–83.

36. Elias WJ, Huss D, Voss T, et al. A pilot study of focused ultrasound thalamotomy for essential tremor. N Engl J Med 2013;369(7):640–8.

37. Jolesz FA. Neurosurgical suite of the future. II. Neuroimaging Clin N Am 2001; 11(4):581–92.

38. McDannold NJ, Jolesz FA. Magnetic resonance image-guided thermal ablations. Top Magn Reson Imaging 2000;11(3):191–202.

39. Anzai Y, Lufkin R, DeSalles A, et al. Preliminary experience with MR-guided thermal ablation of brain tumors. AJNR Am J Neuroradiol 1995;16:39–48.

40. Kahn T, Bettag M, Ulrich F, et al. MRI-guided laser-induced interstitial thermo-therapy of cerebral neoplasms. J Comput Assist Tomogr 1994;18:519–32.

41. Kettenbach J, Kuroda K, Hata N, et al. Laser-induced thermotherapy of cerebral neoplasia under MR tomographic control. Minim Invasive Ther Allied Technol 1998;7:589–98.

42. Hata N, Morrison PR, Kettenbach J, et al. Computer-assisted intra-operative magnetic resonance imaging monitoring of interstitial laser therapy in the brain: a case report. J Biomed Opt 1998;3(3):304–11.

43. Meyers R, Fry WJ, Fry FJ, et al. Early experiences with ultrasonic irradiation of the pallidfugal and nigral complexes in hyperkinetic and hypertonic disorders. J Neurosurg 1959;16:32–54.

44. Fry WJ, Fry FJ. Fundamental neurological research and human neurosurgery using intense ultrasound. IRE Trans Med Electron 1960;(ME-7):166–81.

45. Oka M, Okumura T, Yokoi H, et al. Surgical application of high intensity focused ultrasound. Med J Osaka Univ 1960;10:427–42.

46. Heimburger RF. Ultrasound augmentation of central nervous system tumor ther-apy. Indiana Med 1985;78:469–76.

47. Guthkelch AN, Carter LP, Cassady JR, et al. Treatment of malignant brain tumors with focused ultrasound hyperthermia and radiation: results of a phase I trial. J Neurooncol 1991;10:271–84.

48. Park JW, Jung S, Junt TY, et al. Focused ultrasound surgery for the treatment of recurrent anaplastic astrocytoma: a preliminary report. In: Therapeutic Ultrasound. 5th International Symposium on Therapeutic Ultrasound. New York: American Institute of Physics; 2006. p. 238–40.

49. Jolesz FA, Hynynen K. Magnetic resonance image-guided focused ultrasound surgery. Cancer J 2002;8(Suppl 1):S100–12.

50. Clement GT, Sun J, Giesecke T, et al. A hemisphere array for non-invasive ultra-sound brain therapy and surgery. Phys Med Biol 2000;45:3707–19.

51. Thomas J, Fink MA. Ultrasonic beam focusing through tissue inhomogeneities with a time reversal mirror: applicaton to transskull therapy. IEEE Trans Ultrason Ferroelectrics Freq Contr 1996;43:1122–9.

52. Ishihara Y, Calderon A, Watanabe H, et al. A precise and fast temperature map-ping using water proton chemical shift. Magn Reson Med 1995;34:814–23.

53. Hynynen K, Vykhodtseva NI, Chung AH, et al. Thermal effects of focused ultra-sound on the brain: determination with MR imaging. Radiology 1997;204:247–53.

54. Vykhodtseva NI, Sorrentino V, Jolesz FA, et al. MRI detection of the thermal ef-fects of focused ultrasound on the brain. Ultrasound Med Biol 2000;26:871–80.

55. Pernot M, Aubry JF, Tanter M, et al. In vivo transcranial brain surgery with an ul-trasonic time reversal mirror. J Neurosurg 2007;106:1061–6.

56. Alexandrov AV, Molina CA, Grotta JC, et al. Ultrasound-enhanced systemic thrombolysis for acute ischemic stroke. N Engl J Med 2004;351:2170–8.

57. Bulsara KR, Al-Mefty O. Skull base surgery for benign skull base tumors. J Neurooncol 2004;69(1–3):181–9.

58. Leighton TG. The acoustic bubble. San Diego (CA): Academic Press Limited; 1994.

59. Edmonds PD, Sancier KM. Evidence for free radical production by ultrasonic cavitation in biological media. Ultrasound Med Biol 1983;9:635–9.

60. Flynn HG. Generation of transient cavities in liquids by microsecond pulses of ultrasound. J Acoust Soc Am 1982;72:1926–32.

61. Apfel RE. Acoustic cavitation: a possible consequence of biomedical uses of ul-trasound. Br J Cancer Suppl 1982;45:140–6.

62. Miller DL. Particle gathering and microstreaming near ultrasonically activated gas-filled micropores. J Acoust Soc Am 1988;84:1378–87.
63. Holt RG, Roy RA. Measurements of bubble-enhanced heating from focused, mhz-frequency ultrasound in a tissue-mimicking material. Ultrasound Med Biol 2001;27:1399–412.
64. Sokka SD, King R, Hynynen K. MRI-guided gas bubble enhanced ultrasound heating in in vivo rabbit thigh. Phys Med Biol 2003;48:223–41.
65. Pardridge WM. Blood-brain barrier delivery. Drug Discov Today 2007;12:54–61.
66. Eichler AF, Chung E, Kodack DP, et al. The biology of brain metastasestranslation to new therapies. Nat Rev Clin Oncol 2011;8:344–56.
67. Fukumura D, Jain RK. Tumor microenvironment abnormalities: causes, consequences, and strategies to normalize. J Cell Biochem 2007;101:937–49.
68. Demeule M, Regina A, Jodoin J, et al. Drug transport to the brain: key roles for the efflux pump P-glycoprotein in the blood-brain barrier. Vascul Pharmacol 2002;38:339–48.
69. Regina A, Demeule M, Laplante A, et al. Multidrug resistance in brain tumors: roles of the blood-brain barrier. Cancer Metastasis Rev 2001;20:13–25.
70. Pardridge WM. Drug and gene delivery to the brain: the vascular route. Neuron 2002;36:555–8.
71. Pardridge WM. Drug and gene targeting to the brain with molecular Trojan horses. Nat Rev Drug Discov 2002;1:131–9.
72. Pardridge WM. Blood-brain barrier genomics and the use of endogenous transporters to cause drug penetration into the brain. Curr Opin Drug Discov Devel 2003;6:683–91.
73. Doolittle ND, Miner ME, Hall WA, et al. Safety and efficacy of a multicenter study using intraarterial chemotherapy in conjunction with osmotic opening of the blood-brain barrier for the treatment of patients with malignant brain tumors. Cancer 2000;88(3):637–47.
74. Guerin C, Olivi A, Weingart JD, et al. Recent advances in brain tumortherapy: local intracerebral drug delivery by polymers. Invest New Drugs 2004;22: 27–37.
75. Hynynen K, McDannold N, Sheikov NA, et al. Local and reversible blood-brain barrier disruption by non-invasive focused ultrasound at frequencies suitable for trans-skull sonications. Neuroimage 2005;24:12–20.
76. NIH, National institute of neurological disorders and stroke, and National Cancer Institute, report of the brain tumor progress review group. 2000. NIH Publication Number 01-4902, November 2000.
77. Hynynen K, McDannold N, Vykhodtseva N, et al. Focal disruption of the blood–brain barrier due to 260-kHz ultrasound bursts: a method for molecular imaging and targeted drug delivery. J Neurosurg 2006;105:445–54.
78. McDannold N, Vykhodtseva N, Raymond S, et al. MRI-guided targeted blood-brain barrier disruption with focused ultrasound: histological findings in rabbits. Ultrasound Med Biol 2005;31:1527–37.
79. McDannold N, Vykhodtseva N, Hynynen K. Use of ultrasound pulses combined with Definity for targeted blood-brain barrier disruption: a feasibility study. Ultrasound Med Biol 2007;33:584–90.
80. McDannold N, Vykhodtseva N, Hynynen K. Effects of acoustic parameters and ultrasound contrast agent dose on focused-ultrasound induced blood-brain barrier disruption. Ultrasound Med Biol 2008;34:930–7.
81. McDannold N, Vykhodtseva N, Hynynen K. Blood-brain barrier disruption induced by focused ultrasound and circulating preformed microbubbles

appears to be characterized by the mechanical index. Ultrasound Med Biol 2008;34:834–40.

82. McDannold N, Vykhodtseva N, Hynynen K. Targeted disruption of the blood-brain barrier with focusedultrasound: association with cavitation activity. Phys Med Biol 2006;51:793–807.

83. Sheikov N, McDannold N, Jolesz F, et al. Brain arterioles show more active vesiculartransport of blood-borne tracer molecules than capillaries and venules opening of the blood-brain barrier. Ultrasound Med Biol 2006;32:1399–409.

84. Sheikov N, McDannold N, Sharma S, et al. Effect of focused ultrasound applied with an ultrasoundcontrast agent on the tight junctional integrity of the brain microvascular endothelium. Ultrasound Med Biol 2008;34:1093–104.

85. Kinoshita M, McDannold N, Jolesz FA, et al. Targeted delivery of antibodies through the bloodbrain barrier by MRI-guided focused ultrasound. Biochem Biophys Res Commun 2006;340:1085–90.

86. Kinoshita M, McDannold N, Jolesz FA, et al. Non-invasive localized delivery of Herceptin to the mouse brain by MRI-guided focused ultrasound-induced blood-brain barrier disruption. Proc Natl Acad Sci U S A 2006;103:11719–23.

87. Treat LH, McDannold N, Zhang Y, et al. Targeted delivery of doxorubicin to the rat brain at therapeutic levels using MRI-guided focused ultrasound. Int J Cancer 2007;121:901–7.

88. Treat LH, McDannold N, Zhang Y, et al. Improved anti-tumor effect of liposomal doxorubicin after targeted blood-brain barrier disruption by MRI-guided focused ultrasound in rat glioma. Ultrasound Med Biol 2012;38(10):1716–25.

89. Park J, Zhang Y, Vykhodtseva N, et al. The kinetics of blood brain barrier permeability and targeted doxorubicin delivery into brain induced by focused ultrasound. J Control Release 2012;162(1):134–42.

90. Huber PE, Pfisterer P. In vitro and in vivo transfection of plasmid DNA in the Dunning prostate tumor R3327-AT1 is enhanced by focused ultrasound. Gene Ther 2000;7:1516–25.

91. Park EJ, Zhang YZ, Vykhodtseva N, et al. Ultrasound-mediated blood-brain/blood-tumor barrier disruption improves outcomes with trastuzumab in a breast cancer brain metastasis model. J Control Release 2012;163(3):277–84.

92. McDannold N, Arvanitis CD, Vykhodtseva N, et al. Temporary disruption of the blood-brain barrier by use of ultrasound and microbubbles: safety and efficacy evaluation in rhesus macaques. Cancer Res 2012;72(14):3652–63.

93. Arvanitis CD, Livingstone MS, Vykhodtseva N, et al. Controlled ultrasound-induced blood-brain barrier disruption using passive acoustic emissions monitoring. PLoS One 2012;7(9):e45783.

94. Tyler WJ, Tufail Y, Finsterwald M, et al. Remote excitation of neuronal circuits using low-intensity, low-frequency ultrasound. PLoS One 2008;3(10):e3511.

95. Colucci V, Strichartz G, Jolesz F, et al. Focused ultrasound effects on nerve action potential in vitro. Ultrasound Med Biol 2009;35(10):1737–47.

96. Min BK, Bystritsky A, Jung KI, et al. Focused ultrasound-mediated suppression of chemically-induced acute epileptic EEG activity. BMC Neurosci 2011;12:23.

Index

Note: Page numbers of article titles are in **boldface** type.

A

Abscess(es)
    neuroimaging of, 133–139
AD. *See* Alzheimer disease (AD)
Alzheimer disease (AD), 63–69
    described, 63–65
    imaging modalities in, 65–69
Angiography
    in cerebral ischemia evaluation, 197–200
    CT
        whole-brain
            with perfusion imaging
                in AVM evaluation, 226–227
    digital subtraction
        in AVM evaluation, 228–231
    MR
        in AVM evaluation, 227–228
    in vascular lesions evaluation, 197–200
Angiomatosis
    encephalotrigeminal
        neuroimaging of, 183–185
Array coils
    in MRI, 7
Arterial spin labeling (ASL)
    in MRI, 9
Arteriovenous malformations (AVMs)
    diagnosis and evaluation of
        multimodality imaging techniques in, **225–236**
            digital subtraction angiography, 228–231
            dynamic MRA, 227–228
            intraoperative indications, 233–234
            introduction, 226
            in rupture risk assessment, 231–233
            whole-brain CTA and perfusion imaging, 226–227
    incidence of, 226
    introduction, 226
    natural history of, 226
ASL. *See* Arterial spin labeling (ASL)
AVMs. *See* Arteriovenous malformations (AVMs)

Neurol Clin 32 (2014) 271–282
http://dx.doi.org/10.1016/S0733-8619(13)00131-X
0733-8619/14/$ – see front matter © 2014 Elsevier Inc. All rights reserved.

Printed and bound by CPI Group (UK) Ltd, Croydon, CR0 4YY

03/10/2024

01040493-0010